VOLUME EIGHTY SIX

ADVANCES IN PHARMACOLOGY

VOLUME EIGHTY SIX

ADVANCES IN PHARMACOLOGY

Neuropsychotherapeutics

Edited by

JEFFREY M. WITKIN

Witkin Consulting Group, Carmel, IN; Department of Neurological Surgery, Indiana University School of Medicine, Indianapolis, IN; Department of Chemistry & Biochemistry, University of Wisconsin-Milwaukee, Milwaukee, WI, United States

Serial Editor

S.J. ENNA

University of Kansas Medical Center, Kansas City, KS, United States

Managing Editor

LYNN LeCOUNT

University of Kansas Medical Center, School of Medicine, Kansas City, KS, United States

ELSEVIER

ACADEMIC PRESS

An imprint of Elsevier

Academic Press is an imprint of Elsevier
50 Hampshire Street, 5th Floor, Cambridge, MA 02139, United States
525 B Street, Suite 1650, San Diego, CA 92101, United States
The Boulevard, Langford Lane, Kidlington, Oxford OX5 1GB, United Kingdom
125 London Wall, London, EC2Y 5AS, United Kingdom

First edition 2019

ISBN: 978-0-12-816668-0
ISSN: 1054-3589

For information on all Academic Press publications
visit our website at https://www.elsevier.com/books-and-journals

Publisher: Zoe Kruze
Acquisition Editor: Zoe Kruze
Editorial Project Manager: Shellie Bryant
Production Project Manager: Denny Mansingh
Cover Designer: Christian J. Bilbow

Typeset by SPi Global, India

Contents

Contributors *ix*
Preface *xi*

1. GPCR drug discovery-moving beyond the orthosteric to the allosteric domain 1

Christian C. Felder

1. Introduction 2
2. GPCR proteins as drug development targets 3
3. Evolution of GPCR target identification and screening to improve hit selectivity 4
4. Increased attention on allosteric modulators 6
5. The development of M1 and M4 PAMs as a drug development example 9
6. The promise of xanomeline 10
7. Muscarinic receptor subtype explorations 11
8. The hunt for muscarinic receptor subtype selective ligands 12
9. The future of allosteric drug development 13
10. Conclusion 16

Conflict of interest 17
References 17
Further reading 20

2. Lipid rafts in psychiatry 21

Nathan H. Wray and Mark M. Rasenick

1. Introduction 21
2. Studying lipid rafts 23
3. Monoaminergic signaling 25
4. Signal transduction proteins and lipid rafts 32
5. Depression, lipid rafts and $G\alpha_s$ 33
6. Conclusion 37

Acknowledgments 37
Conflict of interest statement 37
References 37
Further reading 45

3. Rapid-acting antidepressants **47**

Jeffrey M. Witkin, Anna E. Martin, Lalit K. Golani, Nina Z. Xu, and Jodi L. Smith

1. Introduction 48
2. NMDA receptor antagonists 51
3. Muscarinic receptor antagonists 54
4. Psychedelic drugs 58
5. Mechanisms awaiting clinical testing 62
6. Mechanisms of action 67
7. Conclusions 80

Acknowledgments 81
Conflict of interest 81
References 81

4. mGlu2/3 receptor antagonists **97**

Shigeyuki Chaki

1. Introduction 98
2. mGlu2/3 receptors—Localization and molecular properties 99
3. Pharmacology of mGlu2/3 receptor antagonists 101
4. Depression and role of mGlu2/3 receptors in depression 103
5. Antidepressant effects of mGlu2/3 receptor antagonists 104
6. Anxiolytic effects of mGlu2/3 receptor antagonists 110
7. Pro-cognitive effects of mGlu2/3 receptor antagonists 112
8. Conclusions 113

Acknowledgments 113
Conflict of interest statement 113
References 114

5. Nitric oxide: Antidepressant mechanisms and inflammation **121**

Mehdi Ghasemi

1. Introduction 122
2. Nitrergic neurotransmission in the central nervous system 123
3. A role for NO signaling in MDD 124
4. Animal behavioral studies 125
5. Effects of antidepressants on nitrergic transmission 127
6. NO signaling and inflammatory processes in MDD 134
7. Conclusion 137

Acknowledgment 138
Conflict of interest 139
References 139

6. Selective allosteric modulation of muscarinic acetylcholine receptors for the treatment of schizophrenia and substance use disorders **153**

Laura B. Teal, Robert W. Gould, Andrew S. Felts, and Carrie K. Jones

1. Introduction 155
2. Cholinergic innervation and regions implicated in schizophrenia and SUD 160
3. Muscarinic acetylcholine receptors and schizophrenia 162
4. Muscarinic acetylcholine receptors and substance use disorders 173
5. Potential challenges with mAChR allosteric modulation 179
6. Conclusion 181

Acknowledgments 182
Conflict of interest statement 182
References 182
Further reading 196

7. Medications development for food-based and drug use disorders **197**

Fernando B. de Moura, Stephen J. Kohut, and Jack Bergman

1. Introduction 198
2. Drug and food addiction 201
3. Gut-brain axis peptides in addiction 203
4. Neurotransmitter systems as modulators of food and drug reward processes 209
5. Non-pharmacological approaches to the management of substance use disorders 219
6. Conclusion 220

Acknowledgment 220
Conflict of interest statement 221
References 221
Further reading 235

8. Obsessive compulsive disorder (OCD): Current treatments and a framework for neurotherapeutic research **237**

Erik Z. Woody, Kurt Leroy Hoffman, and Henry Szechtman

1. Introduction 238
2. Toward a new perspective on psychiatric disorder 245
3. Toward a new perspective on treatment for OCD 253
4. Conclusion 262

Conflict of interest 263
References 263

9. Positive allosteric modulators of the dopamine D1 receptor: A new mechanism for the treatment of neuropsychiatric disorders **273**

Kjell A. Svensson, Junliang Hao, and Robert F. Bruns

1. Introduction 275
2. D1 PAM pharmacology 276
3. Potential therapeutic applications of D1 PAMs 293
4. Conclusion 300

Acknowledgment 300
Conflicts of interest 300
References 300

Contributors

Jack Bergman
Behavioral Biology Program, McLean Hospital; Department of Psychiatry, Harvard Medical School, Boston, MA, United States

Robert F. Bruns
Discovery Chemistry and Research Technologies, Lilly Research Laboratories, Eli Lilly & Co, Lilly Corporate Center, Indianapolis, IN, United States

Shigeyuki Chaki
Research Headquarters, Taisho Pharmaceutical Co., Ltd., Yoshino-cho, Saitama, Japan

Fernando B. de Moura
Behavioral Biology Program, McLean Hospital; Department of Psychiatry, Harvard Medical School, Boston, MA, United States

Christian C. Felder
Karuna Therapeutics, Boston, MA, United States

Andrew S. Felts
Department of Pharmacology; Vanderbilt Center for Neuroscience Drug Discovery, Vanderbilt University, Nashville, TN, United States

Mehdi Ghasemi
Department of Neurology, University of Massachusetts Medical School, Worcester; Department of Neurology, Massachusetts and General Hospital, Boston, MA, United States

Lalit K. Golani
Department of Chemistry & Biochemistry, University of Wisconsin-Milwaukee, Milwaukee, WI, United States

Robert W. Gould
Department of Pharmacology; Vanderbilt Center for Neuroscience Drug Discovery, Vanderbilt University, Nashville, TN, United States

Junliang Hao
Discovery Chemistry and Research Technologies, Lilly Research Laboratories, Eli Lilly & Co, Lilly Corporate Center, Indianapolis, IN, United States

Kurt Leroy Hoffman
Centro de Investigación en Reproducción Animal (CIRA), Universidad Autónoma de Tlaxcala—CINVESTAV, Tlaxcala, Mexico

Carrie K. Jones
Department of Pharmacology; Vanderbilt Center for Neuroscience Drug Discovery, Vanderbilt University, Nashville, TN, United States

Stephen J. Kohut
Behavioral Biology Program, McLean Hospital; Department of Psychiatry, Harvard Medical School, Boston, MA, United States

Anna E. Martin
Witkin Consulting Group, Carmel, IN, United States

Mark M. Rasenick
University of Illinois College of Medicine, Department of Physiology & Biophysics; The Graduate Program in Neuroscience; Department of Psychiatry; The Jesse Brown VAMC, Chicago, IL, United States

Jodi L. Smith
Laboratory of Antiepileptic Drug Discovery, St. Vincent's Hospital, Indianapolis, IN, United States

Kjell A. Svensson
Neuroscience Discovery, Lilly Research Laboratories, Eli Lilly & Co, Lilly Corporate Center, Indianapolis, IN, United States

Henry Szechtman
Department of Psychiatry and Behavioural Neurosciences, McMaster University, Hamilton, ON, Canada

Laura B. Teal
Department of Pharmacology; Vanderbilt Center for Neuroscience Drug Discovery, Vanderbilt University, Nashville, TN, United States

Jeffrey M. Witkin
Witkin Consulting Group, Carmel, IN; Department of Neurological Surgery, Indiana University School of Medicine, Indianapolis, IN; Department of Chemistry & Biochemistry, University of Wisconsin-Milwaukee, Milwaukee, WI, United States

Erik Z. Woody
Department of Psychology, University of Waterloo, Waterloo, ON, Canada

Nathan H. Wray
University of Illinois College of Medicine, Department of Physiology & Biophysics; The Graduate Program in Neuroscience, Chicago, IL, United States

Nina Z. Xu
Witkin Consulting Group, Carmel, IN, United States

Preface

Neuropsychopharmacology is the field of scientific inquiry focused on effects of drugs on psychiatric disorders. The ultimate goal of research efforts in neuropsychopharmacology is the creation of improved medicines. A host of technologies in both the preclinical and clinical research laboratories are utilized to achieve this goal. Preclinical research methods include molecular pharmacology and molecular modeling, functional assessments of compounds in recombinant and native tissue preparations, and whole-animal responses to new molecules. Evaluation of new compounds in humans, based upon predictions from the preclinical laboratory, makes use of biological sampling, genetic analysis, and neuroimaging methods. Tests of the potential efficacy and safety of compounds in patients rely on the skilled clinical assessment tools long-honed in clinical research laboratories.

Neuropsychopharmacology exists as a discipline because there is a tremendous need for improved medicines for psychiatric patients. Surprised, you say? Medicines exist for the treatment of the major psychiatric disorders of schizophrenia, anxiety, substance use disorder, and depression. Indeed, there are many medicines approved for these patients. Scientists and clinicians alike could readily provide a list of approved drugs for each indication. And, in the past several years, many pharmaceutical companies have decided not to work on psychiatric drugs. So, why the need? In psychiatry, like in most medical disease areas, there are two insufficiencies with our modern medicine cabinets: efficacy and safety of the drugs prescribed. On the efficacy side, not all patients respond to the medicine, and of those that do respond, some do not get completely better (remission). A third class of patient does not respond to any current medicine (treatment-refractory). Treatment-refractory patients are not a small percentage of patients with estimates on the order of 30%.

A key need for improvement in psychiatric drugs is in the area of residual symptom treatment. Full remission of disease cannot be established without symptom control. Antipsychotic drugs for schizophrenic patients can impact positive symptoms such as hallucinations and delusions but do not treat other symptoms (e.g., cognitive processing or social functioning). Antidepressants, when effective, can improve mood but do not generally treat the anhedonia or cognitive symptoms of depression. Improvements in other aspects of drug action are also needed. Onset of action is but one example. Selective serotonin reuptake inhibitors (SSRIs) are the first-line therapy for anxiety disorders.

However, unlike drugs like valium, they do not immediately help anxious patients. The same is true for selective SSRI antidepressants that require weeks of daily administration to produce full treatment response for depressed patients.

Safety profiles of medicines used in psychiatry have improved over time, but still remain imperfect. Safety and side effects limit the doses that be used and this can negatively impact symptom treatment. Side effects can also impact patient compliance leading to consequences of morbidity and mortality. For example, tricyclic antidepressants produce side effects of dry mouth and sedation, and monoamine oxidase inhibitors have been lethal. First-line, standard of care antidepressants used today such as the SSRIs do not produce these side effects. However, some produce other side effects that impact patient compliance such as weight gain and sexual dysfunction. The 1,4-benzodiazepine class of anxiolytic drugs (e.g., diazepam or valium) have issues of safety surrounding sedation, dependence, and abuse liability.

In the present volume on neuropsychotherapeutics, new medicines and new approaches to the discovery of medicines for psychiatric disorders are reviewed. The psychiatric disorders that are included in this volume are depression, substance abuse, food addiction, schizophrenia, cognition, and anxiety. Since there are few treatment options for patients suffering from obsessive–compulsive disorder (OCD), the inclusion of a chapter in a psychopharmacology text is rare. OCD is a highly prevalent and severely disabling disorder. In the present volume, Woody and colleagues provide a review of the biological underpinnings of this disorder and the pharmacological substrates that might yield new therapies. Drug abuse disorders are addressed by Teal and colleagues with a review of novel muscarinic receptor ligands. de Moura and his coauthors provide a broad approach to addiction disorders by examining the overlap in biological substrates of food and drug addictions with ideas for the evolution of novel medications. There are other areas of neuropsychotherapeutics that are not covered in this book (e.g., agitation and aggression).

The design of compounds that bind to allosteric domains of drug receptors has enabled important steps forward in improving patient care. The chapter by Felder in this volume outlines new thinking on allosteric approaches to drug design. Although only two compounds have been approved for patients, allosteric compounds are likely to be the new wave of therapeutic breakthroughs. Allosterism is further highlighted in the writings of Teal and colleagues where they provide a review of elegant work in the area of muscarinic receptor ligands for schizophrenia and substance abuse disorder. Svensson and Bruns illustrate the value of allosteric receptor modulation in their chapter highlighting one of the first potentiators of dopamine D_1 receptors. One D_1 receptor potentiator is currently in Phase 2 development for the treatment of dementia in Parkinson's patients.

Antidepressant and anxiolytic drug discovery have also made advances in recent years. The first truly novel antidepressant in decades was approved for patients in February 2019, (*S*)-ketamine (esketamine). This new class of antidepressants, rapid-acting antidepressants, is reviewed by Witkin and colleagues. The drugs now considered in this class include psychedelic agents such as psilocybin. Although glutamate is involved in the etiology and maintenance of symptoms of psychiatric disorders, little headway in using this system for therapeutic gain has been made. Chaki summarizes the metabotropic 2/3 ($mGlu_{2/3}$) receptors as a potential drug target for depression, anxiety, and cognition. His chapter also integrates this mechanism into the realm of rapid-acting antidepressant drugs. It has been known since the pioneering work of Solomon Snyder and colleagues that nitric oxide plays a neurotransmitter role. The chapter by Ghasemi reviews the evidence that nitric oxide plays a role in depression, antidepressant drug action, inflammatory responses, and the interface of inflammation and depression. The lipid bilayer of neurons has undergone new conceptualizations in recent years. This work has been pioneered by and highlighted by Wray and Rasenick. They utilize the lipid raft hypothesis to integrate understanding of drug action at this level and document its importance by illustrating its impact upon antidepressant drugs.

This volume of *Advances in Pharmacology* would not been possible without the dedicated time and efforts of the authors who wrote their chapters after their day jobs; thank you dear authors. I am also grateful to Lynn LeCount who managed the submissions and the interface between authors and the publisher. She also managed to manage me with good humor and patience. Without her dedication, support, and guidance, this volume would not exist. I also thank Sam Enna, the series editor of *Advances in Pharmacology*. Thank you, Sam, for inviting me to put this volume together. I am also thankful for my wife Zosia who allowed me the time to work on this volume and brought me great food to eat.

JEFFREY M. WITKIN, PHD
Witkin Consulting Group
Carmel, IN, United States
Department of Neurological Surgery
Indiana University School of Medicine
Indianapolis, IN, United States
Department of Chemistry & Biochemistry
University of Wisconsin-Milwaukee
Milwaukee, WI, United States

CHAPTER ONE

GPCR drug discovery-moving beyond the orthosteric to the allosteric domain

Christian C. Felder*
Karuna Therapeutics, Boston, MA, United States
*Corresponding author: e-mail address: christianfelder@gmail.com

Contents

1. Introduction 2
2. GPCR proteins as drug development targets 3
3. Evolution of GPCR target identification and screening to improve hit selectivity 4
4. Increased attention on allosteric modulators 6
5. The development of M1 and M4 PAMs as a drug development example 9
6. The promise of xanomeline 10
7. Muscarinic receptor subtype explorations 11
8. The hunt for muscarinic receptor subtype selective ligands 12
9. The future of allosteric drug development 13
10. Conclusion 16
Conflict of interest 17
References 17
Further reading 20

Abstract

Allosteric modulation of G protein coupled receptors (GPCRs) is rapidly becoming a standard option for development of therapeutics headed to the clinic. Although GPCRs represent about 35% of marketed drugs, to date only two allosteric modulators have been approved for human use. However, many are now in early clinical development are can provide unique regulation of GPCRs including high selectivity along with physiologic temporal and spatial signaling. These molecules bind to a site that is distinct from the site where the endogenous agonist binds yet can provide robust modulation effects that span from the positive to the negative. Along with classical chemogenomic techniques, newer technology is being directly applied to their development including three dimensional biophysical structure-function analysis and in silico molecular dynamic simulations. The goal is to provide rationally designed molecules from well informed physical and in silico data to speed the discovery and development of the next generation therapeutics. In this chapter an example of the evolution of allosteric drug discovery targeting the muscarinic receptor family should serve to inform of progress in this exciting area of research and early drug development.

Advances in Pharmacology, Volume 86
ISSN 1054-3589
https://doi.org/10.1016/bs.apha.2019.04.002

1. Introduction

Bringing badly needed drugs to patients whose conditions are poorly or altogether unaddressed has been particular difficult in the area of CNS disorders (Harrison, 2016). For example, no significant treatments for the schizophrenia have been discovered in over 50 years (Ceskova & Silhan, 2018; Kesselheim, Hwang, & Franklin, 2015). While a number of plausible hypotheses have been proffered, the etiology of this devastating condition affecting 1% of the world's population remains unknown. Progress is being made using GWAS of very large merged datasets and specific genes are emerging as plausible targets but are yet to be fully explored (Greenwood et al., 2018). Current pharmaceutical standards of care are wrought with side effects that only add to the disease burden such as metabolic syndrome, significant weight gain, as well as blood and movement disorders. However, promising new targets are emerging that stimulate GPCRs that show early signs of efficacy without the burden of side effects such as the acetylcholine muscarinic receptor family detailed below (Stone and Pilowsky, 2007). Similar bad news continues to plaque those desperately attempting to change the course of neurological diseases such as Alzheimer's and Parkinson's diseases, or at minimum, reduce the symptoms that make managing these patients an expensive and emotionally difficult task for all involved. Again, the acetylcholine muscarinic family of receptors has shown early promise to moderate symptoms and possibly modify disease progression. What lies at the root cause of this lack of general industry progress and these specific project failures? Small molecule therapeutic drug discovery evolves across the pharmaceutical and biotechnology arena at a remarkably uniform and steady pace across the industry. Transformative discoveries that impact the process do occur at relatively high frequency, but truly disruptive technologies that could vastly improve the success of drug discovery are rather rare. A number of excellent analyses have been done in recent years to uncover the root causes of lack of success to outright dismal failures of a number of high profile drug discovery efforts (Hwang et al., 2016; Waring et al., 2015). These failures become increasingly more expensive the further along the effort moves along the development path (DiMasi, Grabowski, & Hansen, 2016). Failing fast has been a catch-phrase to attempt to reach a logical go/no-go decision as quickly as possible. A comprehensive look at each of the components that make up successful drug discovery indicates that a number of areas fall short across the process including ADME, toxicology, market projections, and choice of target, but overall efficacy in the late phase 2 and 3 segments account for the majority of failures. The lack of efficacy indicates a poor choice of target for the disease indication, flawed hypothesis, mismatch of drug dose for the indication, lack of required target engagement or incorrect choice of target modulation and a number of other issues. The following chapter attempts to provide insight into both transformative and disruptive technologies and processes that have impacted GPCR drug development in the last 20 years through the description of muscarinic acetylcholine drug development, a particularly challenging GPCR platform. Also discussed will be reasons for progress or failure of this target class for several CNS diseases which should be informative in general for other GPCR drug discovery examples.

2. GPCR proteins as drug development targets

GPCRs remain highly relevant, viable, and attractive therapeutic targets in many industrial, government and academic portfolios. Estimates remain at approximately 25% of marketed drugs are targeted to GPCRs across all top therapeutic areas including CNS, cancer, immunology, muscoskeletal, etc. (Hauser, Gloriam, Attwood, Rask-Andersen, & Schiöth, 2017; Sriram & Insel, 2018). This class of proteins is one of the best studied and understood at the molecular and atomic level (Shimada, Ueda, Kofuku, Eddy, & Wüthrich, 2019). They reside at the cell surface with domains regulated by small molecules and therapeutic proteins externally accessible and not requiring cell permeation. Their function is to control and regulate a wide range of physiologic processes both acute and metabotropic such as cell maintenance and division. Thus GPCRs can be modulated by drugs to restore imbalanced function or recruited inappropriately in specific diseases. For example, tumor cells hijack their expressed GPCRs to help avoid normal immune function offering a rich set of target to arrest angiogenesis, proliferation, and metastasis (Gutierrez & McDonald, 2018). Genetics linkage of GPCR mutations to a wide variety of diseases is well substantiated at least to the level of contributing to disease etiology, but what has gone awry is still not known in most targets (Maier et al., 2015). Recent success in creating GPCR crystals in concert with molecular dynamic simulations to all three GPCR protein classes provides insight into drug binding, drug binding conformational state dependency, and ultimate regulation of intracellular signaling cascades. The challenges remain as to how one can engineer better ligand selectivity along with fine tuning the required pharmacology desirable to impact disease. How can we preserve and spatial and temporal signaling while dialing up or down the required physiological response? What does choice of ligand class such as small molecule or antibody offer to improve the project outcome? Only relatively recently has it been more deeply appreciated that ligand dependent GPCR conformational flexibility through multiple energy states provide a wide range of possible pharmacological outcomes for signaling and physiologic control (Hollingsworth & Dror, 2018; Kruse et al., 2013).

3. Evolution of GPCR target identification and screening to improve hit selectivity

When selecting a GPCR target for development for a CNS indication, a number of key criteria must be met to increase the likelihood of success. (1) Most obvious is that the target has a direct link to the disease. In very rare cases, the target protein has a functional gain or loss mutation that leads to a disease phenotype. Such a target is the NaV1.7 sodium channel with mutations that leave a patient either insensitive or hypersensitive to pain stimuli (Wadhawan et al., 2017). (2) Also obvious is that the target should be expressed in brain and linked to disease through its modulation at the cellular or circuit level. Studies will need to exist showing brain and peripheral distribution to provide a relationship to possible disease modification or safety concern. (3) Ideally the target is druggable in that the protein can be modulated in the appropriate way to elicit the desired pharmacological response. Type 1 and 3 GPCRs in general are highly druggable targets with small molecules though less success has been realized with type 2 GPCRs. Antibodies are much more difficult ligands to develop for GPCR targets though some success has been realized more recently (Edvinsson, 2018; Mujić-Delić, de Wit, Verkaar, & Smit, 2014). Delivery to deep brain structures is the key hurdle as less than 0.1% of therapeutic antibodies cross the blood brain barrier indicating a need for specific delivery technology (Gabathuler, 2010; Yu & Watts, 2013).

The prosecution of the muscarinic acetylcholine receptor (MAChR) family of 5 receptors (M1-M5) embodied these basic starting point principles yet present unique challenges. Selection of the appropriate mAChR subtype associated with disease was the first challenge as no selective ligands were available when muscarinic projects began to probe receptor subtype physiology. Good pharmacological tools help drive drug target through the complexities of physiology especially when combined with genetic models such as knockout mice. Though highly druggable, the mAChR family are highly homologous in their nucleotide and amino acid sequences and thus have relatively strong structural similarities at their ligand binding domains. Poorly selective tool compounds emerged in the 1980s from a number of companies although the goal was to develop M1 selective compounds to treat Alzheimer's disease (AD) (Felder, Bymaster, Ward, & DeLapp, 2000). It was not until after 2000 that partially selective tool compounds began to emerge that were primarily agonists (Heinrich et al., 2009). Unlike many GPCR families, the selective mAChr agonists preceded the discovery of selective antagonists with the later only very recently being described (Calcutt et al., 2017). As they became available, selective tool compounds with appropriate pharmacology allowed labs to probe the physiological response of target engagement and modulation in rodents with assays that report efficacy across any number of desired end points. For example, M1 agonists were used to probe effects on rodent and monkey cognition for use in Alzheimer's disease (Bubser, Byun, Wood, & Jones, 2012) or an M3 antagonist to probe modulation of respiration or bladder control for COPD or leaky bladder syndrome, respectively (Eglen, Choppin, Dillon, & Hegde, 1999). For CNS indications one would naturally prefer a GPCR target localized exclusively or at least predominantly in the CNS to avoid peripheral side effects. Using a chemo-genetic approach to validate the relationship of target modulation to physiological response is supported with the use of constitutive or conditional knockout mice probed with selective ligands (Wess, Eglen, & Gautam, 2007).

Classical small molecule drug discovery is based on screening large libraries of drug-like molecules in a robust bioassay involving the protein target of interest. Based on the size of the library screened and level of automation applied, usually one or two relatively high concentrations (e.g., 1 and 10 μM) are used for the initial screen. Having two relatively high and single log concentration differences apart allows one to not miss potential weaker compounds as well as providing a two point concentration rise. The resulting dose response should it occur adds confidence that the hit is valid. Once an active readout above an pre-determined threshhold is met, the active compounds are generally re-evaluated in the primary screen over a full concentration range to verify that the active compound is a bona fide hit. The classical sigmoidal shaped curve whether it be for agonism or antagonism spanning two orders of magnitude adds further validity that the hit is a well behaved single binding site interaction at the target protein. Physical chemistry analysis of the ligand is then applied to verify that the molecule is true to the vial label and not a breakdown product of the original material or incorrectly labeled.

The hits are then counter-screened for selectivity within the target family and across other anti-targets that may lead to safety issues later in development. In general, selective antagonists provide a much more simple discovery path than agonists and allosteric modulators. Measuring the pharmacology of agonists can be complex as the nuances of agonistic responses can range from partial, full, to super-agonism above what the stimulation level of the native neurotransmitter and in some cases results in a bell shaped curve. The pharmacology can also vary significantly across species and translation from animal behavioral testing, animal toxicology, to human dosing needs to be carefully verified (https://www.ncbi.nlm.nih.gov/books/NBK53196/) (Felder et al., 2011). With the increased use of small molecule allosteric modulators, GPCR drug discovery is in the beginning of a transformation in tailored ligand design and choices of useful pharmacological complexity.

4. Increased attention on allosteric modulators

To place small molecule drug screening in perspective, classical high throughput screening allowed a range of full and partial agonists and antagonists can be discovered from a diverse library of small molecules. Antagonists appear as competitive, non- or un-competitive as well as inverse agonists (reducing native receptor activity below baseline levels). Though theoretically possible, the emergence of allosteric modulators as a viable pharmacological profile for novel drug design did not broadly enter drug discovery programs until after 2000. Only two allosteric modulators have been approved to date though there are many in early clinical trials. The two include cinacalcet (first GPCR allosteric modulator to be approved in 2004), a positive allosteric modulator of the calcium-sensing GPCR receptor for the treatment of hyperparathyroidism and maraviroc (approved in 2007), a negative allosteric modulator of the chemokine GPCR receptor CCR5 for the prevention of cellular entry of HIV-1. These entities greatly expand the potential for tailored regulation of target biology (May & Christopoulos, 2003). The challenge to their emergence into mainstream therapeutics is likely due to several impediments: (1) Traditional orthosteric site agonists and antagonists were thought to satisfy the demands of target modulation to deliver a marketable drug with sufficient usefulness for therapeutic use. (2) Drug screening was well served with radioligand binding assays while high throughput functional screening for allosteric compounds was considered complex and an inefficient process. (3) Initial screens revealed that allosteric modulators with good drug like properties were rather rare and with no history in allosteric drug development activities logically revealed their extremely low representation in many medicinal chemistry libraries. (4) Few examples existed of successful GPCR allosteric drugs in the industry. Beginning in the late 1990s, more sophisticated and flexible high throughput screening technology emerged allowing more complex assay design for functional signal transduction assays.

Allosteric protein regulation is defined as the ability of proteins to be placed in various conformationally restricted states when interacted upon by another protein or ligand (Monod, Wyman, & Changeux, 1965). This type of protein regulation as it turns out is particularly useful for the highly desirable GPCR drug targets. GPCRs are regulated by their natural neurotransmitter when it binds to a site directly at the center of the cylindrically shaped receptor. The center neurotransmitter binding pocket is called the orthosteric domain (entomology: correct atom orientation in space). Allosteric modulators bind at an allosteric binding site distinct from the orthosteric binding domain (entomology: other than) (Fig. 1). Allosteric modulators alter the pharmacology of the interaction of the orthosteric ligand with its

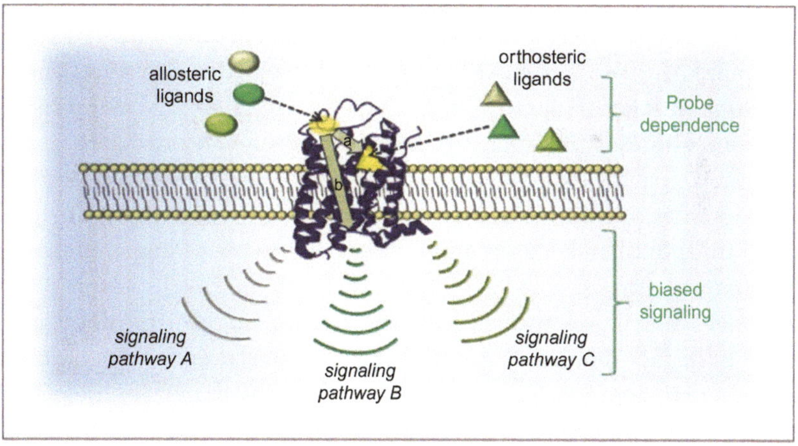

Fig. 1 Schematic of GPCR signal transduction: Green spheres represent allosteric modulator ligands that bind to the outer vestibule allosteric pocket (yellow sphere). Green triangles represent natural orthosteric neurotransmitters such as acetylcholine or synthetic orthosteric ligands that bind to the orthosteric domain (yellow triangle). Allosteric modulators can modulate binding affinity (path a) and/or efficacy (path b) of orthosteric ligands in a positive (PAM) or negative (NAM), or simply occupy the site inducing no downstream activity (SAM). The modulation is often reciprocally affected by the specific orthosteric ligand (probe dependence) and can potentially preferentially alter receptor activation of specific signaling pathways (biased signaling). *Adapted from Wild, C., Cunningham, K. A., & Zhou, J. (2014). Allosteric modulation of G protein-coupled receptors: An emerging approach of drug discovery.* Austin Journal of Pharmacology and Therapeutics, 2, *1–3.*

GPCR target. For example, at the most basic level, positive allosteric modulators (PAMs) can greatly enhance the potency of acetylcholine binding to its orthosteric site in the muscarinic receptor and the resulting signal transduction through either G protein or beta arrestin coupling proteins. Conversely negative allosteric modulators (NAMs) can diminish the potency of acetylcholine. Silent modulators (SAMs) bind but fail to modulate subsequent signal transduction. Screening for allosteric modulators requires bioassays to be designed to allow addition of an orthosteric ligand while introducing small test molecules to then modulate the expected orthosteric response. In more complex assays established on robotic systems, multiple additions of ligands are performed over time to resolve agonism, antagonism, and modulation (Bertekap, Burford, Li, & Alt, 2015). Next comes the challenging task of resolving the potentially complex pharmacology of each hit which requires multiple assays designed to resolve the ligands final pharmacological character.

Relatively recently GPCRs were thought to reside predominantly in either high affinity or low affinity binding states and these two conformations could be resolved using radioligand binding assays. Biophysical technological advances such as GPCR protein crystallography with agonist and antagonist ligands docked in various poses has allowed visualization of these ligand bound states (Hilger, Masureel, & Kobilka, 2018). Now more than 59 unique GPCR crystals have been published though only about a third are in the active conformation bound with agonists (DeVree et al., 2016). More recently a muscarinic M2 receptor protein crystal was resolved to 2.8 Å with agonist and PAM bound simultaneously providing useful insight into complex GPCR activation states (Kruse et al., 2013). Upon agonist and PAM binding, a G protein and Beta-arrestin are subsequently engaged to transduce the stimulatory event to the intracellular environment. Cryo-electron microscopic analysis and crystal structures with both or these accessory proteins bound have been solved for a relatively few GPCRs to date. However, these techniques are static representations of bound and unbound GPCRs. What is needed is to follow over time the process of ligand binding to its most energetically stable binding site and the transitions states of the GPCR through activation and coupling to transduction accessory G proteins and Beta-arrestin, and finally inactivation. High speed and capacity GUI-based computers have been built recently that allow in silico mapping of every atom within a GPCR, along with surrounding membrane lipid and water molecules over time. These remarkable visualizations are called molecular dynamic simulations which provide a new level of awareness of GPCR transitions and key molecular interactions and signaling (Hollingsworth & Dror, 2018).

5. The development of M1 and M4 PAMs as a drug development example

Development of muscarinic ligands, whether agonist or antagonist has historically been fraught with a general lack of selectivity across the five muscarinic receptor subtypes. Of the families of GPCRs, the muscarinic family has a very high sequence similarity at the nucleotide and amino acid levels. Ligands would interact with at least two of the subtypes and usually all five to some degree despite screening for selective ligands across over a million compound libraries. A series of compounds with modest selectivity profiles were advanced to early clinical studies (Heinrich). The therapeutic strategy for the most part focused on Alzheimer's patients in an attempt to reverse or at least stabilize cognitive decline (Felder et al., 2000). The hypothesis emerged from earlier studies demonstrating cholinergic deafferentation from the medial septum and diagonal band which projects to key memory circuits to prefrontal cortical and hippocampal areas (Coyle, Price, & Delong, 1983). These acetylcholine replacement strategies for the most part failed primarily due to the intolerable side effect profile driven by parasympathomimetic physiology (SLUDGE: salivation, lacrimation, urination, and gastrointestinal effects). Why would so many large corporations bring less than ideal drugs this far forward? During the early decade of the 1990s the selectivity profile of muscarinic agonists were measured primarily by contraction of resected and suspended organ tissue in physiologic bath preparations. For example, heart tissue was thought to express primarily M2 receptors and a contraction of an atrial slice in an organ bath preparation represented the bradycardic effect of muscarinic agonists in rats. M1 was measured in suspended vas deferens and M3 in suspended ileum preps. There were no organ bath assays for M4 and M5 receptors at that time. However, many muscarinic subtypes are expressed together within various organs and tissues making these organ baths less than ideal for solving the selectivity issue. Having each receptor gene isolated and in a form that is expressible in cell lines which allows each to be studied or screened for ligands in isolation. All five receptors were finally cloned and expressed in cell lines in the late 1980s and signal transduction assays beginning to be studied. Radioligand binding assays were normally used to measure ligand displacement at each receptor subtype using high affinity non-selective antagonists such as *N*-methyl scopolamine. High throughput functional in vitro second messenger assays did not become widely available until the most of these early drugs were well on their way to clinical development. For this receptor family the predominant desirable and targeted pharmacology are ligands with various levels of partial and full agonistic properties. Truly selective muscarinic agonists did not emerge until after 2000 and was solved primarily through targeting allosteric sites also described in more detail below. But why did pharma continue to invest in the muscarinic platform in the shadow of such failures? One compound in particular showed remarkable efficacy in patients suffering from Alzheimer's disease and schizophrenia along with side effect concerns.

6. The promise of xanomeline

Xanomeline was studied in a phase 2 clinical trial involving 343 patients diagnosed with Alzheimer's disease (Bodick et al., 1997). Active treatment of three doses were continued 23 weeks after enrollment and various instruments for measuring cognition and activities of daily living were used including the primary measures ADAS-Cog and CIBIC + and secondary measures of behavioral ADDS and NOSGER. There was a strong suggestion of cognitive benefit in AD patients at the higher doses (150 and 225 mg/day). Of interest was the dose dependent reduction in onset of psychosis symptoms such as hallucinations, compulsiveness, delusions, suspiciousness, agitation, fearfulness, and wandering as well as significant improvements in activities of daily living. However, significant patients dropped out of the studies due to typical cholinergic syndrome side effects including sweating, nausea, vomiting, diarrhea and excess salivation as well as orthostasis and syncope. Based on the constellation of symptoms showing improvements in Alzheimer's patients beyond the primary goal of providing cognitive benefit, a second study was designed and conducted in schizophrenic patients and healthy control subjects (Shekhar et al., 2008). The study was inspired by the symptom domain overlap between neurological and neuropsychiatric disorders such as those observed in AD and schizophrenia with respect to psychosis, agitation, cognitive decline, and mood disorders. Though the study included a relatively small cohort (10 schizophrenics and 10 health control subjects), dropouts were few likely due to the drug tolerance of schizophrenic patients in general and younger ages of the subject compared to the prior AD study. There were surprising and promising improvements across the three main domains of schizophrenia including cognitive, positive (e.g., psychosis), and negative (e.g., flat affect). When the results of these two proof of concept trials were evaluated together, a compelling hypothesis emerged suggesting that M1 and M4 receptor stimulation may be an optimal approach for the treatment of symptoms associated these and possibly other neuropsychiatric and neurological diseases.

7. Muscarinic receptor subtype explorations

Were the benefits observed for these difficult to treat AD and schizophrenic patients due to activation of one or more receptor subtypes and which single subtype or combination might maintain the benefits and reduce the side effects? Several decades of intense studies followed using both a chemogenomic approach as well as a focus on creating selective tool compounds with both agonistic and antagonistic properties. A few labs invested in the development of MR subtype knockout mouse lines in which the locus was deleted in the germline so animals developed never expressing a particular subtype and in the case of double knockouts, that pair of receptors. The next step after genotyping the offspring and selecting the wild type controls and separating them from heterozygotes and homozygotes is to freeze embryos and sperm to cryopreserve the lines. The animals were raised to young adulthood and then tested in a variety of un-evoked (e.g., normal behaviors including locomotion, sleep, feeding, socialization) and evoked responses (e.g., cognitive impairment, pain, psychosis models). These studies have been extensively reviewed (Bymaster, McKinzie, Felder, & Wess, 2003). In general each single or double conditional muscarinic receptor subtype knockout animal had no or very modest phenotypes. All were viable and could feed, move, breed, and sleep relatively normally. The M1 receptor knockout was spontaneously hyperactive but with few other spontaneous phenotypes. The M2 receptor knockout was generally devoid of spontaneous phenotypes but was linked to smooth muscle and cardiac function in the periphery and to neurotransmitter release regulation in the CNS being primarily a presynaptic auto-receptor for acetylcholine. It was also linked to regulation of analgesia in the spinal cord. The M3 receptor knockout was hypophagic and lean and the receptor was linked to smooth muscle function and exocrine gland secretion driving a significant amount of salivation, sweating, and pancreatic function. The M4 receptor knockout was slightly hyperactive but hyper-responsive to dopamine agonists. Further studies implicated this receptor subtype in the circuits involved in psychosis, cognition, and pain (Thomsen, Sørensen, & Dencker, 2018). The M5 receptor was found to be expressed primarily in the vasculature and the striatal areas of the CNS and regulated vasoconstriction and dopamine release in the VTA. Muscarinic distribution can also be resolved when selective antibodies or radioligands are not available (Ito et al., 2009). Interestingly, when challenged with a psychoactive agent, for example, the M1 and M4 knockout lines had evidence of phenotypes that overlapped with compounds with pharmacology that favored those subtypes. One such compound was xanomeline suggesting that an M1 and or M4 preferring agonist would be useful in AD and schizophrenia and possibly other diseases exhibiting these symptoms (Woolley, Carter, Gartlon, Watson, & Dawson, 2009). In all the investment in these animals as well as conditional tissue specific knockout lines continues to refine what is known about muscarinic physiology.

8. The hunt for muscarinic receptor subtype selective ligands

In the case of muscarinic receptors, the orthosteric pocket binds and is activated in full with acetylcholine. However, the muscarinic receptor orthosteric domain accepts muscarinic ligands (being selective for the muscarinic family of receptors over other GPCR families), compounds of quite diverse scaffolds readily across all five subtypes. While some ligands show preference for one or more subtypes, none are truly selective. For drug development to be successful one requires at least a potency margin of fivefold over the side effect dose ratios to efficacy and that should translate to at least fivefold higher potency at the receptor of interest over the M2 and M3 receptors which are most implicated in driving the parasympathomimetic physiology in animals and humans. Xanomeline and many of the compounds from that era do not meet this basic criteria. A clever solution is currently being explored by Karuna Therapeutics in which a peripherally restricted pan muscarinic antagonist is being dosed with xanomeline to quell the peripheral side effects. An allosteric approach focused on both M1-PAM and M4-PAM development for schizophrenia was initiated in 1997 by Eli Lilly and subsequently by other groups.

The advantage of this type of GPCR regulation over an orthosteric site targeted ligand is that it will preserve the spatial and temporal regulation of the receptor yet either enhance or diminish its activity. Neurotransmitters are released is pulsatile in response to action potentials. When targeting synaptic receptors and it would seem logical to preserve as much natural signaling response as possible. The amount of gain control over the GPCR can also be finely regulated by altering the design of the allosteric ligand. When first conceived, allosteric ligands for the muscarinic receptors were a hypothetical endeavor with no GPCR crystal structures or other biophysical guides to rationally design such entities. Therefore, large high throughput screens were initiated to empirically discover starting points.

For example, an M4 receptor allosteric screen was initiated in 1997 and out of approximately 500,000 compound library, 4 hits were discovered and only one was truly drug like. The assay was designed to measure calcium mobilization coupled to the M4 receptor with a promiscuous G protein co-expressed with the human M4 receptor. Hits were discovered by co-incubation with 20% efficacious concentration of acetylcholine. If a hit augmented the acetylcholine response it was either another orthosteric agonist or a PAM. Secondary screening to resolve the true pharmacology was designed as the ability of the test ligand to shift a full concentration curve of acetylcholine and not displace a antagonist radioligand. The SAR campaign took approximately 2 years and over 500 M4-PAM molecules were synthesized and lead-like molecules emerged. LY2033298 shifted the acetylcholine concentration response curve several orders of magnitude to the left in a parallel fashion and did not modify antagonist binding at the orthosteric domain establishing it as a true PAM of the M4 receptor. While still not ready for clinical development, it met the key criteria of high selectivity for the M4 receptor subtype and was sufficiently drug-like to allow testing in vitro and in vivo in comparison with less selective orthosteric muscarinic agonists such as xanomeline. LY2033298 was shown to possess similar efficacy to xanomeline in models predictive of antipsychotic efficacy such as reversal of psychotropic agent-induced prepulse inhibition of the acoustic startle response and conditioned avoidance responding (Chan et al., 2008). Thus a selective modulator could recapitulate similar attractive anti-psychotic ligand behaviors of the more complex ligand xanomeline. Moreover, this ligand did not induce the parasympathomimetic side effects seen with xanomeline and other non-selective agents. As all compounds yearning to be drugs, this one was not perfect and issues with solubility and safety relegated this platform to experimental and not therapeutic purposes.

9. The future of allosteric drug development

The proof of principal embodied in LY2033298 was not the only effort in the allosteric drug development arena. A number of groups initiated similar programs once the data from these leads began to emerge in symposia and subsequently the pharmacology journals (Fig. 2). Efforts across a number of GPCRs were being explored with varying levels of success (Felder et al., 2018). In particular, likely based on the positive clinical data from xanomeline, many groups were focused on development of

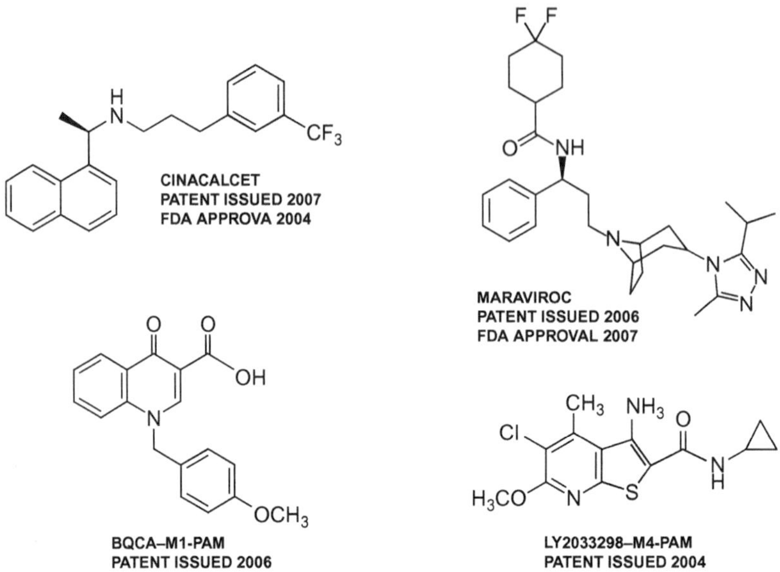

Fig. 2 Structures of first in class PAMs. Cinacalcet was the first approved PAM and maraviroc the first approved NAM. Of the muscarinic family, LY2033298 the first patented muscarinic PAM and BQCA was the first patented M1-PAM.

M1-PAM leads. These compounds provided high selectivity and very potent leftward shifts of orthosteric agonist responses. Virtually all the early examples led to GI hypersensitivity and seizure liability in dog toxicology studies, a species particularly sensitive to muscarinic agonists. One group steered around the seizure liability by selecting M1-PAMs without intrinsic agonist activity and pre-screening for this response early in mice to weed out seizurogenic PAMs and have advanced to through safety testing (Rook et al., 2018). Another group also passed the phase 1 gauntlet with a weak partial M1 selective PAM that separated nicely from side effects preclinically (Kurimoto et al., 2018; Sako et al., 2018). Due to the role of PAM predominantly in modulation and not direct activation it was thought that they had a natural limit to their ability to overdrive neural circuits and would be much less seizurogenic as well as less able to drive peripheral side effects. In retrospect this does not appear to be the case and PAMs appear to be capable of overdriving neural circuits as much as orthosteric full or highly efficacious orthosteric agonists.

The creation of full or partial PAMs or NAMs with or without intrinsic agonist or antagonist activity would benefit from rational design to make their development less time and resource intensive. Application of rational design techniques based on molecular dynamic simulations are being applied to provide a much more narrow scope of ligands to synthesize and test (McCorvy et al., 2018; Wang et al., 2017). These efforts have been greatly accelerated with the application of specific protein generation and purification techniques adapted for membrane bound GPCRs. In a tour de force, the Kobilka lab was able to co-crystalize the M2 receptor simultaneously bound with an high affinity orthosteric agonist ligand iperoxo and a M2/4-PAM LY2119620 (Kruse et al., 2013). This static structure provided insight into orthosteric site movements and how they created synergy with allosteric outer vestibule site movement to generate cooperativity of binding and signal transduction. This structure was then embellished with molecular dynamic simulations in the Dror lab to refine the movements over time with their predictions (Dror et al., 2013). Clearly there is a close structural relationship between the allosteric and orthosteric site that seem to be recapitulated in other GPCR where the PAM binds to the outer vestibule domain. Curiously there appears to be allosteric domains at various locations in GPCRs which can have influence over the orthosteric binding events and subsequently signal transduction. For example, in the case of the D1-PAM the binding appears to occur at the intracellular face of the receptor to influence signaling (Wang et al., 2018). GPCRs signal primarily through their interaction with heterotrimeric G proteins. They also recruit beta arrestin to initiate internalization to either endocytic and lysosomal compartments for recycling back to the plasma membrane or for degradation, respectively. Opiate receptor ligands that bias the receptor to either G protein or beta arrestin pathways have been described (Rankovic, Brust, & Bohn, 2016; Siuda, Carr III, Rominger, & Violin, 2017). These biased stimulatory events can greatly alter the outcome of the physiology of receptor activated pathways leading to either desirable or undesirable outcomes. For example, mu opiate receptor biased ligands can engender therapeutically desirable outcomes if G protein biased and undesirable and potentially lethal outcomes if purely arrestin biased. However, these ligands are not completely biased and measurement of the level of relative bias is highly assay dependent and variable across labs and assay conditions employed for its assessment. Whether orthosteric and potentially allosteric bias signaling will be therapeutic useful is yet to be determined.

GPCR internalization was originally thought to provide a mechanism to slow or soften the action of agonists by downregulation of signaling by reducing potentially activatable receptor levels at the plasma membrane, and if in significant over abundance, then shunt them to degradative destinies.

More recent evidence indicates that GPCRs continue to actively signal once internalized with their native or synthetic ligand or utilize their constitutive activity to drive intracellular signaling physiology. For example, in the case of CGRP receptors, a persistent and less prone to side effect pain response has been linked to intracellular signaling events (Yarwood et al., 2017). This potentially transformative signaling pathway is on the frontier of drug development opportunities. How will orthosteric or allosteric drugs differentially regulate the intracellular GPCR signaling domain?

10. Conclusion

GPCRs provide a pliable substrate rich in novel binding pockets, pleiotropic landscape of functional regulation opportunities leading to a wealth of potential therapeutic outcomes. Described as one of the more difficult GPCR families to drug selectively, the muscarinic receptor family has provided a useful platform to discover and test novel approaches for GPCR drug discovery. Creation of muscarinic receptor subtype selective ligands has been challenging but not impossible. Significant progress has been achieved developing highly selective allosteric modulators although none has yet progressed through POC to test the hypothesis. The ability to directly target the orthosteric domain and still achieve selectivity in a drug-like molecule has been questioned. Such a ligand has been generated previously. A selective M1 orthosteric agonist was developed and taken through safety into early clinical development. LY593093 was terminated but remained a useful and early example of a highly selective partial agonist that bound at the orthosteric domain. With the progressive technological advances, it was later determined to be a bitopic agonist (Fig. 3) (Valant et al., 2008). binding at both the allosteric domain conferring high selectivity, as well as at the orthosteric domain with 80% maximal efficacy providing robust yet safe pharmacology (Liu et al., 2015; Watt et al., 2011). Therefore, introducing combinations of desired properties within a single molecular entity is possible to achieve a clinically viable molecule. Harnessing in silico, biophysical, and structural knowledge of the target of interest to then rationally design the desired combination of properties to drive correction of pathophysiology will certainly be possible if not routine in the not too distant future. One has to wonder what other yet undiscovered secrets GPCRs and protein targets in general still hold allowing precision medicines to reach patients in need.

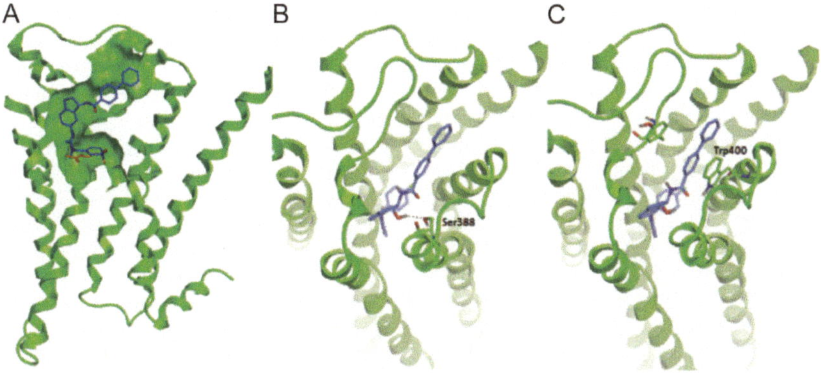

Fig. 3 Homology model of the M1 receptor docked to acetylcholine (orange) and a selective multi-topic M1 agonist, LY593093 (blue). (A) Ribbon diagram of the M1 receptor (green) with the ligand binding pocket visualized as a VDW surface. (B) 90-degree rotation of (A). (C) 90 degree rotation of (A). *Adapted from Liu, B., Croy, C.H., Hitchcock, S.A., Allen, J.R., Rao, Z., Evans, D., et al. (2015). Design and synthesis of N-[6-(substituted aminoethylideneamino)-2-hydroxyindan-1-yl] arylamides as selective and potent muscarinic M1 agonists.* Bioorganic & Medicinal Chemistry Letters, *25(19), 4158–4163.*

Conflict of interest

C.C.F. is employed by Karuna Therapeutics, Boston, MA, USA.

References

Bertekap, R. L., Burford, N. T., Li, Z., & Alt, A. (2015). High-throughput screening for allosteric modulators of GPCRs. In M. Filizola (Ed.), *G protein-coupled receptors in drug discovery. Methods in molecular biology, Vol. 1335,* New York, NY: Humana Press.

Bodick, N. C., Offen, W. W., Levey, A. I., Cutler, N. R., Gauthier, S. G., Satlin, A., et al. (1997). Effects of xanomeline, a selective muscarinic receptor agonist, on cognitive function and behavioral symptoms in Alzheimer disease. *Archives of Neurology, 54,* 465–473.

Bubser, M., Byun, N., Wood, M. R., & Jones, C. K. (2012). Muscarinic receptor pharmacology and circuitry for the modulation of cognition. In A. Fryer, A. Christopoulos, & N. Nathanson (Eds.), *Muscarinic receptors. Handbook of experimental pharmacology, Vol. 208,* Berlin, Heidelberg: Springer.

Bymaster, F. P., McKinzie, D. L., Felder, C. C., & Wess, J. (2003). Use of M 1–M 5 muscarinic receptor knockout mice as novel tools to delineate the physiological roles of the muscarinic cholinergic system. *Neurochemical Research, 28,* 437–442.

Calcutt, N. A., Smith, D. R., Frizzi, K., Sabbir, M. G., Chowdhury, S. K. R., Mixcoatl-Zecuatl, T., et al. (2017). Selective antagonism of muscarinic receptors is neuroprotective in peripheral neuropathy. *The Journal of Clinical Investigation, 127,* 608–622.

Ceskova, E., & Silhan, P. (2018). Novel treatment options in depression and psychosis. *Neuropsychiatric Disease and Treatment, 14,* 741.

Chan, W. Y., McKinzie, D. L., Bose, S., Mitchell, S. N., Witkin, J. M., Thompson, R. C., et al. (2008). Allosteric modulation of the muscarinic M4 receptor as an approach to treating schizophrenia. *Proceedings of the National Academy of Sciences of the United States of America, 105,* 10978–10983.

Coyle, J. T., Price, D. L., & Delong, M. R. (1983). Alzheimer's disease: A disorder of cortical cholinergic innervation. *Science*, *219*, 1184–1190.
DeVree, B. T., Mahoney, J. P., Vélez-Ruiz, G. A., Rasmussen, S. G., Kuszak, A. J., Edwald, E., et al. (2016). Allosteric coupling from G protein to the agonist-binding pocket in GPCRs. *Nature*, *535*(7610), 182–198.
DiMasi, J. A., Grabowski, H. G., & Hansen, R. W. (2016). Innovation in the pharmaceutical industry: New estimates of R & D costs. *Journal of Health Economics*, *47*, 20–33.
Dror, R. O., Green, H. F., Valant, C., Borhani, D. W., Valcourt, J. R., Pan, A. C., et al. (2013). Structural basis for modulation of a G-protein-coupled receptor by allosteric drugs. *Nature*, *503*, 295–299.
Edvinsson, L. (2018). CGRP antibodies as prophylaxis in migraine. *Cell*, *175*, 1719.
Eglen, R. M., Choppin, A., Dillon, M. P., & Hegde, S. (1999). Muscarinic receptor ligands and their therapeutic potential. *Current Opinion in Chemical Biology*, *3*, 426–432.
Felder, C. C., Bymaster, F. P., Ward, J., & DeLapp, N. (2000). Therapeutic opportunities for muscarinic receptors in the central nervous system. *Journal of Medicinal Chemistry*, *43*, 4333–4353.
Felder, C. C., Goldsmith, P. J., Jackson, K., Sanger, H. E., Evans, D. A., Mogg, A. J., et al. (2018). Current status of muscarinic M1 and M4 receptors as drug targets for neurodegenerative diseases. *Neuropharmacology*, *136*, 449–458.
Felder, C. C., Tu, Y., Schober, D., Quets, A., Xiao, H., Watt, M., et al. (2011). Native tissue pharmacology of the mGluR2 selective agonist, LY2812223. *Current Neuropharmacology*, *9*, 19–20.
Gabathuler, R. (2010). Approaches to transport therapeutic drugs across the blood–brain barrier to treat brain diseases. *Neurobiology of Disease*, *37*, 48–57.
Greenwood, T., Lazzeroni, L., Calkins, M. E., Freedman, R., Green, M. F., Gur, R. E., et al. (2018). Genome-wide association of endophenotypes for schizophrenia from the consortium on the genetics of schizophrenia (COGS) study. *Biological Psychiatry*, *83*, S44.
Gutierrez, A. N., & McDonald, P. H. (2018). GPCRs: Emerging anti-cancer drug targets. *Cellular Signalling*, *41*, 65–74.
Harrison, R. K. (2016). Phase II and phase III failures: 2013–2015. *Nature Reviews. Drug Discovery*, *15*, 817–818.
Hauser, A. S., Gloriam, D. E., Attwood, M. M., Rask-Andersen, M., & Schiöth, H. B. (2017). Trends in GPCR drug discovery: New agents, targets and indications. *Nature Reviews. Drug Discovery*, *16*, 829–842.
Heinrich, J. N., Butera, J. A., Carrick, T., Kramer, A., Kowal, D., Lock, T., et al. (2009). Pharmacological comparison of muscarinic ligands: Historical versus more recent muscarinic M1-preferring receptor agonists. *European Journal of Pharmacology*, *1*, 53–56.
Hilger, D., Masureel, M., & Kobilka, B. K. (2018). Structure and dynamics of GPCR signaling complexes. *Nature Structural & Molecular Biology*, *25*, 4–12.
Hollingsworth, S. A., & Dror, R. O. (2018). Molecular dynamics simulation for all. *Neuron*, *99*, 1129–1143.
Hwang, T. J., Carpenter, D., Lauffenburger, J. C., Wang, B., Franklin, J. M., & Kesselheim, A. S. (2016). Failure of investigational drugs in late-stage clinical development and publication of trial results. *JAMA Internal Medicine*, *176*, 1826–1833.
Ito, Y., Oyunzul, L., Seki, M., Oki, T. F., Matsui, M., & Yamada, S. (2009). Quantitative analysis of the loss of muscarinic receptors in various peripheral tissues in M1–M5 receptor single knockout mice. *British Journal of Pharmacology*, *156*, 1147–1153.
Kesselheim, A. S., Hwang, T. J., & Franklin, J. M. (2015). Two decades of new drug development for central nervous system disorders. *Nature Reviews. Drug Discovery*, *14*, 815.
Kruse, A. C., Ring, A. M., Manglik, A., Hu, J., Hu, K., Eitel, K., et al. (2013). Activation and allosteric modulation of a muscarinic acetylcholine receptor. *Nature*, *504*(7478), 101–106.

Kurimoto, E., Matsuda, S., Shimizu, Y., Sako, Y., Mandai, T., Sugimoto, T., et al. (2018). An approach to discovering novel muscarinic M1 receptor positive allosteric modulators with potent cognitive improvement and minimized gastrointestinal dysfunction. *Journal of Pharmacology and Experimental Therapeutics*, *364*, 28–37.

Liu, B., Croy, C. H., Hitchcock, S. A., Allen, J. R., Rao, Z., Evans, D., et al. (2015). Design and synthesis of N-[6-(substituted aminoethylideneamino)-2-hydroxyindan-1-yl] arylamides as selective and potent muscarinic M1 agonists. *Bioorganic & Medicinal Chemistry Letters*, *25*(19), 4158–4163.

Maier, R., Moser, G., Chen, G. B., Ripke, S., Absher, D., Agartz, I., et al. (2015). Joint analysis of psychiatric disorders increases accuracy of risk prediction for schizophrenia, bipolar disorder, and major depressive disorder. *The American Journal of Human Genetics*, *96*, 283–294.

May, L. T., & Christopoulos, A. (2003). Allosteric modulators of G-protein-coupled receptors. *Current Opinion in Pharmacology*, *3*(5), 551–556.

McCorvy, J. D., Butler, K. V., Kelly, B., Rechsteiner, K., Karpiak, J., Betz, R. M., et al. (2018). Structure-inspired design of β-arrestin-biased ligands for aminergic GPCRs. *Nature Chemical Biology*, *14*, 126.

Monod, J., Wyman, J., & Changeux, J. P. (1965). On the nature of allosteric modulators: A plausible model. *Journal of Molecular Biology*, *12*, 88–118.

Mujić-Delić, A., de Wit, R. H., Verkaar, F., & Smit, M. J. (2014). GPCR-targeting nanobodies: Attractive research tools, diagnostics, and therapeutics. *Trends in Pharmacological Sciences*, *35*, 247–255.

Rankovic, Z., Brust, T. F., & Bohn, L. M. (2016). Biased agonism: An emerging paradigm in GPCR drug discovery. *Bioorganic & Medicinal Chemistry Letters*, *26*, 241–250.

Rook, J. M., Bertron, J. L., Cho, H. P., Garcia-Barrantes, P. M., Moran, S. P., Maksymetz, J. T., et al. (2018). A novel M1 PAM VU0486846 exerts efficacy in cognition models without displaying agonist activity or cholinergic toxicity. *ACS Chemical Neuroscience*, *9*, 2274–2285.

Sako, Y., Kurimoto, E., Mandai, T., Suzuki, A., Tanaka, M., Suzuki, M., et al. (2018). TAK-071, a novel M 1 positive allosteric modulator with low cooperativity, improves cognitive function in rodents with few cholinergic side effects. *Neuropsychopharmacology*, *1*, 1–11.

Shekhar, A., Potter, W. Z., Lightfoot, J., Lienemann, D., Pharm, J., Dubé, S., et al. (2008). Selective muscarinic receptor agonist xanomeline as a novel treatment approach for schizophrenia. *American Journal of Psychiatry*, *165*, 1033–1039.

Shimada, I., Ueda, T., Kofuku, Y., Eddy, M. T., & Wüthrich, K. (2019). GPCR drug discovery: Integrating solution NMR data with crystal and cryo-EM structures. *Nature Reviews. Drug Discovery*, *18*, 59–82.

Siuda, E. R., Carr, R., III, Rominger, D. H., & Violin, J. D. (2017). Biased mu-opioid receptor ligands: A promising new generation of pain therapeutics. *Current Opinion in Pharmacology*, *32*, 77–84.

Sriram, K., & Insel, P. A. (2018). G protein-coupled receptors as targets for approved drugs: How many targets and how many drugs? *Molecular Pharmacology*, *93*, 251–258.

Stone, J. M., & Pilowsky, L. S. (2007). Novel targets for drugs in schizophrenia. *CNS & Neurological Disorders Drug Targets*, *6*, 265–272.

Thomsen, M., Sørensen, G., & Dencker, D. (2018). Physiological roles of CNS muscarinic receptors gained from knockout mice. *Neuropharmacology*, *136*, 411–420.

Valant, C., Gregory, K. J., Hall, N. E., Scammells, P. J., Lew, M. J., Sexton, P. M., et al. (2008). A novel mechanism of G protein-coupled receptor functional selectivity muscarinic partial agonist McN-A-343 as a bitopic orthosteric/allosteric ligand. *Journal of Biological Chemistry*, *283*, 29312–29321.

Wadhawan, S., Pant, S., Golhar, R., Kirov, S., Thompson, J., Jacobsen, L., et al. (2017). NaV channel variants in patients with painful and nonpainful peripheral neuropathy. *Neurology. Genetics*, *3*, 207.

Wang, X., Heinz, B. A., Qian, Y. W., Carter, J. H., Gadski, R. A., Beavers, L. S., et al. (2018). Intracellular binding site for a positive allosteric modulator of the dopamine D1 receptor. *Molecular Pharmacology, 94*, 1232–1245.

Wang, S., Wacker, D., Levit, A., Che, T., Betz, R. M., McCorvy, J. D., et al. (2017). D4 dopamine receptor high-resolution structures enable the discovery of selective agonists. *Science, 358*, 381–386.

Waring, M. J., Arrowsmith, J., Leach, A. R., Leeson, P. D., Mandrell, S., Owen, R. M., et al. (2015). An analysis of the attrition of drug candidates from four major pharmaceutical companies. *Nature Reviews. Drug Discovery, 14*, 475–487.

Watt, M. L., Schober, D. A., Hitchcock, S., Liu, B., Chesterfield, A. K., McKinzie, D., et al. (2011). Pharmacological characterization of LY593093, an M1 muscarinic acetylcholine receptor-selective partial orthosteric agonist. *Journal of Pharmacology and Experimental Therapeutics, 338*, 622–632.

Wess, J., Eglen, R. M., & Gautam, D. (2007). Muscarinic acetylcholine receptors: Mutant mice provide new insights for drug development. *Nature Reviews. Drug Discovery, 6*, 721–733.

Woolley, M. L., Carter, H. J., Gartlon, J. E., Watson, J. M., & Dawson, L. A. (2009). Attenuation of amphetamine-induced activity by the non-selective muscarinic receptor agonist, xanomeline, is absent in muscarinic M4 receptor knockout mice and attenuated in muscarinic M1 receptor knockout mice. *European Journal of Pharmacology, 603*, 147–149.

Yarwood, R. E., Imlach, W. L., Lieu, T., Veldhuis, N. A., Jensen, D. D., Herenbrink, C. K., et al. (2017). Endosomal signaling of the receptor for calcitonin gene-related peptide mediates pain transmission. *Proceedings of the National Academy of Sciences of the United States of America, 114*, 12309–12314.

Yu, Y. J., & Watts, R. J. (2013). Developing therapeutic antibodies for neurodegenerative disease. *Neurotherapeutics, 10*, 459–472.

Further reading

Changeux, J. P., & Edelstein, S. J. (2005). Allosteric mechanisms of signal transduction. *Science, 308*, 1424–1428.

CHAPTER TWO

Lipid rafts in psychiatry

Nathan H. Wray[a,b], Mark M. Rasenick[a,b,c,d,*]

[a]University of Illinois College of Medicine, Department of Physiology & Biophysics, Chicago, IL, United States
[b]The Graduate Program in Neuroscience, Chicago, IL, United States
[c]Department of Psychiatry, Chicago, IL, United States
[d]The Jesse Brown VAMC, Chicago, IL, United States
*Corresponding author: e-mail address: raz@uic.edu

Contents

1. Introduction 21
2. Studying lipid rafts 23
3. Monoaminergic signaling 25
   3.1 GPCRs 25
   3.2 Monoamine transporters 26
   3.3 Serotonergic signaling 27
   3.4 Dopaminergic signaling 30
   3.5 Noradrenergic signaling 31
4. Signal transduction proteins and lipid rafts 32
   4.1 G proteins 33
   4.2 Adenylyl cyclase 33
5. Depression, lipid rafts and Gα_s 33
6. Conclusion 37
Acknowledgments 37
Conflict of interest statement 37
References 37
Further reading 45

Abstract

Lipid microenvironments in the plasma membrane are known to influence many signal transduction pathways. Several of those pathways are critical for both the etiology and treatment of depression. Further, several signaling proteins are modified, covalently, by lipids, a process that alters their interface with the microenvironments mentioned above. This review presents a brief discussion of the interface of the above elements as well as a discussion about the participation of lipids and lipid moieties in the action of antidepressants.

1. Introduction

The original Singer-Nicolson model of the plasma membrane postulated the lipid bilayer as a fluid and homogenous two-dimensional plane

Advances in Pharmacology, Volume 86
ISSN 1054-3589
https://doi.org/10.1016/bs.apha.2019.04.001

where proteins could diffuse freely (Singer & Nicolson, 1972). This model has been extensively reimagined and updated as we continue to learn more about the complexity and heterogeneity of the lipid and protein composition of the membrane. In fact, shortly after the publication of the landmark paper positing the fluid mosaic model, various observations suggested that plasma membranes may be composed of laterally heterogeneous microdomains (Ahmed, Brown, & London, 1997; Varma & Mayor, 1998; Yu, Fischman, & Steck, 1973). The lipid raft hypothesis first put forth by Simons and Ikonen (1997), posited that molecular interactions between cholesterol and saturated fatty acids in the two-dimensional plane that is the plasma membrane, drive the formation of ordered membrane domains that organize and recruit proteins. It is now known that the inner and outer leaflet of the plasma membrane are composed of hundreds of different lipids and proteins, which augur heterogeneity for the term "lipid raft" (Ingólfsson et al., 2014). Two basic types of lipid rafts have been proposed. One type enriched in the scaffolding protein caveolin (caveolin 1, 2 and 3 isoforms) which causes membrane invaginations named, caveolae (Latin for little caves). The other being planar lipid rafts which contain flotillin in lieu of caveolin, and therefore do not invaginate. Interestingly, neurons express caveolin but do not display the classical caveolae invaginations (Liu et al., 2018). For the purposes of this article, we define lipid rafts as small (25–100 nm diameter) temporally dynamic and ordered domains of the membrane dependent on cholesterol, rich in saturated fatty acids, sphingolipids, glycosylphosphatidylinositol (GPI)-anchored proteins and associated with cytoskeletal components. These ordered domains organize proteins, influence signal propagation and mediate endocytosis. Caveolin mediated endocytosis requires caveolin and cavin proteins but not clathrin (Kovtun, Tillu, Ariotti, Parton, & Collins, 2015). Planar lipid rafts can also engage in endocytosis albeit with flotillin (Kokubo, Helms, Ohno-iwashita, & Shimada, 2003). Given that a variety of proteins (receptors, transporters, G-proteins, signaling enzymes, scaffolding proteins) involved in neurotransmission localize to lipid rafts, they have been implicated in a variety of mental diseases including unipolar depression, bipolar affective disorder, schizophrenia, Alzheimer's disease, and Parkinson's disease (Allen, Halverson-Tamboli, & Rasenick, 2007; Ehehalt, Keller, Haass, Thiele, & Simons, 2003; Eisensamer et al., 2005; Hashimoto, Takenouchi, Rockenstein, & Masliah, 2003). Here, we focus on the relevance of lipid rafts in psychiatric disorders, particularly lipid raft modulation of monoaminergic receptor signaling and transport activity and the relevance to depression.

2. Studying lipid rafts

Given the challenges studying lipid rafts and early conflicting data regarding the composition and function of lipid rafts investigators have debated their function and even their very existence (Munro, 2003). One of the first lines of evidence for lipid rafts was the observation that membrane proteins and lipids would solubilize into two distinct fractions (Yu et al., 1973). Preparation of membranes using non-ionic detergents such as Triton X-100 (TX100) at 4 °C yields detergent resistant membrane (DRM) fractions containing lipid raft components such as cholesterol, GPI-anchored proteins and sphingomyelin. Unfortunately, this method would often produce inconsistent, even conflicting results as slight variations in detergent concentration, detergent ratios or temperature would alter the protein and lipid composition of the fractions (Babiychuk & Draeger, 2006; Song et al., 1996). Other methods using mechanical separation and sucrose gradient centrifugation have also been developed but suffer from conflicting results from slight changes in protocols (Song et al., 1996). It is noteworthy that some of these methods employ alkaline treatment of membranes, a process inducing saponification, which creates "detergent" without adding it. These initial conflicting observations sparked a controversy calling into question existence of lipid rafts. Some investigators went as far to say that rafts are merely artifacts created by the detergents used to study them (Kraft & Bement, 2013; Sevcsik & Schutz, 2015). Super resolution microscopy is beginning to resolve these controversies (Stone, Shelby, & Veatch, 2017).

Clearly, raft localization is not sufficient evidence to show raft involvement in a given biochemical process. Cholesterol chelation and removal by methyl-β-cyclodextrin (MβCD), filipin, or nystatin has been used to provide evidence for raft involvement in signaling events, operating under the assumption that the resulting altered signaling event is due to loss of lipid rafts. Genetic manipulations using caveolin siRNA and caveolin-1 knockout mice have also been employed to disrupt rafts and examine subsequent altered signaling events (Allen et al., 2009; Bhatnagar, Sheffler, Kroeze, Compton-Toth, & Roth, 2004; Trushina, Du Charme, Parisi, & McMurray, 2006). Unfortunately, these methods are inherently pleiotropic, and data derived from such experiments require further validation (Kwik et al., 2003).

Observing lipid raft protein localization and signaling events has been problematic given their submicroscopic scale and temporally dynamic nature. Caveolae's distinct invaginations have been observed via electron microscopy but studying planar lipid rafts and lipid raft protein composition has been elusive (Thorn et al., 2003). In fact, fluorescently tagged proteins thought to localize in rafts appear homogenously diffuse across the plasma membrane (Czysz, Schappi, & Rasenick, 2015; Yu & Rasenick, 2002). However, recent advances in super-resolution have shown promise in investigating the nanoscale structure and dynamics in rafts such as stimulated emission depletion (STED), photoactivated localization microscopy (PALM), and k-space image correlation spectroscopy (kICS) (Abu-arish et al., 2015; Sengupta et al., 2011). Older confocal techniques such as fluorescent recovery after photobleaching (FRAP), and fluorescent resonance energy transfer (FRET) have also successfully observed raft protein dynamics (Agudo-Ibáñez, Herrero, Barbacid, & Crespo, 2015; Czysz et al., 2015).

It is quite clear that the physiochemical evidence suggests that heterogenous populations of lipids self-organize in artificial biomimetic membranes. Early investigations, using lipid monolayers composed of endogenous membrane lipids at air-water interfaces, revealed liquid-lipid phase separation, which suggested membrane heterogeneity (Rice & Mcconnell, 1989). These observations were later confirmed and characterized in artificial lipid bilayers (Dietrich et al., 2001). These insights have provided in-depth observations of phase separation revealing distinct liquid-ordered (L_o) and liquid-disordered (L_d) domains. L_o (i.e., lipid raft-like) domains display more saturated (extended) lipid acyl chains, lower diffusivity, and more dense molecular packing compared to L_d domains. Interestingly, these characteristics are maintained over a wide range of temperatures and endogenous lipid populations (Feigenson & Buboltz, 2001; Veatch & Keller, 2002, 2003). Despite these observations providing strong observable evidence for raft-like domains, artificial membranes lack integral membrane proteins and the immense lipid heterogeneity found in endogenous plasma membranes.

To overcome these shortcomings, investigators have recently begun validating older observations in membranes prepared from living cells, either as plasma membrane spheres (PMS), or giant plasma membrane vesicles (GPMVs) (Baumgart et al., 2007; Sezgin et al., 2012). These membranes can be induced with DTT, formaldehyde or *N*-ethylmaleimide (Sevcsik & Schutz, 2015). These free plasma membrane vesicles, or blebs, can then provide insights into the behavior and composition of endogenous plasma membrane domains. Many of the insights gathered from blebs are consistent with earlier, inchoate observations of lipid rafts. That is, distinct domains emerge with differing orders, diffusiveness and compositions (Baumgart et al., 2007; Levental, Grzybek, & Simons, 2011; Sengupta, Hammond, Holowka, & Baird, 2008). Furthermore, raft or more ordered domains are enriched in glycosphingolipids, palmitoylated transmembrane proteins, GPI-anchored proteins and proteins with longer transmembrane domains (Diaz-rohrer, Levental, Simons, & Levental, 2014; Levental, Lingwood, Grzybek, Coskun, & Simons, 2010; Sengupta et al., 2008). Unfortunately, blebs generate their own pitfalls, such as a lack of control over their composition and detachment from the cytoskeleton. However, they have proven to be a useful tool in studying lipid rafts.

The aforementioned methods have both advantages and pitfalls, and the best approach is to employ multiple techniques when studying lipid rafts. Despite debates surrounding lipid rafts it is presently accepted they are central to many cell processes such as protein scaffolding, endocytosis, trafficking and modulating the activity of proteins. In fact, at the Keystone Symposium of Lipid Rafts and Cell Function in 2006 a consensus defined lipid rafts as "small (<200nm) heterogenous, highly dynamic, sterol- and sphingolipid-enriched domains that compartmentalize cellular processes" thereby cementing lipid rafts as a permanent fixture in the field of cellular biology (Pike, 2006).

3. Monoaminergic signaling

3.1 GPCRs

The majority of the lipid-raft-associated receptors discussed herein are G-protein coupled receptors (GPCRs). With approximately 800 human genes encoding GPCRs, they are one of the largest family of proteins in the human genome (Oldham & Hamm, 2008). More importantly, GPCRs offer a prime target for pharmaceuticals as it is possible to design highly specific, high affinity ligands for a single receptor. Consequently, approximately 30% of drugs on the market target GPCRs (Hopkins & Groom, 2002). However, in psychiatry many are indirectly targeted by inhibiting neurotransmitter transporters, thus increasing extracellular concentrations of endogenous ligands.

GPCRs transduce a plethora of extracellular stimuli such as odorants, light, hormones, neurotransmitters and then activate intracellular signaling cascades. All GPCRs are composed of seven transmembrane-spanning alpha-helices, an intracellular carboxyl terminus, an extracellular amino terminus and three helical loops on either side of the plasma membrane. GPCRs activate intracellular signaling cascades by coupling with and ultimately activating GTP binding proteins (G-proteins). Heterotrimeric G-proteins are composed of α, β, and γ subunits. Upon ligand activation of the GPCR the receptor will undergo a conformation change that will cause the Gα subunit to exchange a guanosine diphosphate (GDP) for a guanosine triphosphate (GTP), which "activates" the heterotrimeric protein. G-proteins primarily, but not solely, act through the Gα subunit, which once activated, will bind to and modulate a variety of downstream targets deemed second effectors.

Heterotrimeric G-proteins are targeted and tethered to the plasma membrane by numerous fatty acid post-translational modifications. These covalent lipid modifications are sometimes reversible and influence GPCR signaling (Escribá, Wedegaertner, Goñi, & Vögler, 2007). The Gα subunit also has a polybasic positively charged amino-terminus which aids in its association to the negatively charged plasma membrane. Interestingly, the Gα subunits undergo a diverse range of acylation modifications, which target the protein to lipid raft and non-raft regions of the membrane, and influence protein-protein interactions (Oldham & Hamm, 2008).

Heterotrimers are defined by the primary function of their Gα subunit with respect to a G protein effector. The $G\alpha_q$ subunit activates phospholipase C, which cleaves phosphatidylinositol 4,5-bisphosphate (PIP_2) into diacylglycerol (DAG) and inositol trisphosphate (IP_3). The $G\alpha_{12/13}$ subunit primarily modulates actin dynamics. The stimulatory subunit ($G\alpha_s$) and inhibitory subunit ($G\alpha_i$) cause adenylyl cyclase to either stimulate or inhibit adenylyl cyclase to produce (or not) cyclic adenosine mono-phosphate (cAMP) (Milligan & Kostenis, 2006).

3.2 Monoamine transporters

Monoaminergic reuptake transporters (MATs) selectively uptake monoamines from the extracellular space to replenish internal stores within intracellular presynaptic bouton. Thus, expression of transporters is restricted to presynaptic regions in neurons. All MATs are neurotransmitter-sodium symporters composed of 12 alpha-helical transmembrane spanning regions of the solute carrier 6 (SLC6) family. Both the N- and C-terminals protrude in the intracellular space (Aggarwal & Mortensen, 2017). MATs are often anchored to lipid raft microdomains by binding to PIP_2, which also mediates transporter oligomerization and regulates monoamine efflux (Buchmayer et al., 2013).

The three monoamine transporters discussed within are the serotonin transporter (SERT), norepinephrine transporter (NET), and dopamine transporter (DAT). These MATs play a critical role in altering extracellular neurotransmitter concentration. Thus, they also influence signal amplitude and duration of monoaminergic signal transmission. They have been implicated in depression, schizophrenia, ADHD, schizophrenia, and anxiety. Many drugs are thought to act by binding and inhibiting MATs, thus increasing the amount of extracellular endogenous levels of monoamines in the synapse. Selective SERT inhibitors (SSRIs) such as escitalopram, fluoxetine, paroxetine, and sertraline are often prescribed for depression, anxiety and panic disorders. Curiously, 3,4-methylenedioxymethamphetamine (MDMA) or ecstasy, which acts by causing SERT, DAT, and NET efflux of associated monoamines has recently entered phase three clinical trials for the treatment of post-traumatic stress disorder (PTSD; Feduccia & Mithoefer, 2018). Tricyclic antidepressants (TCAs) less selectively inhibit SERT and NET (or selective SERT + NET blockers) are used to treat depression and pain. The selective DAT inhibitor bupropion is prescribed for depression and as an aid in smoking cessation. Methylphenidate and D-amphetamine also inhibit DAT and are used to manage attention deficit hyperactivity disorder (ADHD). Non-selective MAT efflux compounds such a racemic mixture of amphetamine is also prescribed for ADHD. However, at least one antidepressant, tianeptine, increases 5HT transport. Furthermore, 5HT transport is inhibited, rapidly, by many antidepressant drugs even though they do not achieve clinical efficacy for several weeks.

3.3 Serotonergic signaling

Serotonergic signaling has been routinely implicated in depression, alcoholism, anxiety, and schizophrenia (Mann, 2013). Serotonin is synthesized from L-tryptophan in neurons in the raphe nuclei which project to a wide array of brain regions. Currently 14 serotonin receptors have been identified and characterized into the subclasses: 5-HT_{1A}, 5-HT_{2A}, 5-HT_3, 5-HT_4, 5-HT_5, 5-HT_6 and 5-HT_7. The majority of these receptors are metabotropic GPCRs; thus, they act through second messenger systems either by stimulating or inhibiting the production of cAMP or increasing inositol triphosphate and diacylglycerol. The lone exception being the 5-HT_3 subclass, an ionotropic receptor which mediates K^+, Na^+, or Ca^{2+} influx. Many of these receptors localize to specific microdomains of the plasma membrane where their activity is modulated, adding another layer of regulation to this already complex signaling system.

3.3.1 Serotonergic GPCRS

The 5-HT_{1A} receptors are coupled to $G\alpha_i$ and inhibit the activation of adenylyl cyclase and production of intracellular cAMP. They have been shown to colocalize in DRM fractions with caveolin in murine brain tissue. Localization is dependent on palmitoylation, as this modification targets and anchors proteins to lipid raft microdomains (Renner et al., 2007). Further evidence for raft 5-HT_{1A} signaling involvement was observed by disrupting rafts by chelating cholesterol with MβCD, which inhibits G-protein coupling and ligand binding (Pucadyil & Chattopadhyay, 2004). These deficits are restored with the addition of cholesterol (Kalipatnapu & Chattopadhyay, 2009; Sjögren, Hamblin, & Svenningsson, 2006). Furthermore, genetic evidence also suggests receptor cholesterol interactions as the 5-HT_{1A} receptor contains a cholesterol amino acid binding motif (Liu et al., 2018).

The 5-HT_{2A} autoreceptor is highly expressed throughout the brain and couples to $G\alpha_{q,}$ increasing diacylglycerol, inositol triphosphate and intracellular Ca^{2+} concentrations. The receptor colocalizes with caveolin in variety of cell types (Bhatnagar et al., 2004; Dreja et al., 2002; Mialet-Perez et al., 2012). In C6 glioma cells 5-HT_{2A} receptors colocalize with caveolin-1 in intracellular vesicles and on the cell surface. In fact, 5-HT_{2A} binds to caveolin-1, which is a prerequisite for $G\alpha_q$ coupling to the receptor. Consequently, lipid raft disruption by cholesterol depletion or caveolin knockdown diminishes endogenous 5-HT_{2A} signaling (Bhatnagar et al., 2004; Mialet-Perez et al., 2012). This suggests that all molecules responsible for 5HT1a signaling (GPCR, Gq and PLC) are contained within the lipid raft.

The only $G\alpha_s$ coupled (cAMP stimulating) serotonin receptor suggested to reside in lipid rafts is the 5-HT_7 receptor. Indeed, the receptor colocalizes with caveolin-1 in DRMs (Sjogren, 2007). Interestingly, the lipid raft components cholesterol, sphingomyelin, caveolin-1, and gangliosides work in concert to regulate serotonin and exogenous ligand binding to the receptor. Specifically, chelating or inhibiting the synthesis of cholesterol reduces ligand binding and consequently downstream cAMP mediated CREB phosphorylation (Sjögren et al., 2006). Moreover, depleting sphingomyelin and gangliosides or knocking down the expression of caveolin-1 also attenuates ligand binding to the 5-HT_7 receptor in HeLA cells, independent of cholesterol chelation (Sjogren, 2007). Taken together, these studies suggest a role for rafts in the proper functioning of the 5-HT_7.

3.3.2 Serotonergic ligand-gated ion channels

The 5-HT_3 receptor is an ionotropic ligand-gated ion channel and a member of the Cys-loop family of ion channels. It acts by triggering fast signal transduction opening presynaptic Ca^{2+} channels or postsynaptic K^+, Na^+, or Ca^{2+} ion channels upon agonist binding (Wu, Cheng, Jiang, Melcher, & Xu, 2015). The ionotropic receptor localizes exclusively to lipid raft fractions enriched in caveolin-2 and flotillin-1 in studies using both neuroblastoma (N1E-115) and HEK-293 cells. Of particular interest, antidepressant (desipramine, fluoxetine, and reboxetine) and antipsychotic (fluphenazine, haloperidol, and clozapine) compounds also localize with the receptor in lipid raft fractions. Note, however, that the association of antidepressants with lipid rafts occurs on a slower timescale that that of antipsychotics (vide infra). Concentrations of these various compounds correlate highly with non-competitive inhibition of 5-HT_3 mediated cation currents (Eisensamer et al., 2005). Interestingly, lipid raft disruption does not interfere with antidepressant 5-HT_3 antagonism, thus this effect appears to be independent of lipid raft localization (Eisensamer et al., 2005). However, lipid raft depletion by MβCD reduces 5-HT_3 peak amplitude and the kinetics of cation currents demonstrating a role in lipid raft integrity and ion channel function (Nothdurfter et al., 2010).

3.3.3 Serotonin transporters

SERT is inhibited by nearly all antidepressants to varying degrees. Inhibiting SERT increases the amount serotonin available in the synapse, which in turn leads to downstream cellular and molecular adaptations that are thought to mediate antidepressant's efficacy. Interestingly, SERT resides in two distinct populations in the plasma membrane. One group localizes to non-raft regions and displays increased motility compared to its less mobile counterpart present in ganglioside rich (specifically GM1) lipid rafts (Chang et al., 2012). Cholesterol chelation and reduction by MβCD increases lateral motility of SERT in RN46A serotonergic neuronal cells, which is accompanied by a 50% reduction in mean transporter activity. Moreover, SERT's affinity for serotonin decreases after cholesterol depletion (Magnani, Tate, Wynne, Williams, & Haase, 2004; Scanlon, Williams, & Schloss, 2001). These studies suggest a role for lipid rafts promoting a high-affinity, high-activity state of SERT. In fact, upregulation of SERT activity occurs on SERT localized to lipid raft domains via p38 MAPK (Chang et al., 2012). Conversely, downregulation of SERT activity via protein kinase C (PCK) occurs by translocating SERT from lipid raft microdomains to non-raft regions (Samuvel, Jayanthi, Bhat, & Ramamoorthy, 2005). These studies suggest a significant role in lipid rafts modulating SERT activity, and ultimately serotonergic signal propagation.

3.4 Dopaminergic signaling

Dopaminergic signaling has been implicated in many major psychiatric disorders including depression, PTSD, addiction, and schizophrenia (Catapano & Manji, 2007). In fact, many antipsychotics including typical and atypical antipsychotics antagonize dopamine GPCRs, to varying degrees. Conversely, the dopamine agonists bromocriptine and pramipexole show antidepressant effects (Catapano & Manji, 2007). Dopaminergic receptors are separated into D1- or D2-classes depending on their coupling to $G\alpha_s/G\alpha_{olf}$ or $G\alpha_i/G\alpha_o$, respectively (Ilani et al., 2002). Interestingly, the D_3 receptor (D2-class) primarily couples to $G\alpha_i$ but to a lesser degree can act through $G\alpha_s$ (Obadiah et al., 1999). In the brain, D2-class receptors are found both pre- and post-synaptically, whereas D1-class receptors are restricted to post-synaptic regions of neurons (Jaber, Robinson, Missale, & Caron, 1996).

3.4.1 Dopaminergic GPCRs

In the D1 class, the D_1 receptor primarily localizes to lipid raft microdomains in both preparations of rat brain and HEK293 cells (Voulalas, Schetz, & Undieh, 2011; Yu et al., 2004). Strengthening these data, the receptor co-localizes with lipid raft associated and signal transduction proteins such as caveolin-2, flotillin, $G\alpha_s$, and adenylyl cyclase (Yu et al., 2004). Interestingly, disruption of lipid raft integrity by cholesterol depletion with MβCD attenuates basal adenylyl cyclase activity in HEK-293 and human renal proximal tubule (hRPT) cells (Yu et al., 2014). Unlike the D_1 receptor, the D_1 class, D_5 receptor, does not localize to lipid raft fractions, but primarily to cytosolic fractions in preparations of rat frontal cortex (Paspalas & Goldman-rakic, 2004; Yu et al., 2004).

Of the D2 class (D_2,D_3, D_4), the D_2 receptor is detected in both lipid raft and non-raft domains, depending on the technique utilized and the cell type studied. Sucrose gradient preparations of the rat frontal cortex show ubiquitous distribution of the receptor in raft, non-raft and cytosolic regions (Voulalas et al., 2011). However, TX100 detergent preparations of HEK-293T cells show the D_2 principally localizing to DRMs (Celver, Sharma, & Kovoor, 2012; Sharma, Celver, Octeau, & Kovoor, 2013). Curiously, cholesterol depletion decreases localization of raft associated proteins in DRMs, as expected, but not the D_2 receptor (Sharma et al., 2013). The D_3 receptor is found in small quantities in lipid raft fractions, but predominantly in non-raft regions of the plasma membrane in hRPT cells. Unlike the D_2 receptor, cholesterol depletion causes the entirety of D_3 receptor population to redistribute to non-raft regions (Villar et al., 2009).

3.4.2 Dopaminergic transporters

The DAT is expressed ubiquitously along the plasma membrane in raft and non-raft regions, despite cholesterol influencing its function (Foster, Adkins, Lever, & Vaughan, 2008). Total membrane cholesterol depletion with MβCD reduces mean DAT uptake and efflux rate (Jones, Zhen, & Reith, 2012). Moreover, DAT's affinity for dopamine is also attenuated by cholesterol chelation (Adkins et al., 2007). Interestingly, cholesterol chelation with nystatin or filipin, which targets lipid raft cholesterol, has no effect on DAT efflux or uptake rate (Schnitzer, Oh, & Pinney, 1994). Restoration of membrane cholesterol levels also restored DAT function and affinity for dopamine (Jones et al., 2012). Moreover, PKC-mediated internalization of DAT occurs by a lipid raft independent, clathrin dependent mechanism (Sorkina, Hoover, Zahniser, & Sorkin, 2005). These studies suggest that non-raft localized cholesterol may promote a high activity state of the dopamine transporter when localized to non-raft regions of the plasma membrane.

3.5 Noradrenergic signaling

3.5.1 Noradrenergic GPCRs

Both β1 and β2 adrenergic receptors (β-AR) are coupled to $G\alpha_s$ which activates adenylyl cyclase to increase intracellular levels of cAMP. A cholesterol binding motif is present in the β2-AR and cholesterol binding has been shown to increase the stability of the receptor (Zocher, Zhang, Rasmussen, Kobilka, & Müller, 2012). The effect of cholesterol binding on the receptor's function has yet to be fully characterized since there are many conflicting reports (Dipilato & Zhang, 2009; Oner, Kaya, Onaran, Ozcan, & Ugur, 2010; Ostrom, Bundey, & Insel, 2004; Pontier et al., 2008). Inconsistencies may result from the aforementioned technical difficulties associated with studying lipid rafts or cell type differences. Unfortunately, many of the studies investigating lipid rafts' role on adrenergic receptor function have been performed in cardiomyocytes, which may provide limited insight into the impact of lipid raft on β-AR functioning in the brain and psychiatric disorders. That said, β1-AR is exclusively localized in non-raft regions of the membrane, whereas β2-AR is located in caveolae in cardiomyocytes (Xiang, Rybin, Steinberg, & Kobilka, 2002). In HEK293 and C6 glioma cells β2-AR are also localized to lipid rafts (Allen, Yu, Donati, & Rasenick, 2005; Pontier et al., 2008). In cardiomyocytes agonist activation of the β2-AR induces translocation of the receptor out of lipid raft regions where it is less likely to activate adenylyl cyclase, thus reducing downstream signaling events (Ostrom et al., 2001). However, both *Rybin* and *Head* say that disruption of the cytoskeleton or lipid rafts increased β2-activated cAMP signaling in cardiomyocytes, a finding consistent with that of Allen et al. (2005, 2009) in C6 cells (Head et al., 2006).

The $\alpha_{1\text{-}A}$ adrenergic receptor (α_{1A}AR) (Gα_q coupled) is localized to lipid raft microdomains in rat-1 fibroblasts and cardiomyocytes (Morris, Huynh, Vasilevski, & Woodcock, 2006; Morris, Lei, Wu, Michelotti, & Schwinn, 2008). After agonist stimulation the α_{1A}AR translocates to non-raft regions where it is ultimately internalized in a clathrin-dependent manner in rat-1 fibroblasts (Morris et al., 2008). Lipid raft disruption with MβCD promotes receptor internalization, suggesting a role for lipid raft translocation and receptor endocytosis (Morris et al., 2008). Interestingly, lipid raft localization inhibits activation of the receptor by preventing the exposure of the high affinity G-protein binding site to the extracellular space. Thus, rafts promote the inactive conformation of the receptor (Lei, Morris, Smith, & Schwinn, 2009).

3.5.2 Noradrenergic transporters

The NET is localized to lipid raft microdomains. Similar to SERT, NET is downregulated via a PKC dependent pathway. Unlike SERT, activity downregulation is accomplished by lipid raft mediated internalization (Jayanthi, Samuvel, & Ramamoorthy, 2004). NET downregulation is dependent on binding with neurokinin-1 receptor. Interestingly, this association occurs in non-raft domains and then translocates into raft regions before internalization (Arapulisamy, Mannangatti, & Jayanthi, 2013). However, unlike DAT and SERT, the effect of cholesterol on NET norepinephrine affinity or transport activity is unknown.

4. Signal transduction proteins and lipid rafts

Many of proteins involved in the biochemical signal propagation of the aforementioned GPCRs such as G-proteins, adenylyl cyclase, phosphodiesterase, ion channels and phospholipase C (PLC) are localized to lipid rafts. Their ability to interact with GPCRs and G-proteins and engage in signal transduction may be attenuated or augmented by lipid raft microdomains (Allen et al., 2007).

4.1 G proteins

Raft targeting and localization of G-proteins to microdomains provides an additional layer of intracellular signal regulation. Depending on whether localization parallels GPCR localization, microdomain specific localization can inhibit or enhance signaling. Moreover, localization may also alter GPCR-G-protein coupling. Given the variety of tissue and membrane preparations, no definitive consensus exists on the membrane localization of G-proteins. However, considerable evidence suggests $G\alpha_s$, $G\alpha_i$, $G\alpha_q$, $G\alpha_o$, $G\alpha_{12}$, $G\alpha_t$, and $G\beta\Upsilon$ are localized to lipid raft domains. Curiously, only $G\alpha_s$ is internalized subsequent to activation, and that internalization is through lipid raft vesicles (Allen et al., 2007, 2009, 2005).

4.2 Adenylyl cyclase

Of the nine membrane associated isoforms of adenylyl cyclase significant evidence suggests that lipid rafts regulate their ability to produce cAMP, create distinct signaling compartments, and allow for specific GPCR and isoform specific adenylyl cyclase association. Specifically, adenylyl cyclase type VI (ACVI) is present in raft and non-raft domains and may display differential activity depending on localization (Fagan, Smith, & Cooper, 2000). In cardiomyocytes, adenylyl cyclase type V is co-immunoprecipitated with caveolin 3 (Head et al., 2005). Adenylyl cyclase type 8 (AC8) is localized to lipid rafts, and pharmacological inhibition of *N*-glycosylation of AC8 prevents lipid raft association (Pagano et al., 2019). Direct activation of AC by forskolin and subsequent cAMP generation is significantly augmented after cholesterol chelation (Rybin, Xu, Lisanti, & Steinberg, 2000). One possible explanation for this would be increased association of $G\alpha_s$ and AC due to raft disruption. When $G\alpha_s$ is complexed with AC, activation by forskolin is enhanced (Sutkowski, Tang, Broome, Robbins, & Seamon, 1994).

5. Depression, lipid rafts and $G\alpha_s$

While many antidepressants effect MAT inhibition, the fact that antidepressant effects often take weeks to months to manifest suggest that

MAT inhibition alone cannot account for the clinical efficacy of these drugs. It is now widely held that neurological and biochemical alterations required for antidepressant efficacy occur only after chronic administration. Consistent with this supposition, our group has shown that $G\alpha_s$ translocates out of lipid raft microdomains into non-raft domains where it has a more stimulatory effect on adenylyl cyclase and consequently cAMP production. In other words, lipid rafts exert an inhibitory effect on $G\alpha_s$ (Fig. 1). Of the aforementioned receptors, the D_1, $5HT_7$, and the β2-AR couple to $G\alpha_s$ and are localized to lipid rafts. $G\alpha_s$ plasma membrane localization has also been proposed as a biomarker of depression and successful antidepressant response (Czysz et al., 2015; Wray, Schappi, Singh, Senese, & Rasenick, 2018), given in the depressed state $G\alpha_s$ is localized in lipid rafts, and in the non-depressed state $G\alpha_s$ localized in non-raft domains (Donati et al., 2008). Moreover, adenylyl cyclase activity is reduced in membranes prepared from the frontal cortex of suicide completers despite total $G\alpha_s$ and $G\alpha_i$ expression not differing from controls (Abu-arish et al., 2014). This same effect is also seen in the periphery as platelets from depressed patients show reduced capability to produce cAMP, yet levels of $G\alpha_s$ remain unchanged compared to control subjects (Hines & Tabakoff, 2005; Mooney et al., 2013). Consistent with these findings, increasing intracellular cAMP by selectively inhibiting the cAMP specific phosphodiesterase type 4 (PDE4) with the high affinity PDE4 inhibitor rolipram, produces antidepressant effects in rodents

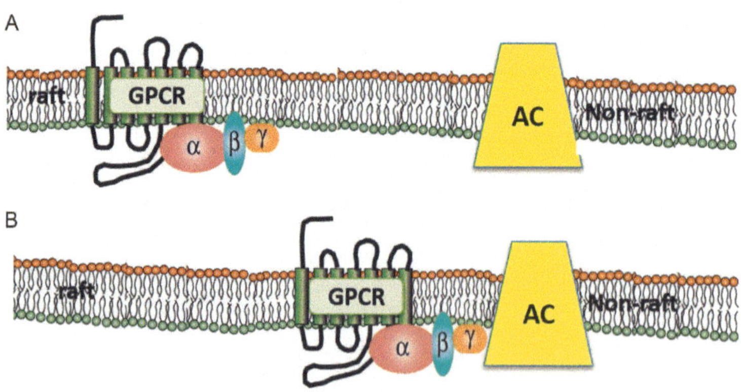

Fig. 1 Lipid rafts modify G protein signaling. (A) In the depressed state $G\alpha_s$ is localized in lipid raft domains where its ability to stimulate adenylyl cyclase and produce cAMP is diminished. (B) Upon chronic antidepressant treatment $G\alpha_s$ translocates to non-raft regions of the plasma membrane where it's capacity to stimulate adenylyl cyclase and generate cAMP is increased.

and humans when administered chronically but not acutely (Itoh, Tokumura, & Abe, 2004). Moreover, decreased PDE4 activity achieved by inhibiting the PDE4 inhibiting protein, Cdk5 in the ventral striatum increases intracellular cAMP and promotes antidepressant-like effects in murine models of depression (Plattner et al., 2015). PDE isoforms PDE4A and PDE4B are upregulated upon chronic antidepressant treatment, also suggesting that cAMP is upregulated after antidepressant administration (Takahashi et al., 1999). Recently, positron emission tomography (PET) studies have shown that cAMP is globally decreased in patients suffering from depression and upon successful remission of symptoms after antidepressant treatment with SSRIs, cAMP increases to levels seen in control patients (Fujita et al., 2017).

The initial evidence for this finding reported increased production of cAMP in membranes prepared from the cortex and hypothalamus of rats treated with tricyclic antidepressant for 15–22 days or treated with ECT (Menkes, Rasenick, Wheeler, & Bitensky, 1983). Moreover, after a 3-day treatment in C6 glioma and 3-week treatment in rats, all classes of antidepressants mediate the translocation of $G\alpha_s$ from lipid raft domains to non-raft domains in a dose-dependent manner (Czysz et al., 2015; Toki, Donati, & Rasenick, 1999). In line with these findings, disruption of lipid rafts by caveolin knockout or MβCD increases intracellular cAMP (Allen et al., 2009). Other psychotropic drugs such as stimulants, anxiolytics, and antipsychotics do not influence the plasma membrane distribution of $G\alpha_s$ (Czysz et al., 2015). Interestingly, the mood stabilizing compounds valproate and lithium have an opposing effect, inducing $G\alpha_s$ redistribution into lipid rafts. Furthermore, the translocation is specific to the $G\alpha_s$ subunit as all other classes of $G\alpha$ are not subject to antidepressant induced translocation (Donati, Thukral, & Rasenick, 2001; Toki et al., 1999). Studies from post-mortem tissue from depressed suicides have shown that $G\alpha_s$ is localized to inhibitory lipid rafts in both the cortex and cerebellum in the depressed state (Donati et al., 2008; Fig. 2).

While an exact mechanism detailing the biochemical events that drive $G\alpha_s$ from lipid rafts to non-rafts is unknown, evidence from our group suggests that it involves a disruption of the $G\alpha_s$ and tubulin complex. Initial evidence implicating tubulin came from the observation that the effect was ablated by the addition of microtubule disrupting agent colchicine (Menkes et al., 1983). It is now well documented that $G\alpha_s$ binds tubulin with an affinity of $\sim$130nm and tubulin is enriched in lipid rafts (Allen et al., 2007; Schappi, Krbanjevic, & Rasenick, 2014). TCAs and SSRIs reduce association of tubulin and $G\alpha_s$, specifically in lipid rafts

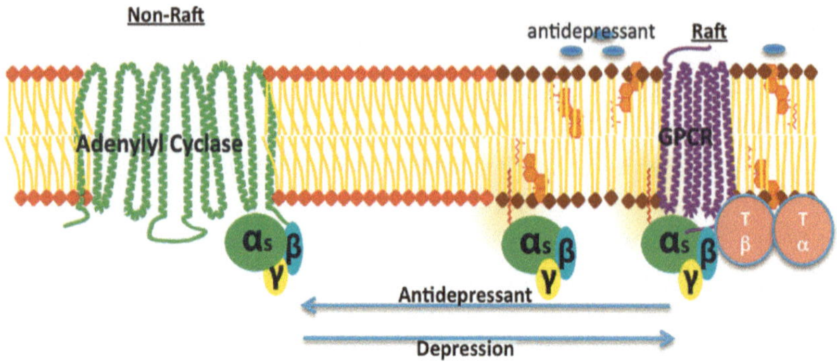

Fig. 2 Depression and antidepressant effects upon $G\alpha_s$ plasma membrane localization. We hypothesize that $G\alpha_s$ is enriched in lipid rafts during depression. Subsequent to chronic treatment with various antidepressant compounds, $G\alpha_s$ is translocated from lipid raft regions of the plasma membrane to non-raft membrane regions that allow greater interaction with/activation of AC (increasing cAMP). This translocation is accompanied by dissociation of $G\alpha_s$ from raft anchors like tubulin (Tα/Tβ)A high ratio of $G\alpha_s$ raft:non-raft localization indicates depression; effective antidepressant treatment lowers this ratio to control levels.

(Singh, Wray, Schappi, & Rasenick, 2018). Interestingly, increasing the acetylation of α-tubulin with histone deacetylase (HDAC) 6 specific inhibitors also reduces the association tubulin and $G\alpha_s$, which results in $G\alpha_s$ translocating out of lipid rafts. Indeed, HDAC 6 inhibitors such as tubastatin show antidepressant effects in animal models of depression (Singh et al., 2018).

Interestingly, our group and others have shown that a variety of antidepressant compounds accumulate in lipid rafts. Eisensamer et al. first reported that TCAs and SSRIs accumulate in lipid raft fractions when added directly to sucrose density gradient isolated lipid rafts. Our group treated C6 glioma cells over 3 days and isolated lipid rafts, which revealed accumulation of SSRIs, MAOIs and to a lesser extent, tricyclic antidepressants (Erb, Schappi, & Rasenick, 2016). This effect was neither diminished nor enhanced by the presence of SERT (Erb et al., 2016), suggesting another lipid-raft binding site. Other psychotropic compounds with similar lipophilicity did not accumulate (Erb et al., 2016), indicating lipophilicity is not the key driver causing the compounds to accumulate in lipid rafts (Erb et al., 2016). More importantly, the antidepressant escitalopram accumulated in a dose and treatment duration manner and its inactive isomer (*R*)-citalopram did not accumulate in lipid rafts, indicating the stereospecificity of this effect (Erb et al., 2016). This effect is paralleled by escitalopram driving $G\alpha_s$ from rafts into non-rafts and (*R*)-citalopram being without an effect.

It was recently discovered that the powerful and rapid acting antidepressant ketamine induces Gα_s membrane redistribution. The translocation is accompanied by an increase agonist mediated cAMP production and phosphorylation of downstream targets. In primary astrocytes brain-derived neurotrophic factor (BDNF) was upregulated after ketamine treatment and attenuated to control levels with addition of the cAMP cell permeable antagonist cAMPS-Rp. Interestingly, agonist mediated increase in cAMP was maintained after knocking down the NMDA receptor. Other NMDA antagonist did not influence the membrane distribution of Gα_s. These data suggest that ketamine may be exerting antidepressant effects independently of its presumed target (Wray et al., 2018).

6. Conclusion

The lipid microenvironment, whether modifying neurotransmitter signaling or modifying drug action and interaction, plays a critical role in both depression and the actions of antidepressant drugs. Add to this the lipid modifications of signaling proteins and a complex array of possibilities are presented. Both appreciation and understanding of this complexity remain immature but are destined to grow as tools for investigation achieve greater and greater sophistication.

Acknowledgments

Support for the authors was derived from NIH R01 AT009169, NIH T32 MH 067631 and VA Merit BX001149, and VA Research Career Scientist BX004475.

Conflict of interest statement

M.M.R. is a VA Research Career Scientist. N.H.W. has no conflicts of interest.

References

Abu-arish, A., Pandzic, E., Goepp, J., Matthes, E., Hanrahan, J. W., & Wiseman, P. W. (2015). Cholesterol modulates CFTR confinement in the plasma membrane of primary epithelial cells. *Biophysical Journal, 109*(1), 85–94. https://doi.org/10.1016/j.bpj.2015.04.042.

Abu-arish, A., Pandzic, E., Goepp, J., Matthes, E., Hanrahan, J. W., Wiseman, P. W., et al. (2014). Adenylyl cyclase activity and G-protein subunit levels in postmortem frontal cortex of suicide victims. *Molecular Pharmacology, 9*(1), 34614–34623. https://doi.org/10.1074/jbc.M404673200.

Adkins, E. M., Samuvel, D. J., Fog, J. U., Eriksen, J., Jayanthi, L. D., Vaegter, C. B., et al. (2007). Membrane mobility and microdomain association of the dopamine transporter studied with fluorescence correlation spectroscopy and fluorescence recovery. *Biochemistry*, *46*, 10484–10497.

Aggarwal, S., & Mortensen, O. V. (2017). Overview of monoamine transporters. *Current Protocols in Pharmacology*, *79*(December), 1–17. https://doi.org/10.1002/cpph.32.

Agudo-Ibáñez, L., Herrero, A., Barbacid, M., & Crespo, P. (2015). H-Ras distribution and signaling in plasma membrane microdomains are regulated by acylation and Deacylation events. *Molecular and Cellular Biology*, *35*(11), 1898–1914. https://doi.org/10.1128/MCB.01398-14.

Ahmed, S. N., Brown, D. A., & London, E. (1997). On the origin of sphingolipid/cholesterol-rich detergent-insoluble cell membranes: Physiological concentrations of cholesterol and sphingolipid induce formation of a detergent-insoluble, liquid-ordered lipid phase in model membranes. *Biochemistry*, *2960*(97), 10944–10953.

Allen, J. A., Halverson-Tamboli, R. A., & Rasenick, M. M. (2007). Lipid raft microdomains and neurotransmitter signalling. *Nature Reviews Neuroscience*, *8*(2), 128–140. https://doi.org/10.1038/nrn2059.

Allen, J. A., Yu, J. Z., Dave, R. H., Bhatnagar, A., Roth, B. L., & Rasenick, M. M. (2009). Caveolin-1 and lipid microdomains regulate Gs trafficking and attenuate Gs/adenylyl cyclase signaling. *Molecular Pharmacology*, *76*, 1082–1093.

Allen, J. A., Yu, J. Z., Donati, R. J., & Rasenick, M. M. (2005). Beta-adrenergic receptor stimulation promotes G alpha s internalization through lipid rafts: A study in living cells. *Molecular Pharmacology*, *67*, 1493–1504.

Arapulisamy, O., Mannangatti, P., & Jayanthi, L. D. (2013). Regulated norepinephrine transporter interaction with the neurokinin-1 receptor establishes transporter subcellular localization. *The Journal of Biological Chemistry*, *288*(40), 28599–28610. https://doi.org/10.1074/jbc.M113.472878.

Babiychuk, E. B., & Draeger, A. (2006). Biochemical characterization of detergent-resistant membranes: A systematic approach. *The Biochemical Journal*, *397*(3), 407–416.

Baumgart, T., Hammond, A. T., Sengupta, P., Hess, S. T., Holowka, D. A., Baird, B. A., et al. (2007). Large-scale fluid/fluid phase separation of proteins and lipids in giant plasma membrane vesicles. *Proceedings of the National Academy of Sciences of the United States of America*, *104*(9), 3165–3170.

Bhatnagar, A., Sheffler, D. J., Kroeze, W. K., Compton-Toth, B., & Roth, B. L. (2004). Caveolin-1 interacts with 5-HT2A serotonin receptors and profoundly modulates the signaling of selected Galphaq-coupled protein receptors. *The Journal of Biological Chemistry*, *279*(33), 34614–34623.

Buchmayer, F., Schicker, K., Steinkellner, T., Geier, P., Hamilton, P. J., Jurik, A., et al. (2013). Amphetamine actions at the serotonin transporter rely on the availability of phosphatidylinositol-4,5-bisphosphate. *Proceedings of the National Academy of Sciences of the United States of America*, *110*(28), 11642–11647. https://doi.org/10.1073/pnas.1220552110.

Catapano, L. A., & Manji, H. K. (2007). G protein-coupled receptors in major psychiatric disorders. *Biochimica et Biophysica Acta*, *1768*, 976–993. https://doi.org/10.1016/j.bbamem.2006.09.025.

Celver, J., Sharma, M., & Kovoor, A. (2012). D(2)-dopamine receptors target regulator of G protein signaling 9-2 to detergent-resistant membrane fractions. *Journal of Neurochemistry*, *120*, 56–69.

Chang, J. C., Tomlinson, I. D., Warnement, M. R., Ustione, A., Carneiro, A. M. D., Piston, D. W., et al. (2012). Single Molecule analysis of serotonin transporter regulation using antagonist-conjugated quantum dots reveals restricted, p38 MAPK-dependent mobilization underlying uptake activation. *The Journal of Neuroscience*, *32*(26), 8919–8929. https://doi.org/10.1523/JNEUROSCI.0048-12.2012.

Czysz, A. H., Schappi, J. M., & Rasenick, M. M. (2015). Lateral diffusion of Gα_s in the plasma membrane is decreased after chronic but not acute antidepressant treatment: Role of lipid raft and non-raft membrane microdomains. *Neuropsychopharmacology: Official Publication of the American College of Neuropsychopharmacology*, *40*(3), 766–773.

Diaz-rohrer, B. B., Levental, K. R., Simons, K., & Levental, I. (2014). Membrane raft association is a determinant of plasma membrane localization. *Proceedings of the National Academy of Sciences of the United States of America*, *111*(23), 8500–8505. https://doi.org/10.1073/pnas.1404582111.

Dietrich, C., Bagatolli, L. A., Volovyk, Z. N., Thompson, N. L., Levi, M., Jacobson, K., et al. (2001). Lipid rafts reconstituted in model membranes. *Biophysical Journal*, *80*(March), 1417–1428.

Dipilato, L. M., & Zhang, J. (2009). The role of membrane microdomains in shaping β2-adrenergic receptor-mediated cAMP dynamics. *Molecular BioSystems*, *5*, 832–837. https://doi.org/10.1039/b823243a.

Donati, R. J., Dwivedi, Y., Roberts, R. C., Conley, R. R., Pandey, G. N., & Rasenick, M. M. (2008). Postmortem brain tissue of depressed suicides reveals increased Gs localization in lipid raft domains where it is less likely to activate adenylyl cyclase. *Journal of Neuroscience*, *28*(12), 3042–3050. https://doi.org/10.1523/JNEUROSCI.5713-07.2008.

Donati, R. J., Thukral, C., & Rasenick, M. M. (2001). Chronic treatment of C6 glioma cells with antidepressant drugs results in a redistribution of Gsalpha. *Molecular Pharmacology*, *59*(6), 1426–1432. Retrieved from http://www.ncbi.nlm.nih.gov/pubmed/11353802.

Dreja, K., Voldstedlund, M., Vinten, J., Tranum-Jensen, J., Hellstrand, P., & Sward, K. (2002). Cholesterol depletion disrupts caveolae and differentially impairs agonist induced arterial contraction. *Arteriosclerosis, Thrombosis, and Vascular Biology*, *22*, 1267–1272.

Ehehalt, R., Keller, P., Haass, C., Thiele, C., & Simons, K. (2003). Amyloidogenic processing of the Alzheimer beta-amyloid precursor protein depends on lipid rafts. *The Journal of Cell Biology*, *160*, 113–123.

Eisensamer, B., Uhr, M., Gimpl, G., Deiml, T., Rammes, G., Lambert, J., et al. (2005). Antidepressants and antipsychotic drugs colocalize with 5-HT3 receptors in raft-like domains. *Journal of Neuroscience*, *25*(44), 10198–10206. https://doi.org/10.1523/JNEUROSCI.2460-05.2005.

Erb, S. J., Schappi, J. M., & Rasenick, M. M. (2016). Antidepressants accumulate in lipid rafts independent of monoamine transporters to modulate redistribution of the G protein, Gα_s. *Journal of Biological Chemistry*, *291*(4). jbc.M116.727263. https://doi.org/10.1074/jbc.M116.727263.

Escribá, P. V., Wedegaertner, P. B., Goñi, F. M., & Vögler, O. (2007). Lipid-protein interactions in GPCR-associated signaling. *Biochimica et Biophysica Acta—Biomembranes*, *1768*(4), 836–852. https://doi.org/10.1016/j.bbamem.2006.09.001.

Fagan, K. A., Smith, K. E., & Cooper, D. M. F. (2000). Regulation of the Ca^{2+}-inhibitable adenylyl cyclase type VI by capacitative Ca^{2+} entry requires localization in cholesterol-rich domains. *Journal of Biological Chemistry*, *275*(34), 26530–26537. https://doi.org/10.1074/jbc.M001369200.

Feduccia, A. A., & Mithoefer, M. C. (2018). Progress in neuropsychopharmacology & biological psychiatry MDMA-assisted psychotherapy for PTSD: Are memory reconsolidation and fear extinction underlying mechanisms? *Progress in Neuropsychopharmacology and Biological Psychiatry*, *84*(October 2017), 221–228. https://doi.org/10.1016/j.pnpbp.2018.03.003.

Feigenson, G. W., & Buboltz, J. T. (2001). Ternary phase diagram of dipalmitoyl-PC/dilauroyl-PC/cholesterol: nanoscopic domain formation driven by cholesterol. *Biophysical Journal*, *80*(June), 2775–2788.

Foster, J. D., Adkins, S. D., Lever, J. R., & Vaughan, R. A. (2008). Phorbol ester induced trafficking independent regulation and enhanced phosphorylation of the dopamine transporter associated with membrane rafts and cholesterol. *Journal of Neurochemistry*, *105*, 1683–1699.

Fujita, M., Richards, E. M., Niciu, M. J., Ionescu, D. F., Zoghbi, S. S., Hong, J., et al. (2017). cAMP signaling in brain is decreased in unmedicated depressed patients and increased by treatment with a selective serotonin reuptake inhibitor HHS public access. *Molecular Psychiatry*, *22*(5), 754–759. https://doi.org/10.1038/mp.2016.171.

Hashimoto, M., Takenouchi, T., Rockenstein, E., & Masliah, E. (2003). α-Synuclein up-regulates expression of caveolin-1 and down-regulates extracellular signal-regulated kinase activity in B103 neuroblastoma cells: Role in the pathogenesis of Parkinson's disease. *Journal of Neurochemistry*, *85*, 1468–1479. https://doi.org/10.1046/j.1471-4159.2003.01791.x.

Head, B. P., Patel, H. H., Roth, D. M., Lai, N. C., Niesman, I. R., Farquhar, M. G., et al. (2005). G-protein-coupled receptor signaling components localize in both sarcolemmal and intracellular caveolin-3-associated microdomains in adult cardiac myocytes. *The Journal of Biological Chemistry*, *280*(35), 31036–31044. https://doi.org/10.1074/jbc.M502540200.

Head, B. P., Patel, H. H., Roth, D. M., Murray, F., Swaney, J. S., Niesman, I. R., et al. (2006). Microtubules and actin microfilaments regulate lipid raft/caveolae localization of adenylyl cyclase signaling components. *The Journal of Biological Chemistry*, *281*(36), 26391–26399.

Hines, L. M., & Tabakoff, B. (2005). Platelet adenylyl cyclase activity: A biological marker for major depression and recent drug use. *Biological Psychiatry*, *58*(12), 955–962.

Hopkins, A. L., & Groom, C. R. (2002). The druggable genome. *Nature Reviews Drug Discovery*, *1*(9), 727–730. https://doi.org/10.1038/nrd892.

Ilani, T., Fishburn, C. S., Levavi-sivan, B., Carmon, S., Raveh, L., & Fuchs, S. (2002). Coupling of dopamine receptors to G proteins: Studies with chimeric D 2/D 3 dopamine receptors. *Cellular and Molecular Neurobiology*, *22*(1), 47–56.

Ingólfsson, H. I., Melo, M. N., van Eerden, F. J., Arnarez, C., Lopez, C. A., Wassenaar, T. A., et al. (2014). Lipid organization of the plasma membrane. *Journal of the American Chemical Society*, *136*(41), 14554–14559.

Itoh, T., Tokumura, M., & Abe, K. (2004). Effects of rolipram, a phosphodiesterase 4 inhibitor, in combination with imipramine on depressive behavior, CRE-binding activity and BDNF level in learned helplessness rats. *European Journal of Pharmacology*, *498*(1–3), 135–142. https://doi.org/10.1016/j.ejphar.2004.07.084.

Jaber, M., Robinson, S. W., Missale, C., & Caron, M. G. (1996). Dopamine receptors and brain function. *Neuropharmacology*, *35*(11), 1503–1519.

Jayanthi, L. D., Samuvel, D. J., & Ramamoorthy, S. (2004). Regulated internalization and phosphorylation of the native norepinephrine transporter in response to phorbol esters. *The Journal of Biological Chemistry*, *279*(18), 19315–19326. https://doi.org/10.1074/jbc.M311172200.

Jones, K. T., Zhen, J., & Reith, M. E. (2012). Importance of cholesterol in dopamine transporter function. *Journal of Neurochemistry*, *123*, 700–715.

Kalipatnapu, S., & Chattopadhyay, A. (2009). Membrane organization of the human serotonin 1A receptor monitored by detergent insolubility using GFP fluorescence. *Molecular Membrane Biology*, *7688*, 539–547. https://doi.org/10.1080/09687860500421738.

Kokubo, H., Helms, J. B., Ohno-iwashita, Y., & Shimada, Y. (2003). Ultrastructural localization of flotillin-1 to cholesterol-rich membrane microdomains, rafts, in rat brain tissue. *Brain Research*, *965*, 83–90.

Kovtun, O., Tillu, V. A., Ariotti, N., Parton, R. G., & Collins, B. M. (2015). Cavin family proteins and the assembly of caveolae. *Journal of Cell Science*, *128*, 1269–1278. https://doi.org/10.1242/jcs.167866.

Kraft, M. L., & Bement, W. (2013). Plasma membrane organization and function: Moving past lipid rafts. *Molecular Biology of the Cell*, *24*, 2765–2768. https://doi.org/10.1091/mbc.E13-03-0165.

Kwik, J., Boyle, S., Fooksman, D., Margolis, L., Sheetz, M. P., & Edidin, M. (2003). Membrane cholesterol, lateral mobility, and the phosphatidylinositol 4,5-bisphosphate-dependent organization of cell actin. *Proceedings of the National Academy of Sciences of the United States of America*, *100*, 13964–13969.

Lei, B., Morris, D. P., Smith, M. P., & Schwinn, D. A. (2009). Lipid rafts constrain basal α 1A-adrenergic receptor signaling by maintaining receptor in an inactive conformation. *Cellular Signaling*, *21*(10), 1532–1539. https://doi.org/10.1016/j.cellsig.2009.06.001.

Levental, I., Grzybek, M., & Simons, K. (2011). Raft domains of variable properties and compositions in plasma membrane vesicles. *Proceedings of the National Academy of Sciences of the United States of America*, *108*(28), 11411–11416.

Levental, I., Lingwood, D., Grzybek, M., Coskun, Ü., & Simons, K. (2010). Palmitoylation regulates raft affinity for the majority of integral raft proteins. *Proceedings of the National Academy of Sciences of the United States of America*, *107*(51), 22050–22054. https://doi.org/10.1073/pnas.1016184107/-/DCSupplemental.www.pnas.org/cgi/doi/10.1073/pnas.1016184107.

Liu, J. J., Hezghia, A., Shaikh, S. R., Cenido, J. F., Sublette, M. E., & Stark, R. E. (2018). Regulation of monoamine transporters and receptors by lipid microdomains: Implications for depression. *Neuropsychopharmacology*, *43*(11), 2165–2179. https://doi.org/10.1038/s41386-018-0133-6.

Magnani, F., Tate, C. G., Wynne, S., Williams, C., & Haase, J. (2004). Partitioning of the serotonin transporter into lipid microdomains modulates transport of serotonin. *Journal of Biological Chemistry*, *279*(37), 38770–38778. https://doi.org/10.1074/jbc.M400831200.

Mann, J. J. (2013). The serotonergic system in mood disorders and suicidal behaviour. *Philosophical Transactions of the Royal Society of London. Series B, Biological Sciences*, *368*, 20120537.

Menkes, D. B., Rasenick, M. M., Wheeler, M. A., & Bitensky, M. W. (1983). Guanosine triphosphate activation of brain adenylate cyclase: Enhancement by long-term antidepressant treatment. *Science (New York, N.Y.)*, *219*(4580), 65–67.

Mialet-Perez, J., D'Angelo, R., Villeneuve, C., Ordener, C., Negre-Salvayre, A., Parini, A., et al. (2012). Serotonin 5-HT2A receptor-mediated hypertrophy is negatively regulated by caveolin-3 in cardiomyoblasts and neonatal cardiomyocytes. *Journal of Molecular and Cellular Cardiology*, *52*, 502–510.

Milligan, G., & Kostenis, E. (2006). Heterotrimeric G-proteins: A short history. *British Journal of Pharmacology*, *147*(Suppl. 1), S46–S55.

Mooney, J. J., Samson, J. A., McHale, N. L., Pappalarado, K. M., Alpert, J. E., & Schildkraut, J. J. (2013). Increased Gsα within blood cell membrane lipid microdomains in some depressive disorders: An exploratory study. *Journal of Psychiatric Research*, *47*(6), 706–711. https://doi.org/10.1016/j.jpsychires.2013.02.005.

Morris, J. B., Huynh, H., Vasilevski, O., & Woodcock, E. A. (2006). α1-Adrenergic receptor signaling is localized to caveolae in neonatal rat cardiomyocytes. *Journal of Molecular and Cellular Cardiology*, *41*, 17–25. https://doi.org/10.1016/j.yjmcc.2006.03.011.

Morris, D. P., Lei, B., Wu, Y., Michelotti, G. A., & Schwinn, D. A. (2008). The α_{1a}-adrenergic receptor occupies membrane rafts with its G protein effectors but internalizes via clathrin-coated pits. *The Journal of Biological Chemistry*, *283*(5), 2973–2985. https://doi.org/10.1074/jbc.M705795200.

Munro, S. (2003). Lipid rafts: Elusive or illusive? *Cell*, *115*(4), 377–388. https://doi.org/10.1016/S0092-8674(03)00882-1.

Nothdurfter, C., Tanasic, S., Di Benedetto, B., Rammes, G., Wagner, E., Kirmeier, T., et al. (2010). Impact of lipid raft integrity on 5-HT 3 receptor function and its modulation by antidepressants. *Neuropsychopharmacology*, *35*(7), 1510–1519. https://doi.org/10.1038/npp.2010.20.

Obadiah, J., Avidor-reiss, T., Fishburn, C. S., Carmon, S., Bayewitch, M., Vogel, Z., et al. (1999). Adenylyl cyclase interaction with the D2 dopamine receptor family; differential coupling to Gi, Gz, and Gs. *Cellular and Molecular Neurobiology*, *19*(5), 653–664.

Oldham, W. M., & Hamm, H. E. (2008). Heterotrimeric G protein activation by G-protein-coupled receptors. *Nature Reviews Molecular Cell Biology*, *9*(1), 60–71. https://doi.org/10.1038/nrm2299.

Oner, S. S., Kaya, A. I., Onaran, H. O., Ozcan, G., & Ugur, O. (2010). beta2-Adrenoceptor, Gs and adenylate cyclase coupling in purified detergent-resistant, low density membrane fractions. *European Journal of Pharmacology*, *630*, 42–52.

Ostrom, R. S., Bundey, R. A., & Insel, P. A. (2004). Nitric oxide inhibition of adenylyl cyclase type 6 activity is dependent upon lipid rafts and caveolin signaling complexes. *The Journal of Biological Chemistry*, *279*(19), 19846–19853. https://doi.org/10.1074/jbc.M313440200.

Ostrom, R. S., Gregorian, C., Drenan, R. M., Xiang, Y., Regan, J. W., & Insel, P. A. (2001). Receptor number and Caveolar co-localization determine receptor coupling efficiency to adenylyl cyclase. *The Journal of Biological Chemistry*, *276*(45), 42063–42069. https://doi.org/10.1074/jbc.M105348200.

Pagano, M., Clynes, M. A., Masada, N., Ciruela, A., Ayling, L., Wachten, S., et al. (2019). Insights into the residence in lipid rafts of adenylyl cyclase AC8 and its regulation by capacitative calcium entry. *American Journal of Physiology Cell Physiology*, *296*, 607–619. https://doi.org/10.1152/ajpcell.00488.2008.

Paspalas, C. D., & Goldman-rakic, P. S. (2004). Microdomains for dopamine volume neurotransmission in primate prefrontal cortex. *Journal of Neuroscience*, *24*(23), 5292–5300. https://doi.org/10.1523/JNEUROSCI.0195-04.2004.

Pike, L. J. (2006). Rafts defined: A report on the keystone symposium on lipid rafts and cell function. *Journal of Lipid Research*, *47*, 1597–1598. https://doi.org/10.1194/jlr.E600002-JLR200.

Plattner, F., Hayashi, K., Hernández, A., Benavides, D. R., Tassin, T. C., Tan, C., et al. (2015). The role of ventral striatal cAMP signaling in stress-induced behaviors. *Nature Neuroscience*, *18*(8), 1094–1100. https://doi.org/10.1038/nn.4066.

Pontier, S. M., Percherancier, Y., Galandrin, S., Breit, A., Gales, C., & Bouvier, M. (2008). Cholesterol-dependent separation of the beta2-adrenergic receptor from its partners determines signaling efficacy: Insight into nanoscale organization of signal transduction. *The Journal of Biological Chemistry*, *283*, 24659–24672.

Pucadyil, T. J., & Chattopadhyay, A. (2004). Cholesterol modulates ligand binding and G-protein coupling to serotonin$_{1A}$ receptors from bovine hippocampus. *Biochimica et Biophysica Acta (BBA)—Biomembranes*, *1663*, 188–200. https://doi.org/10.1016/j.bbamem.2004.03.010.

Renner, U., Glebov, K., Lang, T., Papusheva, E., Balakrishnan, S., Keller, B., et al. (2007). Localization of the mouse 5-hydroxytryptamine(1A) receptor in lipid microdomains depends on its palmitoylation and is involved in receptor-mediated signaling. *Molecular Pharmacology*, *72*, 502–513.

Rice, P. A., & Mcconnell, H. M. (1989). Critical shape transitions of monolayer lipid domains. *Proceedings of the National Academy of Sciences of the United States of America*, *86*(September), 6445–6448.

Rybin, V. O., Xu, X., Lisanti, M. P., & Steinberg, S. F. (2000). Differential targeting of β-adrenergic receptor subtypes and adenylyl cyclase to cardiomyocyte caveolae. *Journal of Biological Chemistry*, *275*(52), 41447–41457. https://doi.org/10.1074/jbc.M006951200.

Samuvel, D. J., Jayanthi, L. D., Bhat, N. R., & Ramamoorthy, S. (2005). A role for p38 mitogen-activated protein kinase in the regulation of the serotonin transporter: Evidence for surface expression. *Journal of Neuroscience*, *25*(1), 29–41. https://doi.org/10.1523/JNEUROSCI.3754-04.2005.

Scanlon, S. M., Williams, D. C., & Schloss, P. (2001). Membrane cholesterol modulates serotonin transporter activity. *Biochemistry*, *40*, 10507–10513.

Schappi, J. M., Krbanjevic, A., & Rasenick, M. M. (2014). Tubulin, actin and heterotrimeric G proteins: Coordination of signaling and structure. *Biochimica et Biophysica Acta—Biomembranes*, *1838*(2), 674–681. https://doi.org/10.1016/j.bbamem.2013.08.026.

Schnitzer, E., Oh, P., & Pinney, E. (1994). Filipin-sensitive caveolae-mediated transport in endothelium: Reduced transcytosis, scavenger endocytosis, and capillary permeability of select macromolecules. *Journal of Cell Biology*, *127*(5), 1217–1232.

Sengupta, P., Hammond, A., Holowka, D., & Baird, B. (2008). Structural determinants for partitioning of lipids and proteins between coexisting fluid phases in giant plasma membrane vesicles. *Biochimica et Biophysica Acta*, *1778*, 20–32. https://doi.org/10.1016/j.bbamem.2007.08.028.

Sengupta, P., Jovanovic-talisman, T., Skoko, D., Renz, M., Veatch, S. L., & Lippincott-schwartz, J. (2011). Probing protein heterogeneity in the plasma membrane using PALM and pair correlation analysis. *Nature Methods*, *8*(11), 969–975. https://doi.org/10.1038/nmeth.1704.

Sevcsik, E., & Schutz, G. J. (2015). Insights & perspectives with or without rafts? Alternative views on cell membranes. *BioEssays: News and Reviews in Molecular, Cellular and Developmental Biology*, *38*, 129–139. https://doi.org/10.1002/bies.201500150.

Sezgin, E., Kaiser, H. J., Baumgart, T., Schwille, P., Simons, K., & Levental, I. (2012). Elucidating membrane structure and protein behavior using giant plasma membrane vesicles. *Nature Protocols*, 7(6), 1042–1051.

Sharma, M., Celver, J., Octeau, J. C., & Kovoor, A. (2013). Plasma membrane compartmentalization of D2 dopamine. *The Journal of Biological Chemistry*, *288*(18), 12554–12568. https://doi.org/10.1074/jbc.M112.443945.

Simons, K., & Ikonen, E. (1997). Functional rafts in cell membranes. *Nature*, *387*(6633), 569–572. https://doi.org/10.1038/42408.

Singer, S. J., & Nicolson, G. L. (1972). The fluid mosaic model of the structure of cell membranes. *Science*, *175*, 720–731.

Singh, H., Wray, N., Schappi, J. M., & Rasenick, M. M. (2018). Disruption of lipid-raft localized $G\alpha_s$/tubulin complexes by antidepressants: A unique feature of HDAC6 inhibitors, SSRI and tricyclic compounds. *Neuropsychopharmacology*, *43*(7), 1481–1491. https://doi.org/10.1038/s41386-018-0016-x.

Sjogren, B. (2007). Caveolin-1 affects serotonin binding and cell surface levels of human 5-HT $_{7(a)}$ receptors. *FEBS Letters*, *581*, 5115–5121. https://doi.org/10.1016/j.febslet.2007.09.059.

Sjögren, B., Hamblin, M. W., & Svenningsson, P. (2006). Cholesterol depletion reduces serotonin binding and signaling via human 5-HT $_{7(a)}$ receptors. *FEBS Letters*, *552*, 1–10. https://doi.org/10.1016/j.ejphar.2006.08.069F.

Song, K. S., Li, S., Okamoto, T., Quilliam, L. A., Sargiacomo, M., & Lisanti, M. P. (1996). Co-purification and direct interaction of Ras with caveolin, an integral membrane protein of caveolae microdomains. *Journal of Biological Chemistry*, *271*(16), 9690–9697.

Sorkina, T., Hoover, B. R., Zahniser, R., & Sorkin, A. (2005). Constitutive and protein kinase C-induced internalization of the dopamine transporter is mediated by a Clathrin-dependent mechanism. *Traffic*, *271*(1), 157–170. https://doi.org/10.1111/j.1600-0854.2004.00259.x.

Stone, M. B., Shelby, S. A., & Veatch, S. L. (2017). Super-resolution microscopy: Shedding light on the cellular plasma membrane. *Chemical Reviews*, *117*(11), 7457–7477.

Sutkowski, E. M., Tang, W. J., Broome, C. W., Robbins, J. D., & Seamon, K. B. (1994). Regulation of forskolin interactions with type I, II, V, and VI adenylyl cyclases by Gs alpha. *Biochemistry*, *33*(43), 12852–12859.

Takahashi, M., Terwilliger, R., Lane, C., Mezes, P. S., Conti, M., & Duman, R. S. (1999). Chronic antidepressant administration increases the expression of cAMP-specific phosphodiesterase 4A and 4B isoforms. *The Journal of Neuroscience: The Official Journal of the Society for Neuroscience*, *19*(2), 610–618. Retrieved from http://www.ncbi.nlm.nih.gov/pubmed/9880581.

Thorn, H., Stenkula, K. G., Karlsson, M., Unn, O., Nystrom, F. H., Gustavsson, J., et al. (2003). Cell surface orifices of caveolae and localization of caveolin to the necks of caveolae in adipocytes. *Molecular Biology of the Cell*, *14*(October), 3967–3976. https://doi.org/10.1091/mbc.E03.

Toki, S., Donati, R. J., & Rasenick, M. M. (1999). Treatment of C6 glioma cells and rats with antidepressant drugs increases the detergent extraction of G(s alpha) from plasma membrane. *Journal of Neurochemistry*, *73*(3), 1114–1120.

Trushina, E., Du Charme, J., Parisi, J., & McMurray, C. T. (2006). Neurological abnormalities in caveolin-1 knockout mice. *Behavioural Brain Research*, *172*(1), 24–32.

Varma, R., & Mayor, S. (1998). GPI-anchored proteins are organized in submicron domains at the cell surface. *Nature*, *394*(August), 798–801.

Veatch, S. L., & Keller, S. L. (2002). Organization in lipid membranes containing cholesterol. *Physical Review Letters*, *89*, 1–4. https://doi.org/10.1103/PhysRevLett.89.268101.

Veatch, S. L., & Keller, S. L. (2003). Separation of liquid phases in giant vesicles of ternary mixtures of phospholipids and cholesterol. *Biophysical Journal*, *85*(November), 3074–3083.

Villar, V. A. M., Jones, J. E., Armando, I., Palmes-saloma, C., Yu, P., Pascua, A. M., et al. (2009). G protein-coupled receptor kinase 4 (GRK4) regulates the phosphorylation and function of the dopamine D 3 receptor. *Biological Chemistry*, *284*(32), 21425–21434. https://doi.org/10.1074/jbc.M109.003665.

Voulalas, P. J., Schetz, J., & Undieh, A. S. (2011). Molecular and cellular neuroscience differential subcellular distribution of rat brain dopamine receptors and subtype-specific redistribution induced by cocaine. *Molecular and Cellular Neuroscience*, *46*(3), 645–654. https://doi.org/10.1016/j.mcn.2011.01.004.

Wray, N. H., Schappi, J. M., Singh, H., Senese, N. B., & Rasenick, M. M. (2018). NMDAR-independent, cAMP-dependent antidepressant actions of ketamine. *Molecular Psychiatry*, *2*, 1. https://doi.org/10.1038/s41380-018-0083-8.

Wu, Z., Cheng, H., Jiang, Y., Melcher, K., & Xu, H. E. (2015). Ion channels gated by acetylcholine and serotonin: Structures, biology, and drug discovery. *Nature Publishing Group*, *36*(8), 895–907. https://doi.org/10.1038/aps.2015.66.

Xiang, Y., Rybin, V. O., Steinberg, S. F., & Kobilka, B. (2002). Caveolar Localization dictates physiologic signaling of β2-adrenoceptors in neonatal cardiac myocytes. *The Journal of Biological Chemistry*, *277*(37), 34280–34286. https://doi.org/10.1074/jbc.M201644200.

Yu, J., Fischman, D. A., & Steck, T. L. (1973). Selective solubilization of proteins and phospholipids from red blood cell membranes by nonionic detergents. *Journal of Cellular Biochemistry*, *1*(3), 233–248.

Yu, J. Z., & Rasenick, M. M. (2002). Real-time visualization of a fluorescent GÖ s: Dissociation of the activated G protein from plasma membrane. *Molecular Pharmacology*, *61*(2), 352–359. https://doi.org/10.1124/mol.61.2.352.

Yu, P., Sun, M., Villar, V. A. M., Zhang, Y., Weinman, E. J., Felder, R. A., et al. (2014). Differential dopamine receptor subtype regulation of adenylyl cyclases in lipid rafts in human embryonic kidney and renal proximal tubule cells. *Cellular Signaling*, *26*(11), 2521–2529. https://doi.org/10.1016/j.cellsig.2014.07.003.

Yu, P., Yang, Z., Jones, J. E., Wang, Z., Owens, S. A., Mueller, S. C., et al. (2004). D1 dopamine receptor signaling involves caveolin-2 in HEK-293 cells. *Kidney International*, *66*, 2167–2180.

Zocher, M., Zhang, C., Rasmussen, S. G., Kobilka, B. K., & Müller, D. J. (2012). Cholesterol increases kinetic, energetic, and mechanical stability of the human β2-adrenergic receptor. *Proceedings of the National Academy of Sciences of the United States of America*, *109*(50), E3463–E3472.

Further reading

Agarwal, S. R., Gratwohl, J., Cozad, M., Yang, P., Clancy, C. E., & Harvey, R. D. (2018). Compartmentalized cAMP signaling associated with lipid raft and non-raft membrane domains in adult ventricular myocytes. *Frontiers in Pharmacology*, *9*(April), 1–14. https://doi.org/10.3389/fphar.2018.00332.

Donati, R. J., Schappi, J., Czysz, A. H., Jackson, A., & Rasenick, M. M. (2015). Differential effects of antidepressants escitalopram versus lithium on Gs alpha membrane relocalization. *BMC Neuroscience*, *16*, 1–9. https://doi.org/10.1186/s12868-015-0178-y.

Svenningsson, P., & Sjogren, B. (2007). Depletion of the lipid raft constituents, sphingomyelin and ganglioside, decreases serotonin binding at human 5-HT $_{7(a)}$ receptors in HeLa cells. *Acta Physiologica*, *190*, 47–53. https://doi.org/10.1111/j.1748-1716.2007.01687.x.

Tiwari, S., & Chattopadhyay, A. (2011). Biochemical and biophysical research communications identification of cholesterol recognition amino acid consensus (CRAC) motif in G-protein coupled receptors. *Biochemical and Biophysical Research Communications*, *404*(1), 569–573. https://doi.org/10.1016/j.bbrc.2010.12.031.

Wright, P. T., Nikolaev, V. O., O'Hara, T., Diakonov, I., Bhargava, A., Tokar, S., et al. (2014). Caveolin-3 regulates compartmentation of cardiomyocyte beta2-adrenergic receptor-mediated cAMP signaling. *Journal of Molecular and Cellular Cardiology*, *67*, 38–48.

CHAPTER THREE

Rapid-acting antidepressants

Jeffrey M. Witkin[a,b,c,*], Anna E. Martin[a], Lalit K. Golani[c], Nina Z. Xu[a], Jodi L. Smith[d]

[a]Witkin Consulting Group, Carmel, IN, United States
[b]Department of Neurological Surgery, Indiana University School of Medicine, Indianapolis, IN, United States
[c]Department of Chemistry & Biochemistry, University of Wisconsin-Milwaukee, Milwaukee, WI, United States
[d]Laboratory of Antiepileptic Drug Discovery, St. Vincent's Hospital, Indianapolis, IN, United States
*Corresponding author: e-mail address: witkinconsult@gmail.com

Contents

1. Introduction 48
2. NMDA receptor antagonists 51
3. Muscarinic receptor antagonists 54
4. Psychedelic drugs 58
5. Mechanisms awaiting clinical testing 62
   5.1 $mGlu_{2/3}$ receptor antagonists 62
   5.2 AMPA receptor potentiators 64
   5.3 α5-containing $GABA_A$ receptors 65
6. Mechanisms of action 67
7. Conclusions 80
Acknowledgments 81
Conflict of interest 81
References 81

Abstract

Conventional antidepressants (biogenic amine mechanisms) are not fully efficacious (e.g., symptoms remain after treatment, not all patients respond), produce effects only after weeks of daily dosing, and do not impact all disease symptoms. In contrast, a new class of antidepressants has been emerging since 2006 that has demonstrated rapid onset, large effect size, activity after only a single or few dose applications, and positive impact in treatment refractory patients and against some treatment-resistant symptoms (e.g., anhedonia). Rapid-acting antidepressant drug action has been demonstrated in controlled clinical studies for ketamine, a few other NMDA receptor antagonists, and scopolamine. Less clinical data are currently available for psychedelic drugs such as psilocybin, lysergic acid diethylamide, and ayahuasca. The mechanisms of action of rapid-acting antidepressants are not fully understood. However, a general triggering mechanism appears to involve the potentiation of AMPA receptor function. Although the durability of antidepressant effects of ketamine and scopolamine is limited, psychedelic drugs have been reported to produce effects for many months. The primary

Advances in Pharmacology, Volume 86
ISSN 1054-3589
https://doi.org/10.1016/bs.apha.2019.03.002

impediment to generating a medicine of this type for depressed patients is side effects and the lack of methods to ensure enduring antidepressant effects. Thus, further exploration of drug possibilities continues. Esketamine ((S)-ketamine) was recently FDA approved. Compounds currently in clinical development include the NMDA receptor antagonist (R)-ketamine, the NMDA receptor modulator, GLYX-13 (Rapastinel), and the AMPA receptor potentiator TAK-653. Additional pharmacological classes have produced effects in the preclinical laboratory to suggest their potential as rapid-acting agents. These include mGlu2/3 receptor antagonists, AMPA receptor potentiators, and negative allosteric modulators of $GABA_A(\alpha5)$ receptors. In all cases, molecules exist that could be used to provide clinical proof of concept testing.

1. Introduction

Major depressive disorder (MDD) is a debilitating and costly neuropsychiatric disorder, associated with high prevalence estimates and high rates of morbidity and mortality (Chiu et al., 2018; de la Vega, Piña, Peralta, Kelly, & Giner, 2018; Doran & Kinchin, 2017). Standard of care antidepressants increase the synaptic availability of biogenic amine neurotransmitters, in particular 5-hydroxytrytamine (5-HT) or serotonin and norepinephrine (NE) (Iversen, 2005). These conventional antidepressants act by blocking the synaptic reuptake of either 5-HT (serotonin reuptake inhibitors or SRIs), NE (norepinephrine uptake inhibitors or NRIs), or function as dual-acting inhibitors (SNRIs). Conventional antidepressants produce response (diminution of some symptoms) in only about 1/3 of patients; remission (full arrest of symptoms) occurs in about 1/3 of patients; and another group of patients (~1/3) do not respond to these drugs (Rush et al., 2006) (treatment-resistant depression).

Conventional antidepressants generally require weeks to produce full treatment response (Katz, Koslow, & Frazer, 1996-1997; Katz et al., 2004) in the patient population for which they have any response efficacy. This is a more serious concern than typically realized. Patients must wait weeks for the possibility of symptom relief. If there is none, adjunct therapies are typically initiated. If antidepressant switching is needed, the patient again must wait weeks for potential relief, all the time leaving the patient vulnerable to disease-related health and well-being issues including the possibility of suicide.

The size of treatment effects in studies with conventional antidepressants is generally small (Locher et al., 2017). In contrast, the rapid-acting agents produce symptom impact in many cases in patients that have not responded to standard antidepressant therapies. Conventional antidepressants also are limited in the symptoms of depression that they treat. Ketamine, in contrast, has shown efficacy against anhedonia (discussed more below) that has been difficult to treat with conventional agents (Lally et al., 2014, 2015). Ketamine also rapidly impacts suicidal ideation (one dose) (Wilkinson et al., 2018), an outcome of importance to high-risk patients.

There have been hints in the literature that some drugs might have more rapid-acting effects than others. In the case of the biogenic-amine-based antidepressants for example, some symptoms are affected sooner than others and this is compound dependent (Katz et al., 2004). Furthermore, for some drugs, data, albeit limited in nature, have suggested that they might impact treatment-refractory depression better than standard of care agents. Currently, for treatment-resistant depression, there is only one drug approved—Symbyax, a combination of the antidepressant fluoxetine with the antipsychotic drug olanzapine (Haridas et al., 2003). Tianeptine has shown antidepressant efficacy after 1 week of dosing (Novotný & Faltus, 2003). In open label studies, tianeptine has shown efficacy in treatment-resistant depressed patients (Tobe & Rybakowski, 2013; Woo et al., 2013). Buprenorphine has also produced treatment responses in patients unresponsive to conventional antidepressants (Bodkin, Zornberg, Lukas, & Cole, 1995; Karp et al., 2014; Nyhuis, Gastpar, & Scherbaum, 2008). Buprenorphine produced improvement in mood within 1 week of dosing in one study (Ehrich, Turncliff, Sellers, Jones, & Fava, 2012). Both tianeptine and buprenorphine have the common mechanisms of action involving opioid receptors. Compounds in development for treatment resistant depression (rapid agents) are reviewed in the present paper and summarized elsewhere (Garay et al., 2017).

In the past several years (see Fig. 1), discoveries have launched a new era of antidepressant research (Witkin, 2011). The possibilities raised by the prominent behavioral changes produced by these new drugs bring the same excitement that existed when other life-saving drugs were being discovered (e.g., chlorpromazine in the 1950s) (Witkin, 2015). Surrounding the work with these newer antidepressant molecules is hope. As in the early 1900s films when someone was relieved of bouts of hysteria by a slap across the face (thanks, I needed that). And miraculous in the witnessing of newly revitalized human spirit (one film from the pioneering researcher Helen Mayberg shows a woman that had not responded to other therapies, turning to her daughter after electrical stimulation of area 25 and saying "it's a beautiful day, let's go bowling").

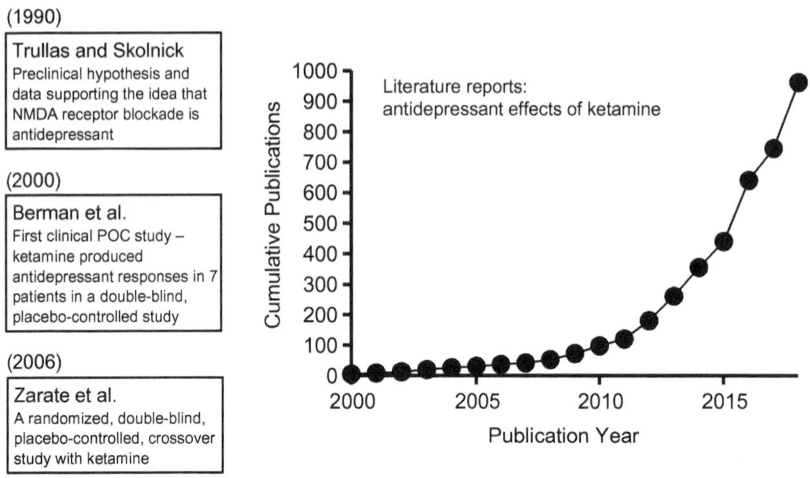

Fig. 1 Time line of literature publications on ketamine as a rapid-acting antidepressant.

A new class of antidepressants, beginning with the NMDA receptor antagonists with ketamine being used as the prototype, has evolved that produce rapid (single dose), large-effect size antidepressant responses in patients, some of whom have previously been treatment refractory (Wilkinson & Sanacora, 2018). Although a formal definition of rapid-acting antidepressant has not been put forward, these compounds are generally so classified for their ability to produce major impact on symptoms and, in some patients, to produce remission, within one or few doses. Further, these antidepressant effects outlast the pharmacokinetics of the drug. Beyond the definition of rapid, these compounds have also impacted symptoms of depression that have generally remained immune to medicinal therapy. This bold new antidepressant concept is also rapidly and exponentially advancing (Fig. 1) as in the era of early discoveries in psychopharmacology (Witkin, 2015). Credit for the remarkable progress in this area must be given to the early pioneers who made leaps from disparate data to hypotheses (as in the case of ketamine with Trullas & Skolnick, 1990) and to the clinical researchers who created the early elegant data (as with Berman et al., 2000 and Zarate et al., 2006). In some cases, serendipity, the great leader of scientific advances (Meyers, 2007), is to be recognized; scopolamine as a rapid-acting antidepressant was discovered accidently in the course of ancillary work on the compound (Furey & Drevets, 2006). Another important driver to the large headway that has been gained in a short period with rapid-acting antidepressants is due to the large and rapid, and in the case of treatment-refractory patients, frankly remarkable, behavioral changes that are produced by these drugs. Because of the large pharmacological effects of rapidly acting antidepressants, clinical trials can be fast and markedly less expensive than the multiweek, multipatient, multisite studies generally used to define efficacy for conventional antidepressants. Too, patients suffering from depression have been willing to enroll in clinical studies on these new agents that are in some cases beyond the categorization of conventional (e.g., psychedelic drugs).

2. NMDA receptor antagonists

The hypothesis of Trullas and Skolnick (1990) that NMDA receptor antagonists would be antidepressant was substantiated with data from pre-clinical behavioral despair models using NMDA receptor antagonists that could individually modulate the range of NMDA receptor binding sites. Competitive, uncompetitive, polyamine-site, and glycine-site antagonists all generated antidepressant-like effects in rodent models that detect activity of conventional antidepressants (Skolnick, Popik, & Trullas, 2009). The clinical proof of concept study reported by Berman et al. (2000) and its systematic and elegant replication by Zarate et al. (2006) would ultimately lead to a revolution in the field of antidepressant drug discovery (Fig. 1). Several current reviews on the antidepressant effects of ketamine and other rapid-acting antidepressants are available (Gerhard & Duman, 2018; Gould, Zarate, & Thompson, 2019; Machado-Vieira, Henter, & Zarate, 2017; Wilkinson & Sanacora, 2018; Witkin, Knutson, Rodriguez, & Shi, 2018).

The initial clinical data with ketamine (Fig. 2) demonstrated the following key features that differentiated its pharmacological effects from those of conventional biogenic-amine-based antidepressants. (1) Rapid activity: ketamine produced effects within minutes after a single intravenous infusion, (2) Treatment-resistant depression: ketamine produced symptom relief in patients that did not respond to conventional antidepressants, (3) Duration of action: antidepressant effects of ketamine outlasted the plasma levels of ketamine, and (4) Effect size: large effects on depressed symptoms were observed. Further differentiation was to be identified in subsequent clinical studies. For example, (5) Other patient populations: ketamine produced antidepressant efficacy in other populations of depressed patients (e.g., bipolar depression) (Diazgranados et al., 2010) and other groups (e.g., posttraumatic stress disorder (Feder et al., 2014). In addition, (6) SRI and

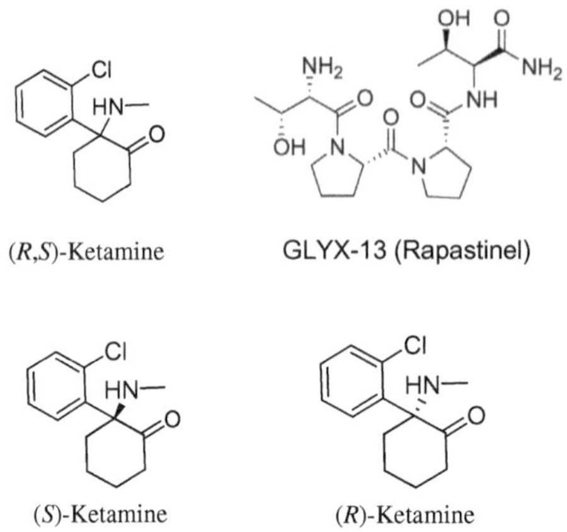

Fig. 2 Structures of some NMDA receptor antagonists. Ketamine is a rapid-acting antidepressant. (S)-ketamine (esketamine) has just been FDA approved as an antidepressant. (R)-ketamine might have a reduced side-effect profile. GLYX-13 (Rapastinel) is an NMDA receptor modulator and is in Phase 3 development for depression.

SNRI-unresponsive symptoms: ketamine produced effects on symptoms of depression (Lally et al., 2014, 2015) that are often difficult to decrease with conventional antidepressants (e.g., anhedonia) (Argyropoulos & Nutt, 2013).

There are no approved drugs for the treatment of anhedonia (see Cao et al., 2019 for a review of drugs that might impact this diseases symptom). Clinical investigation of ketamine in treatment-resistant depressed patients revealed the ability of ketamine to impact this residual and key symptom of depression. Lally et al. (2014) studied ketamine in a randomized, double-blind, placebo-controlled, crossover study in 36 patients with treatment-resistant bipolar depression. Patients were either bipolar I or II and continued to express major depressive disorders symptoms despite ongoing treatment with either valproate or lithium as mood stabilizers. Ketamine rapidly reduced the degree of anhedonia symptoms in these patients. A systematic replication of this work in patients diagnosed with major depressive disorder was reported (Lally et al., 2015). As summarized in Fig. 3, ketamine produced these antianhedonic effects independently of its general antidepressant efficacy. Brain metabolic activity assessed through measures of glucose utilization revealed that activation of dorsal anterior cingulate cortex and putamen was correlated with anhedonia symptom relief.

Clinical observations with ketamine resulted in the fast-paced efforts to identify other NMDA receptor antagonists that might also produce rapid

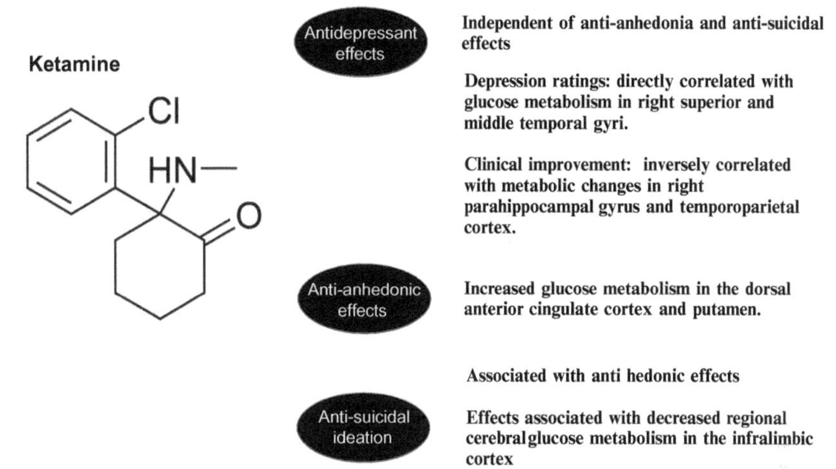

Fig. 3 Some clinical effects of ketamine in depressed patients and some biological correlates. *Data are primarily from Carlson, P. J., Diazgranados, N, Nugent, A. C., Ibrahim, L, Luckenbaugh, D. A., Brutsche, N., et al. (2013). Neural correlates of rapid antidepressant response to ketamine in treatment-resistant unipolar depression: A preliminary positron emission tomography.* Biological Psychiatry, *73(12), 1213–1221; Ballard, E. D., Lally, N., Nugent, A. C., Furey, M. L., Luckenbaugh, D. A., Zarate, C. A., Jr. (2014). Neural correlates of suicidal ideation and its reduction in depression.* The International Journal of Neuropsychopharmacology *18(1), pii: pyu069, and Lally, N., Nugent, A. C., Luckenbaugh, D. A., Niciu, M. J., Roiser, J. P., Zarate, C. A., Jr. (2015). Neural correlates of change in major depressive disorder anhedonia following open-label ketamine.* Journal of Psychopharmacology. *29(5), 596–607.*

antidepressant effect. For example, the NMDA receptor antagonist selective for NR2B receptors, CP-101,606, was also effective in TRD patients (Preskorn et al., 2008). Zn^{2+}, a blocker of the NMDA receptor ion channel, augmented the effects of imipramine in treatment resistant depressed patients (Siwek et al., 2009). (S)-ketamine (Esketamine) (Fig. 2) (Molero et al., 2018) was approved for use in depressed patients by the U.S. FDA in February of 2019. The low affinity NMDA receptor antagonist dextromethorphan has demonstrated rapid response efficacy in a treatment-resistant patient (Lauterbach, 2016) and by retrospective analysis in bipolar II patients (Kelly & Lieberman, 2014).

Additional impetus for the discovery of other NMDA receptor antagonists with rapid-acting antidepressant activity derives from the known side effects and toxicity of ketamine that include dissociative effects, psychotomimetic effects, drug abuse, and brain lesions (see discussion and summary in Witkin et al., 2017). Thus, discovery efforts have been directed toward the identification of compounds that retain clinical efficacy but display reduced side-effect potential. One such compound, GLYX-13 (Rapastinel) (Fig. 2), has been characterized as an NMDA receptor modulator that acts outside the ion channel where ketamine produces its blocking effects (Donello et al., 2018). Preclinical studies documented the antidepressant-like efficacy of GLYX-13 in rodent models (Liu et al., 2017). Phase 2 clinical studies demonstrated efficacy in patients that have encouraged the ongoing efforts to develop GLYX-13 as a new rapid-acting antidepressant (Moskal et al., 2017). Compound screening has been utilized to help identify other novel, rapid-acting antidepressants. For example, compound screening for molecules that target the dopamine transporter ultimately identified an ifenprodil analog, Ro-25-6981, that demonstrates rapid-acting antidepressant-like effects (Talbot et al., 2016).

Other suggestions for achieving reduced side-effect burden and toxicity come from studies with (R)-ketamine (Fig. 2) and some ketamine metabolites such as (S)-norketamine (Hashimoto, 2016; Yang et al., 2015; Zhang & Hashimoto, 2018; Zhang, Li, & Hashimoto, 2014). (R)-ketamine has also demonstrated efficacy in some animal models for which (S)-ketamine is not active and has a longer duration of action than (S)-ketamine (Fukumoto et al., 2017). Another NMDA receptor modulator, 4-chlorokynurenine, has also been suggested as such an agent from preclinical studies (Zanos et al., 2015).

Another molecule that has potentially less side-effect burden than ketamine is the NR2B subunit- selective NMDA receptor antagonist Ro 25-6981 (Yellepeddi et al., 2018). The NR2B-selective antagonist AZD-6765 (Lanicemine) has been studied in patients with efficacy demonstrated albiet short lived (Sanacora et al., 2014; Zarate et al., 2013). However, a subsequent study with a different design failed to demonstrate efficacy (Sanacora et al., 2017).

Another issue that surrounds the use of NMDA receptor antagonists for depression is the durability of their antidepressant effects. For patients responding to ketamine, the duration of action is on the order of weeks post-dosing. Procedures for sustaining efficacy continue to be evaluated.

3. Muscarinic receptor antagonists

First proposed by Janowsky and colleagues in 1972, the cholinergic-adrenergic hypothesis of mania and depression correlated depression with increased cholinergic activity. Several tricyclic antidepressants were found to have central anticholinergic properties while drugs with central cholinomimetic properties were found to cause depression symptoms in some people (Janowsky, el-Yousef, Davis, & Sekerke, 1972).

In 2006, Furey and Drevets introduced the muscarinic receptor antagonist scopolamine (Fig. 4) as another drug with rapid-acting antidepressant efficacy. They conducted two studies with depressed outpatients (18–50 years of age) who also met the DSM-IV criteria for recurrent major depressive disorder (MDD) or bipolar disorder. Under standard double-blind conditions, the first study utilized four testing sessions consisting of a 15-min intravenous infusion of a saline placebo and three doses of scopolamine hydrobromide in the following concentrations: 2.0, 3.0, and 4.0 μg/kg. The sessions were performed 3–5 days apart from one another and performed in random order for all four sessions with the exception that the 4.0 μg/kg could not be used as the first dose for any of the patients.

The second study was constructed in a similar manner as in the first study; however, the second study consisted of a single lead-in placebo followed by six randomized sessions in which the patient would have the placebo for three sessions followed by scopolamine at 4.0 μg/kg for three sessions or have scopolamine at 4.0 μg/kg for three sessions followed by the placebo for three sessions. Before each infusion and between infusions, the first study used the Montgomery-Asberg Depression Rating Scale (MADRS) and the Hamilton Anxiety Rating Scale (HARS) to assess antidepressant and anti-anxiety responses to scopolamine. In addition to utilizing MADRS and HARS, the second study used the Young Mania Rating Scale, the Clinical Global Impressions–Improvement scale, the Profile of Mood State (POMS), and visual analog scales (VAS) focusing on the components happy, sad, drowsy, irritated, alert, anxious, and restless. VAS and POMS were performed at the baseline and at 20, 60, 120, and 180 min after each infusion. Both studies also obtained blood samples at baseline and at 30, 45, 60, 90, 120, and 150 min after the infusion began.

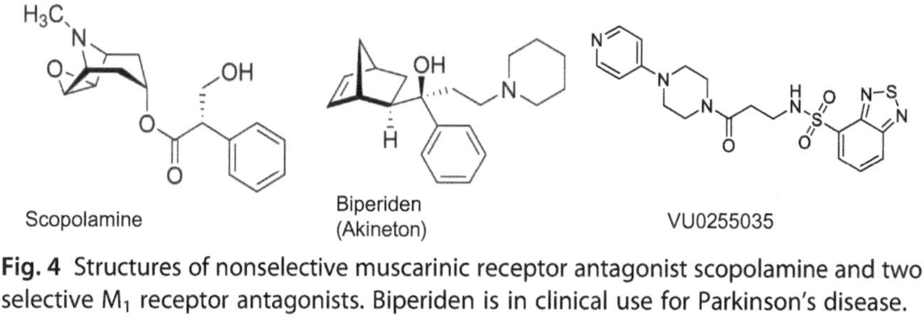

Fig. 4 Structures of nonselective muscarinic receptor antagonist scopolamine and two selective M_1 receptor antagonists. Biperiden is in clinical use for Parkinson's disease.

In both studies, a significant decrease in depression and anxiety rating scale scores were observed after the initial dose of scopolamine at 4.0 μg/kg, and reductions in the scores continued to be observed once the placebo was administered after the previous dose(s) of scopolamine. Unlike conventional antidepressants that commonly do not elicit a response after initial treatment, the muscarinic receptor antagonist scopolamine was found to produce relatively rapid antidepressant effects which were observed following its initial treatment. Such rapid response rates were also evident in the patients who did not respond to conventional antidepressants in the past and were seen in those who suffered from comorbid anxiety disorders.

Since the Furey and Drevets (2006) study, the data have been replicated several times, and similar findings have been reported in a few additional studies utilizing other treatment populations and other muscarinic receptor antagonists (see Dagyte, Den Boer, & Trentani, 2011; Drevets, Zarate, & Furey, 2013; Howland, 2009; Jaffe, Novakovic, & Peselow, 2013; Janowsky, 2011). However, a recent study found a lack of significant antidepressant activity in patients with more severe and drug-resistant depression (Park et al., 2019).

The mechanism of action for scopolamine remained elusive as scopolamine acts relatively equally on all five muscarinic receptor subtypes, M_1 through M_5. In 2014, Witkin et al. reported the results of forced-swim tests utilizing M_1–M_5 receptor deficient mice. Scopolamine produced antidepressant-associated effects in wild-type mice and M_3–M_5 null mice; however, in both M_1 and M_2 null mice, the antidepressant effects of scopolamine were not induced (Witkin et al., 2014) (Fig. 5, top panel). A role for the M_1 receptor subtype was supported by subsequent findings on the mechanisms of action of scopolamine (Navarria et al., 2015; Wohleb et al., 2016). Lending additional support to the presumed role of M_1 and M_2 receptors in scopolamine's mechanism of action, studies have demonstrated a correlation between M_1 and M_2 receptors and mood disorders and mood disorder circuitry (Cannon et al., 2006; Gibbons, Scarr, McLean, Sundram, & Dean, 2009; Huang & Hsu, 2010; Meredith, Blank, & Groenewegen, 1989; Navarria et al., 2015; Wohleb, Gerhard, Thomas, & Duman, 2017). Biperiden (Fig. 4) and pirenzepine, selective for M_1 over M_2 receptors, produced similar antidepressant signatures to that of scopolamine in wild-type mice (Witkin et al., 2014; Zhou et al., 2017). The antidepressant-associated effects of biperiden and pirenzepine were significantly attenuated in M_1 null mice (Witkin et al., 2014). A selective M_1 receptor antagonist VU0255035 (Fig. 4) also produced positive effects in the antidepressant-detecting mouse forced-swim assay (Witkin et al., 2014).

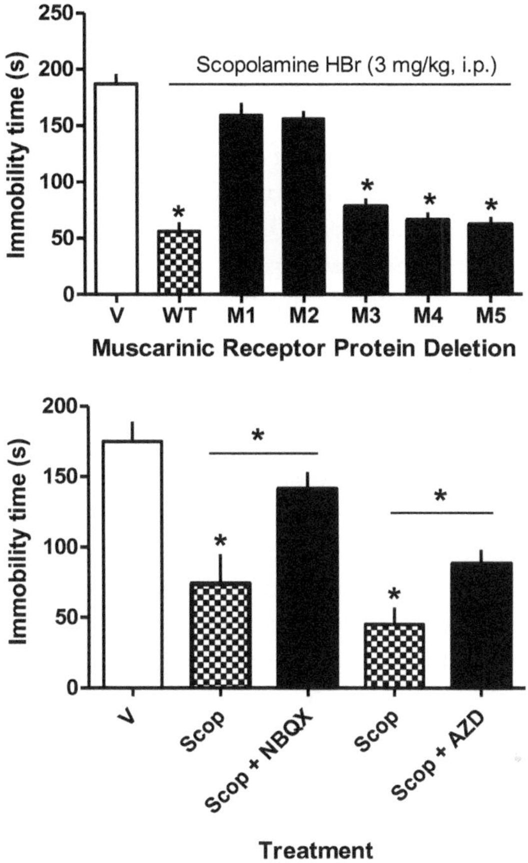

Fig. 5 Top Panel: Effects of congenic deletion of muscarinic receptor subtype genes on the antidepressant-like effects of scopolamine (3 mg/kg, i.p.) in the mouse forced-swim test. Bottom Panel: Attenuation of the antidepressant-like effects of scopolamine by the AMPA receptor antagonist NBQX or the mTOR inhibitor AZD8055. *$P<0.05$; **$P<0.01$; ***$P<0.001$ compared to vehicle control (top panel) or compared to another treatment group (bottom panel) as indicated. *Data are replotted from Witkin, J. M., Overshiner, C., Li, X., Catlow, J. T., Schober, D. A., Heinz, B. A., et al. (2014). The M_1 and M_2 muscarinic receptor subtypes regulate antidepressant-like effects of the rapidly acting antidepressant scopolamine.* The Journal of Pharmacology and Experimental Therapeutics. 351*(2), 448–456, (top panel) or Martin et al. (2017) (bottom panel).*

M_1-selective antagonists await clinical investigation. Biperiden is in clinical use for Parkinson's disease (Brocks, 1999) and could be used for this purpose. To date there is no consensus on the potential antidepressant effects of biperiden; Kasper, Moises, and Beckmann (1981) reported efficacy in patients whereas Gillin et al. (1995) did not. VU0255035 appears to have issues with its ability to adequately expose the central nervous system after systemic dosing (Witkin et al., 2014).

Due to the more severe side effects of ketamine such as dissociations, increased blood pressure and addiction (Ghoneim, Hinrichs, Mewaldt, & Petersen, 1985), scopolamine might be an effective and less problematic alternative. However, scopolamine is not without issues and can cause memory impairments and bradycardia (Qiu et al., 2016). Thus, several studies have attempted to minimize the negative effects of scopolamine by using it in conjunction with another antidepressant. Podkowa, Salat, Lenda, Pilc, and Palucha-Poniewiera (2016) combined scopolamine with the $mGlu_{2/3}$ receptor antagonist LY341495, both at subeffective doses, and observed enhanced antidepressant efficacy without memory impairment in mice. In a similar study, scopolamine was administered simultaneously with the $mGlu_7$ receptor allosteric agonist AMN082, and once again, enhanced antidepressant efficacy and no spatial memory impairment was observed (Podkowa et al., 2018).

As scopolamine's mechanism is further investigated and revealed, drug targets can be narrowed and specified for particular subsets of patients. For example, a 2016 study demonstrated the possibility of predicting the patients who would respond to scopolamine treatment by analyzing amygdalar activity using functional magnetic resonance imaging (fMRI). While undergoing fMRI, the patients were exposed to emotional stimuli, specifically a sad face. Healthy controls and MDD patients who did not respond to scopolamine treatment produced the same amygdalar responses; however, treatment-responsive MDD patients produced a distinct amygdalar response compared to control and to nontreatment-responsive patients. As treatment with scopolamine continued, treatment-responsive patients produced amygdalar responses that resembled the healthy control's responses (Szczepanik, Drevets, Khanna, Zarate, & Furey, 2012).

4. Psychedelic drugs

The ability to quantitatively study behavioral effects of psychedelic drugs in humans enabled clinical studies of their potential therapeutic benefit against a variety of pathophysiological conditions including depression and treatment-resistant depression (Johnson and Griffiths, 2017; Kyzar, Nichols, Gainetdinov, Nichols, & Kalueff, 2017; Rucker, Iliff, & Nutt, 2018) (see Dos Santos, Bouso, Alcázar-Córcoles, & Hallak, 2018 for a review).

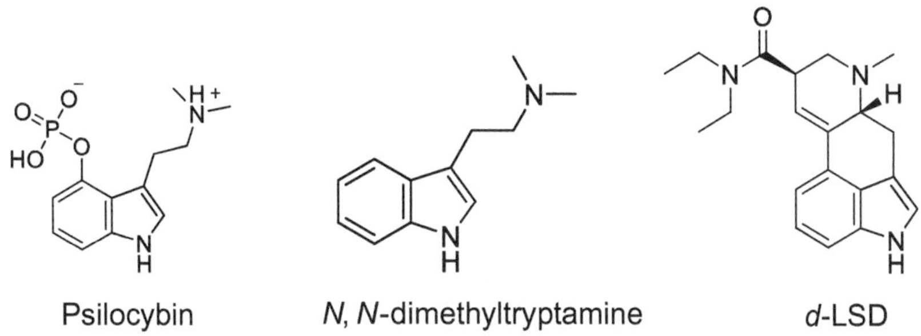

Fig. 6 Structures of some psychedelic drugs that have been studied in patients with major depressive disorder.

A summary of the major research findings of these compounds (Fig. 6) in major depressive disorder is summarized in Table 1 illustrating a range of clinical populations that have been studied in both open label and blinded, placebo-controlled studies. Psilocybin has been most quantitatively studied. The early studies with lysergic acid diethylamide (LSD) focused primarily on anxiety symptoms. Some other drugs like MDMA (ecstasy), generally classified as an entactogen or empathogen (Nichols, 1986), have been minimally investigated. Ibogaine is another compound with potential promise in this area (Wasko, Witt-Enderby, & Surratt, 2018). Carrillo et al. (2018) have recently reported that speech analysis and machine learning can predict which patients are depressed and which of those that will respond to psilocybin. One determinant of the efficacy and durability of the effects of psilocybin are measures of the quality of the psychedelic experience (Roseman, Nutt, & Carhart-Harris, 2018).

Psilocybin has been investigated across a range of doses that have supported its effectiveness as a mood enhancer and potential antidepressant. Higher doses of psilocybin (1 or 3mg/70kg) engendered large, decreases across a range of clinician- and self-rated measures of depressed mood and anxiety (Carhart-Harris et al., 2016;Griffiths et al., 2016; Ross et al., 2016) as well as sustained improvements in perceptions for quality of life, meaning of life, and optimism, accompanied by decreases in death anxiety (Griffiths et al., 2016; Ross et al., 2016). At lower doses, psilocybin's psychological effects become less pronounced, but retained statistical significance over long-term follow-up sessions up to 6months later (Griffiths et al., 2016; Grob et al., 2011). The range of mood-enhancing and antidepressant effects of psilocybin have been found to be sustained for a majority of study participants in long-term follow-up inquiries (Table 1). Psilocybin engenders moderate, transient dose- and time-dependent increases in

Table 1 Clinic studies of some psychedelic drugs in patients.

Patient population	Study design	Results	Reference
Psilocybin			
Late-stage cancer	12 Patients, double-blind, placebo-controlled	Improvement in depression and anxiety scores. Sustained effect for anxiety at 6 months and for depression with one measuring instrument at 6 months	Grob et al. (2011)
Life-threatening cancer with anxiety and depression	51 Patients, double-blind, crossover design. Placebo-like dose (1 or 3 mg/70 kg) and high dose (22 or 30 mg/70 kg), counterbalanced 5 weeks between treatments	Improvement in depression scores and increases in positive attitude about life up to 6 months posttreatment (30 mg/70 kg dose group)	Griffiths et al. (2016)
Life-threatening cancer with anxiety and depression	29 Patients, double-blind, placebo-controlled, crossover design using 0.3 mg/kg	Improvement in depression and anxiety scores on day 1 and at 26-week follow-up	Ross et al. (2016)
Treatment-resistant depression	Open label, no control, 10 and 25 mg, 2 weeks apart	Depression symptoms were decreased 1 week and 3 months after 25 mg with large and enduring reductions in anxiety and anhedonia	Carhart-Harris et al. (2016)
Treatment-resistant depression	19 Patients; 16 receiving fMRI scans	Antidepressant response (100% at 1 week; 47% at week 5); decreased amygdala blood flow positively associated with treatment response	Carhart-Harris et al. (2017)
Treatment-resistant depression	20 Patients from Carhart-Harris et al. (2016)	Continued efficacy at 6 months	Carhart-Harris et al. (2018)
Treatment-resistant depression	Placebo control—10 and 25 mg, 2 weeks apart with psychological support	Enhanced ability to recognize emotional faces—associated with reductions in anhedonia	Stroud et al. (2018)

Table 1 Clinic studies of some psychedelic drugs in patients.—cont'd

Patient population	Study design	Results	Reference
Treatment-resistant depression	20 Patients given drug and psychological support; 19 receiving fMRI scans	Antidepressant efficacy observed with increases in amygdalar responses to emotional faces	Roseman, Demetriou, Wall, Nutt, and Carhart-Harris (2018)
LSD			
Severe depression	15 Patients, open label; 13 completed study	7 Patients (53.8%) exhibited symptom improvement	Savage (1952)
Terminal cancer	22 Patients, open label	2/3 of patients stated a positive change-6 of these patients stated dramatic improvement	Pahnke, Kurland, Goodman, and Richards (1969)
Terminal cancer	31 Patients, open label	Emotional and physical distress markedly improved (29% of patients); 41.9% had mild improvement; 22.6% showed little effect; 6.4% of patients were negatively affected	Grof, Goodman, Richards, and Kurland (1973)
Anxiety from life-threating illness	12 Patients, double-blind, placebo-controlled	Significant decrease in state anxiety	Gasser et al. (2014)
Life-threatening cancer	12 Patients, double-blind, placebo-controlled	Significant decrease in anxiety and increase in quality of life 12 months posttreatment	Gasser, Kirchner, and Passie (2015)
Ayahuasca			
Recurrent depression	6 Patients, open label patients	Significant improvement	Osório Fde et al. (2015)
Recurrent depression	17 Patients, open label	Significant improvement 1, 7, 21 days posttreatment	Sanches et al. (2016)
Treatment-resistant depression	29 Patients, randomized, double-blind, placebo-controlled	Significant improvement 1, 2, and 7 days posttreatment	Palhano-Fontes et al. (2018)

systolic and/or diastolic blood pressure and heart rate (Griffiths et al., 2016; Grob et al., 2011; Ross et al., 2016), but has not created any serious negative effects on cardiovascular function and other aspects of health at the doses studied.

Ayahuasca is a brew made from the *Banisteriopsis caapi* vine and other ingredients and contains the hallucinogen dimethyltryptamine (Hamill, Hallak, Dursun, & Baker, 2018). The results thus far are promising for the antidepressant effects and safety of these molecules under the laboratory conditions studied (Table 1). A recent clinical study was the first to demonstrate efficacy in a population of treatment-resistant patients (Palhano-Fontes et al., 2018). In this study, ayahuasca was dosed in patients under a randomized, placebo-controlled trial where response to treatment was significant at all time points (day 1, 2, and 7 postdosing). At day 7 the response rate was 64% compared to 27% for placebo. Remission rates tended toward significance (36% vs. 7%, $P=0.054$). Ayahuasca increased salivary cortisol levels in both healthy volunteers and in patients with treatment-resistant depression (Galvão et al., 2018).

The potential for abuse liability of psychedelics has generally been considered minimal. In a recent study, lysergic acid diethylamide (LSD), psilocybin, and mescaline were studied with repeat dosing. Limited abuse liability was observed in a model where abused drugs enhance the electrical stimulation of reward pathways. However, LSD attenuated the depression-like effects of a kappa opioid receptor agonist (Sakloth et al., 2019). Johnson, Griffiths, Hendricks, and Henningfield (2018) have also assessed the abuse liability of psilocybin using clinical criteria where they determined it to be a potential Schedule IV drug. The study by Sakloth used repeat dosing in order to mimic the microdosing some people are engaging in. A survey of microdosers of psilocybin and LSD found that they reported improvements in negative emotions and dysfunctional attitudes along with increases in wisdom, open-mindedness, and creativity ($P<0.001$, $r=0.15$) when compared to those that did not microdose (Anderson et al., 2019).

5. Mechanisms awaiting clinical testing

5.1 $mGlu_{2/3}$ receptor antagonists

Convergent findings from behavioral, neurochemical, biochemical, and electrophysiological studies predict that $mGlu_{2/3}$ receptor antagonists will produce rapid antidepressant efficacy in patients (see overviews and

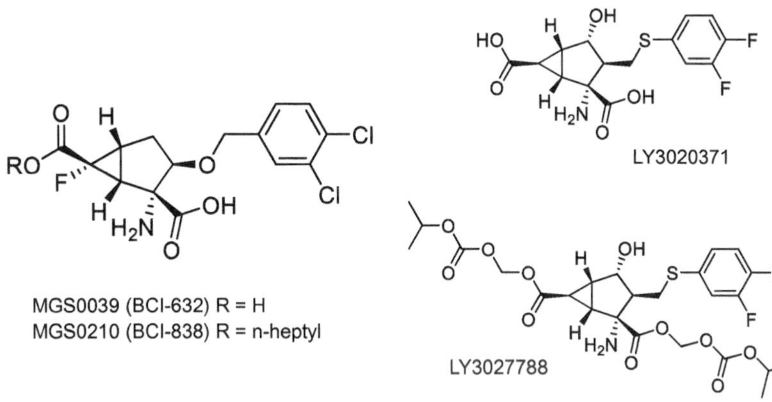

Fig. 7 Structures of some antagonists of mGlu2/3 receptors. MGS0039 and MGS0210 have been in Phase 1 studies in healthy human volunteers. LY3020371 and an orally bioavailable prodrug LY3027788 await clinical investigation.

discussion in Chaki, 2017, 2019; Witkin et al., 2018). For example, the $mGlu_{2/3}$ receptor antagonist LY34149 and LY3020371 (Witkin et al., 2017) (Fig. 7) produce antidepressant phenotypes in rodent models that detect antidepressants and produce a host of associated pharmacological actions that overlap precisely with that of the known rapidly acting antidepressant ketamine (Witkin et al., 2017; see Witkin et al., 2018 for a summary).

At the same time that antidepressant efficacy in humans is predicted from the preclinical data on these compounds, $mGlu_{2/3}$ receptor antagonists are also predicted to have reduced liabilities for producing ketamine-associated safety and tolerability issues associated with ketamine administration. Data from preclinical studies have pointed to a low risk for cognitive, motor, subjective, neurochemical, and electrophysiological effects that might negatively impact patients (Witkin, Monn, et al., 2017; see Witkin et al., 2018 for a summary). In addition, 14-day toxicology studies with LY3020371 in rats and monkeys produced high plasma drug exposures of LY302037 but no critical toxicological findings (Witkin, Monn, et al., 2017). Overall, the data on this mechanism suggest antidepressant efficacy in patients without some of the side effects that are induced by ketamine.

Molecules are available for human testing to provide proof of concept that $mGlu_{2/3}$ receptor antagonism would function as a rapid-acting antidepressant mechanism. MGS0210 (BCI-838) is a prodrug of MGS0039 (BCI-632) (Fig. 7); both compounds have been studied in healthy human volunteers without untoward side effects (Gadient et al., 2012; S. Chaki, personal communication). LY3020271 and a diester prodrug, LY3027788 (Fig. 7), have completed preclinical assessments (Witkin, Monn, et al., 2017; Witkin, Ornstein, et al., 2017; Witkin, Overshiner, et al., 2017) and are additionally suitable for human Phase1 investigation.

5.2 AMPA receptor potentiators

Originally conjectured to be antidepressant by Skolnick in 2001 based upon the BDNF-hypothesis of antidepressant drug action (Skolnick, 2008), data from a host of clinical and preclinical literature sources on conventional and rapid-acting drugs and on the biochemistry of depression point to AMPA receptor potentiation as a primary trigger for rapid-antidepressant drug action as first formally enunciated by Alt, Nisenbaum, Bleakman, and Witkin (2006). Data summarizing the findings on AMPA receptor potentiation as a mechanism of action of rapid-acting antidepressants can be found in Alt et al. (2006) and Nisenbaum and Witkin (2010). Convergent data from biochemical, behavioral, and pharmacological studies lend support to a role for AMPA receptors. These data include effects of AMPA receptor potentiators on biochemical mediators of depression and antidepressant action and on the modulation of AMPA receptors by stress, mood disorders and by drugs that treat mood disorders (Alt et al., 2006; Nisenbaum & Witkin, 2010). Recently, Lian et al. (2018) used metabolomic analysis of ketamine in mouse hippocampus to identify substrates activated by ketamine or ketamine in the presence of an AMPA receptor antagonist; two sets of metabolites were uncovered.

Structures of two AMPA receptor potentiators that have been studied in humans, CX717 (Oertel et al., 2010) and LY451395 (Trzepacz et al., 2013) are shown in Fig. 8. The research community awaits formal investigation of whether AMPA receptor potentiators can transduce rapid-acting antidepressant effects. Test of the hypothesis must be approached with the right molecule for which there is limited understanding. AMPA receptor potentiators vary in their degree of intrinsic efficacy (see Nisenbaum & Witkin, 2010)

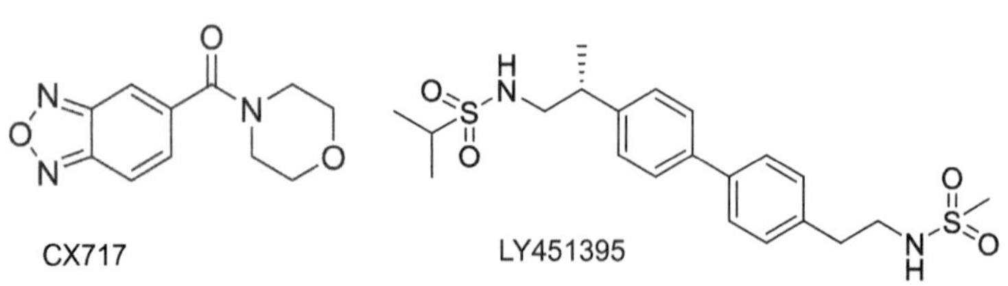

Fig. 8 Structures of two AMPA receptor potentiators that have undergone clinical investigation. Studies in depressed patients have not been reported.

and for higher efficacy ligands, there might be dose limitations that could compromise test of the AMPA potentiation hypothesis (Kunugi, Tajima, Kuno, Sogabe, & Kimura, 2018). TAK-653 (structure not yet disclosed) is an AMPA potentiator devoid of agonist activity that is being considered as a potential therapy for treatment-resistant depression. It is currently in clinical development (https://www.clinicaltrials.gov/ct2/show/NCT03792672?term=TAK-653&rank=3).

5.3 α5-containing $GABA_A$ receptors

This mechanism was formally brought into consideration for rapid-acting antidepressants with the work from Thompson's lab. L-655,708 and MRK-016 (Fig. 9), two negative allosteric modulators α5-containing $GABA_A$ receptors, produced antidepressant and synaptic excitatory effects in two rodent models (Fischell, Van Dyke, Kvarta, LeGates, & Thompson, 2015). These effects emerged within 24h of a single dose. Both of these compounds also produced antidepressant-like effects in the forced-swim assay (Carreno, Collins, Frazer, & Lodge, 2017; Zanos et al., 2017). Activity was observed 1 week after a single dose of L-655,708 and inactivation of the ventral hippocampus with lidocaine prevented the sustained antidepressant-like effects (Carreno et al., 2017). Expression of $GABA_A$(α5) was upregulated in depressed patients and in an animal model of stress that detects antidepressant effects of these molecules (Xiong et al., 2018).

Additional evidence of potential antidepressant effects of this mechanism was reported recently. A series of $GABA_A$(α5)-selective molecules was studied in the mouse forced-swim test. The antagonist Xli-093 was not active, the partial negative allosteric modulator, PWZ-029 (Fig. 9), was modestly active, and the full negative allosteric modulator, RY-080 (Fig. 9) was robustly active in producing an antidepressant-like signature in this assay (Fig. 10, top panel). Further pharmacological analysis provided additional

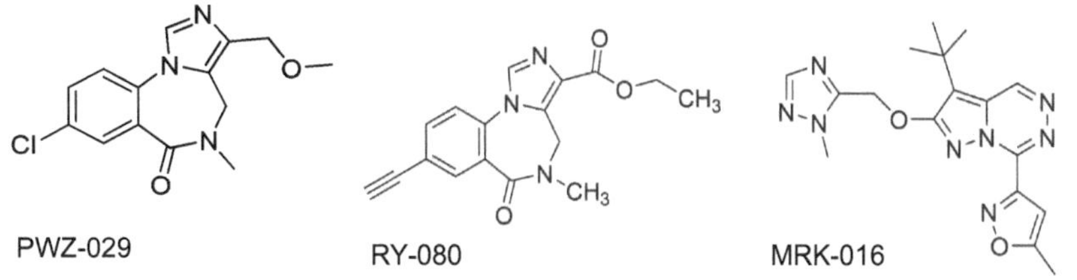

Fig. 9 Structures of some negative allosteric modulators of α5-containing $GABA_A$ receptors. RY-080 has greater negative intrinsic efficacy than PWZ-029. MRK-016 has been studied in humans where it has demonstrated tolerability. No antidepressant data have been reported to date.

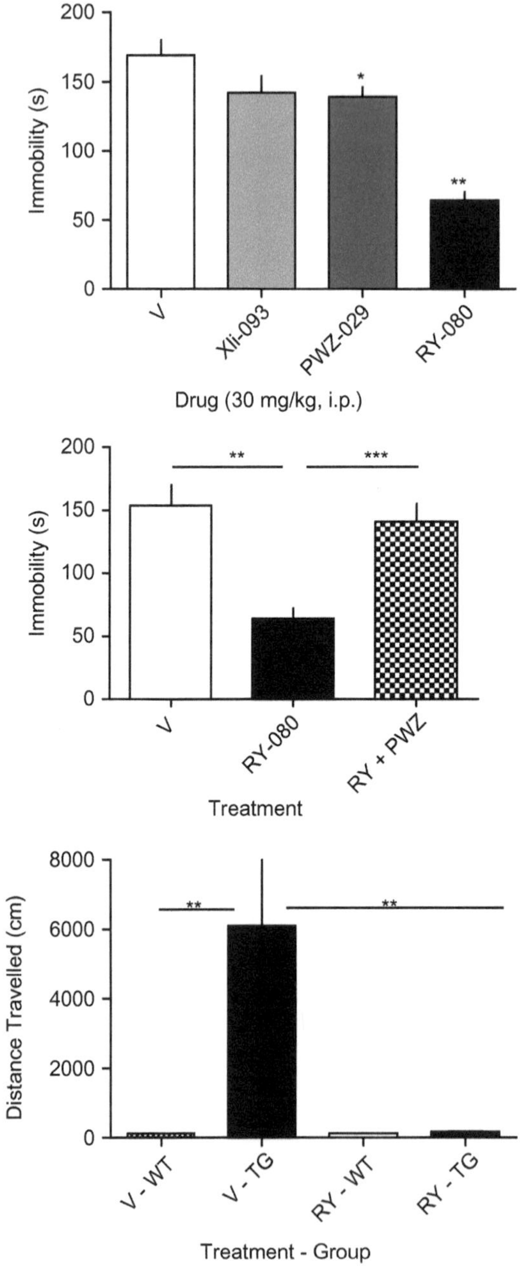

Fig. 10 See legend on opposite page.

documentation that antidepressant efficacy was achieved through negative allosteric modulation of α5-containing $GABA_A$ receptors. The partial inverse agonist, PWZ-029, was able to significantly prevent the antidepressant effects of the full inverse agonist RY-080 (Fig. 10, middle panel) as predicted by receptor theory. Similarly, the antagonist (Xli-093) was also an effective blocker of the antidepressant-like effects of RY-080 (Xu et al., 2018).

rTg4510 mice accumulate pathological tau with age and correspondingly demonstrate an explosive hyperactivity that might be relevant to modeling of agitation and aggression in neurodegenerative disease states. It was shown that RY-080 selectively attenuated the agitated hyperactivity of aged rTg4510 mice (Fig. 10, bottom panel). Data from these transgenic mice suggest the potential for negative allosteric modulators of $GABA_A$(α5) receptors to help downregulate the amotivational, agitated and aggressive states that arise in neurodegenerative disorders where depression is a primary comorbid symptom.

This mechanism does not engender ketamine-associated side effects or produce effects predictive of abuse liability (Carreno et al., 2017; Xu et al., 2018; Zanos et al., 2017). MRK-016 (Fig. 9) is tolerated in humans without induction of anxiogenic, epileptogenic, or hallucinogenic effects (Atack, Maubach, Wafford, et al., 2009). It therefore is a potential compound for clinical investigation in depressed patient patients.

6. Mechanisms of action

This section attempts to provide a very brief overview of the pharmacological and molecular mechanisms associated with and possibly necessary for the antidepressant effects of rapid-acting antidepressants discussed earlier.

Fig. 10 Top Panel: Antidepressant-like effects, as measured in the forced-swim assay, of some negative allosteric modulators of α5-containing $GABA_A$ receptors (PWZ-029 and RY-08) and an antagonist of these receptors (Xli-093) all dosed at 30mg/kg, i.p. in mice. Middle Panel: Prevention of the antidepressant-like effects of RY-080 by PWZ-029. Bottom Panel: Blockade of the agitated hyperactivity of aged rTg4510 mice by RY-080 (10mg/kg, i.p.) at 60min into behavioral monitoring. *$P<0.05$; **$P<0.01$; ***$P<0.001$ compared to vehicle control (top panel) or compared to another treatment group or groups as indicated. WT: wild-type mice; TG: rTg4510 mice. *Data are replotted from Xu, N. Z, Ernst, M., Treven, M., Cerne, R., Wakulchik, M., Li, X., et al. (2018). Negative allosteric modulation of alpha 5-containing $GABA_A$ receptors engenders antidepressant-like effects and selectively prevents age-associated hyperactivity in tau-depositing mice.* Psychopharmacology *235(4), 1151–1161.*

At present, there is not a single universal or all-encompassing theory that accounts for all of the data. However, large structural hypotheses have been proposed that appear to account for significant amounts of basic mechanistic territory.

Clinical efficacy of novel mechanisms, as with the rapid-acting antidepressant drugs, is a huge advance. Not only is there the potential for new medicines for depressed patients, but the robust clinical efficacy of novel mechanisms enables back-translation to the mechanisms underlying these antidepressant effects. The reader is referred to several recent experimental and review papers discussing potential mechanisms by which rapid-acting antidepressant achieve differentiation from standard of care drugs (Abdallah, Sanacora, Duman, & Krystal, 2018—glutamate; De Gregorio, Enns, Nuñez, Posa, & Gobbi, 2018—psychedelics; Duman, Aghajanian, Sanacora, & Krystal, 2016—synaptic plasticity; Gerhard & Duman, 2018—molecular; Jeon, Dean, Scarr, & Gibbons, 2015—cholinergic; Johnson, Hendricks, Barrett, & Griffiths, 2018—psychedelics; Kadriu et al., 2018—glutamate; Kroes & Nilsson, 2017—pathways; Lepack, Bang, Lee, Dwyer, & Duman, 2016—molecular; Ly et al., 2018—psychedelics and neural plasticity; Musazzi, Tornese, Sala, & Popoli, 2017—stress; Pałucha-Poniewiera, 2018—glutamate; Rantamäki & Yalcin, 2016—neural networks; Song, Martinowich, & Lee, 2017—BDNF; Strasburger et al., 2017—general; Thomas & Duman, 2017—molecular; Wohleb et al., 2017—molecular; Workman, Niere, & Raab-Graham, 2018—neural remodeling; Yuan, Wauson, & Duric, 2016—kinase signaling; Zanos & Gould, 2018—general; Zanos et al., 2018—ketamine metabolites).

Ketamine is the primary drug that has been so evaluated and there is very little data on some of the other molecules (e.g., $GABA_A$ ligands and psychedelics). Some of the primary biological effects of rapid-acting antidepressants that form the basis for hypotheses regarding mechanisms of action are listed in Table 2. A primary scheme for antidepressant induction posits glutamate release as an initial trigger. As glutamate efflux is not as easy to measure as other biochemical endpoints, these data are limited. However, clinically, noninvasive methods have confirmed this idea (Valentine & Sanacora, 2009). Chowdhury et al. (2017) found that both scopolamine and ketamine rapidly stimulate glutamate cycling at the doses required to produce antidepressant-associated effects. In fact, the rapid increase of glutamate cycling precedes the antidepressant effects. As such, cycling could potentially be used as a biomarker of antidepressant efficacy.

Table 2 Biological correlates and proposed mechanisms underlying the effects of rapid-acting antidepressants[a].

Biological effect	Drug	References
Glutamate efflux	Ketamine	Thelen et al. (2019)
	Scopolamine	Rawls and Mcginty (1998) Yu et al. (2018)
	LY3020371	Witkin, Overshiner, et al. (2017)
Suppression of GABA interneurons	Ketamine	Homayoun and Moghaddam (2007)
	Scopolamine	Wohleb et al. (2016)
AMPA receptor activation	Ketamine	Li et al. (2010) Koike and Chaki (2014) Witkin et al. (2016) Martin et al. (2017) Karasawa, Shimazaki, Kawashima, and Chaki (2005)
	MGS0039	Ago et al. (2013)
	GLYX-13	Burgdorf et al. (2013) Lu et al. (2014) Jiang, Lin, and Salton (2018)
	Scopolamine	Voleti et al. (2013) Martin et al. (2017) Yu, Li, Zhou, et al. (2018)
	LY341495	Karasawa, Kotani, Kambe, and Chaki (2010) Koike and Chaki (2014) Witkin et al. (2016) Witkin, Overshiner, et al. (2017)
	LY3020371	Witkin, Overshiner, et al. (2017)
	MRK-016	Zanos et al. (2017)
mTOR activation	Ketamine	Li et al. (2010) Lepack et al. (2016) Thelen et al. (2019) Yang et al. (2018)
	MGS0039	Koike, Iijima, and Chaki (2011)
	GLYX-13	Lu et al. (2014) Lepack et al. (2016) Jiang et al. (2018)
	Scopolamine	Voleti et al. (2013) Dong et al. (2018) Lepack et al. (2016)
	LY341495	Martin et al. (2017) Witkin, Overshiner, et al. (2017)
	LY3020371	Witkin, Overshiner, et al. (2017)

Continued

Table 2 Biological correlates and proposed mechanisms underlying the effects of rapid-acting antidepressants[a].—cont'd

Biological effect	Drug	References
VTA neuron activation	Ketamine	Witkin et al. (2016)
	LY341495	Witkin et al. (2016)
	LY3020371	Witkin, Overshiner, et al. (2017)
Oxygen increases in ACC	Ketamine	Witkin et al. (2016)
	LY3020371	Witkin, Overshiner, et al. (2017)
Biogenic amine efflux in PFC	Ketamine	Adams, Bradberry, and Moghaddam (2002) Lorrain, Baccei, Bristow, Anderson, and Varney (2003) Cadeddu, Jadzic, and Carboni (2016) Witkin et al. (2016) Pham et al. (2017) Shokry et al. (2018)
	MGS0039	Kawashima et al. (2005) Karasawa et al. (2005)
	Nucleus accumbens	Karasawa, Yoshimizu, and Chaki (2006)
	Scopolamine	Tsukada, Harada, Nishiyama, Ohba, and Kakiuchi (2000) Karasawa et al. (2010)
	LY341495	Witkin et al. (2016) Witkin, Overshiner, et al. (2017)
	LY3020371	Witkin, Overshiner, et al. (2017)
	Psilocybin	Sakashita et al. (2015)
BDNF release	Ketamine	Lepack et al. (2016)
	LY341495	Lepack et al. (2016)
	GLYX-13	Lepack et al. (2016)
	Scopolamine	Ghosal et al. (2018) Yu et al. (2018)
ERK signaling	Ketamine	Lepack et al. (2016)
	LY341495	Lepack et al. (2016)
	GLYX-13	Lepack et al. (2016)

Table 2 Biological correlates and proposed mechanisms underlying the effects of rapid-acting antidepressants[a].—cont'd

Biological effect	Drug	References
eEF2 deactivation	Ketamine	Autry et al. (2011) Monteggia, Gideons, and Kavalali (2013)
	GLYX-13	Lu et al. (2014)
Increase in dendritic spines	Ketamine	Li et al. (2010) Thelen et al. (2019)
	Scopolamine	Voleti et al. (2013)
	GLYX-13	Burgdorf et al. (2015)
	MGS0039	Dong et al. (2018)
Wake promotion	Ketamine	Witkin, Monn, et al. (2017)
	LY3020371	Witkin, Monn, et al. (2017)
CSF: Nicotinamide and Hydroxyisocaproic acid[b]	Ketamine	Witkin, Overshiner, et al. (2017)[c]
	LY3020271	Witkin, Overshiner, et al. (2017)[c]
Hippocampus: Pyruvic acid and hydroxylamine[b]	Ketamine	Witkin, Overshiner, et al. (2017)[c]
	LY3020371	Witkin, Overshiner, et al. (2017)[c]
Predicted activation: GRIA2 and ADORA1[b]	Ketamine	Witkin, Overshiner, et al. (2017)[c]
	LY3020371	Witkin, Overshiner, et al. (2017)[c]
Indole-3-acetate and Methionine[b]	Ketamine	Rotroff et al. (2016)[c]
Citrulline, Arginine and Ornithine[b]	Ketamine	Rotroff et al. (2016)[c] Witkin, Overshiner, et al., 2017[c]
Kynurenine pathway and the arginine pathway	Ketamine	Moaddel et al. (2018)
Clock genes[d]	Ketamine	Orozco-Solis et al. (2017)

[a]Data are for biological processes postinitial receptor binding and thus do not include the target-cellular biology mechanisms.
[b]From metabolomic analysis.
[c]Data are from patient plasma samples (Moaddel et al., 2018; Rotroff et al., 2016) or rat CSF or hippocampus (Witkin, Overshiner, et al., 2017).
[d]Downregulated clock genes included Ciart, Per2, Npas4, Dbp, and Rorb for both ketamine and sleep-deprivation.
ACC, anterior cingulate cortex; *FST*, forced-swim test; *LTP*, long-term potentiation; *PFC*, prefrontal cortex; *VTA*, ventral tegmental area.

Glutamate release can be achieved in different ways. For example, with NMDA receptor ion channel blockers like ketamine, blockade of inhibitory GABAergic interneurons leads to glutamate overflow. With $mGlu_{2/3}$ receptor antagonists, increased synaptic glutamate is generated by the blockade of $mGlu_2$ autoreceptors. The implications of these differences in glutamate triggering are large with characteristic NMDA receptor antagonist side effects on the one hand and a relatively benign side-effect profile engendered by $mGlu_{2/3}$ receptor antagonists on the other. The by-passing of the ion channel mechanism by GLYX-13 provides another clue to the reasons for its relatively low side effect signature. Donello et al. (2018) have characterized GLYX-13 as a partial agonist at NMDA receptors and have identified some key binding targets for the molecule outside of the NMDA receptor ion pore.

Mechanisms not dependent upon NMDA receptors have also recently been advanced based upon the activity of ketamine metabolites that are not NMDA receptor antagonists but otherwise demonstrate antidepressant-like effects (Gould et al., 2019; Zanos et al., 2016). Indeed, the antidepressant-like effects of (S)-norketamine are not dependent upon AMPA receptors as is the case for ketamine (Yang et al., 2018). Furthermore, (2S,6S;2R,6R)-hydroxynorketamine has been described as necessary for the antidepressant-like effects of ketamine (Gould et al., 2019; Zanos et al., 2016). However, whether the metabolite is necessary is debated (Chaki & Yamaguchi, 2018; Yamaguchi et al., 2018). Recently, a ketamine metabolite, (2R,6R)-hydroxynorketamine, was shown to produce rapid antidepressant effects in rodent models without producing ketamine-linked adverse effects or abuse potential (Highland et al., 2018). There are, however, also data that argue against the ketamine metabolite hypothesis (Yamaguchi et al., 2018; Yang et al., 2017; Zhang et al., 2018).

Non-NMDA-related mechanisms of action for ketamine have also been suggested by another line of data. Rasenick and colleagues presented data suggesting a role for a Gαs/cAMP-dependent mechanism involving biochemical processing through lipid rafts (Wray & Rasenick, 2019; Wray, Schappi, Singh, Senese, & Rasenick, 2018).

Early studies (Table 2) were able to identify AMPA receptors as key players in the pharmacological induction of antidepressant efficacy. The AMPA receptor potentiation hypothesis (Alt et al., 2006; Nisenbaum & Witkin, 2010) continues to form the basis for understanding the initial sequence of events leading to rapid antidepressant action, a biochemical mechanism that shares commonality with the chronic administration of biogenic-amine-based antidepressants like fluoxetine (Svenningsson et al., 2002). Zn^{2+} functioning as an NMDA receptor antagonist has augmenting effects in treatment-refractory depressed patients (Siwek et al., 2009) and is susceptible to blockade in rodent models with AMPA receptor antagonists (Szewczyk et al., 2010). The $GABA_A(\alpha5)$-selective negative allosteric modulator L-655,708 also was shown to activate the NMDA- and AMPA-dependent processes. L-655,708 enhanced basal synaptic transmission and the induction of NMDA-dependent long-term potentiation along with the phosphorylation of synaptic NMDA and AMPA receptors (Xue et al., 2017). Activation of AMPA receptors induced enrichment of synaptic $\alpha5$-$GABA_A$ receptors (Hausrat et al., 2015).

In 2010, data consigning a role for mTOR stimulation began to accumulate (Table 2). These findings led to a model that posited that the machinery driving antidepressant efficacy required facilitation of AMPA receptor function to trigger the stimulation of mTOR that could ultimately impact cellular processing of protein synthesis including dendritic outgrowth; functionality of the dendritic spine formations could then replace the lost synaptic connectivity invoking mood dysfunction (see Li et al., 2010 for the first such model for ketamine and Voleti et al., 2013 for scopolamine). An example demonstrating the requirement for these biochemical processes is shown for ketamine and scopolamine in Fig. 5 (bottom panel). These biochemical mechanisms were shown to be critical inducers of dendritic spines and increased functional synaptic communication. The models fit the well-described hypotheses that depression is a consequence of reduced functional connectivity as posited in stress biology (Duman & Monteggia, 2006). A recent example of this idea was shown for GLYX-13 in its ability to enhance long-term potentiation (Moskal et al., 2017). However, a recent clinical study showed that rapamycin prolonged rather than attenuated the antidepressant effects of ketamine (Abdallah et al., 2018). A role for BDNF in antidepressant drugs has been espoused for many years and was incorporated into the mechanistic dialog on rapid-acting antidepressants (Table 2). Clinical studies with ketamine have confirmed BDNF as a key biomarker of antidepressant response (Duncan et al., 2013).

Metabolic activation has been observed with rapid-acting agents (see Fig. 3 for ketamine as an example). In preclinical studies, increased oxygen availability has been detected in the anterior cingulate cortex of rats after ketamine or $mGlu_{2/3}$ receptor antagonist dosing (Table 2). Wake promotion is another prominent biological effect of some rapid-acting agents (Table 2). Electroencephalography (EEG) studies have shown that ketamine produces cortical EEG synchronization; this effect is shared by 3,4-methylenedioxypyrovalerone (Shokry et al., 2018), a hallucinogenic drug that might give clue to activities of the psychedelic drugs shown to be antidepressants. The increase in gamma power induced by ketamine has become recognized as a biosignature of the drug (Shaw et al., 2015). This effect of ketamine was recently reported to predict treatment response in depressed patients (Nugent, Wills, Gilbert, & Zarate, 2019). The amplification of gamma power was also reported for an α5-associated $GABA_A$ receptor NAM that produced antidepressant-like effects in rodents (Zanos et al., 2017).

Rapid-acting antidepressants engender a rich neurochemical activation profile that has been integrated into the mechanistic thinking on these drugs (Table 2). For example, AMPA-dependent neuronal activation (medial prefrontal cortex) of serotonergic neurons in the dorsal raphe is necessary for the antidepressant-like effects of ketamine and the $mGlu_{2/3}$ receptor antagonist LY341495 (Fukumoto, Iijima, & Chaki, 2016; Fukumoto, Iijima, Funakoshi, & Chaki, 2018). The requirement for serotonin release in medial prefrontal cortex by ketamine was further enunciated by the data of Pham et al. (2017). However, a new study showed that 5-HT depletion did not affect the antidepressant effects of (R)-ketamine in a chronic social defeat stress model (Zhang, Dong, Fujita, Fujita, & Hashimoto, 2018).

Dopamine is a prominent mediator of mood. Indeed, a major hypothesis of antidepressant drug action is that conventional antidepressants sensitize dopamine efflux and function (Phillips & Fibiger, 1976; West & Weiss, 2011; Willner, 1997). Ketamine elicits dopamine efflux and enhances dopaminergic neurotransmission in the central nervous system (Moghaddam & Krystal, 2012; Witkin et al., 2016). Meta-analysis of treatment responses suggested that partial agonists could be a good alternative for adjunct treatment in depression (Romeo, Blecha, Locatelli, Benyamina, & Martelli, 2018). Ketamine has been shown to reverse the suppression of ventral tegmental area dopamine neuron activity and to restore hippocampal long-term potentiation associated with learned helplessness induction (Belujon and Grace, 2014). Dopamine cells in the ventral tegmental area are activated by both ketamine and $mGlu_{2/3}$ receptor antagonists and give rise to dopamine efflux in prefrontal cortex (Witkin et al., 2016; Witkin, Overshiner, et al., 2017) (Fig. 11). A psychedelic drug, psilocin, also increases dopamine outflow in the nucleus accumbens (Sakashita et al., 2015). Together, these data suggest a prominent role of mesolimbic dopamine in the efficacy of rapid-acting antidepressants. However compelling, dopamine neurotransmission cannot fully account for the activity of rapid-acting antidepressants. There is something more needed as exemplified by the lack of continued antidepressant efficacy of drugs like cocaine or amphetamines. Dopamine

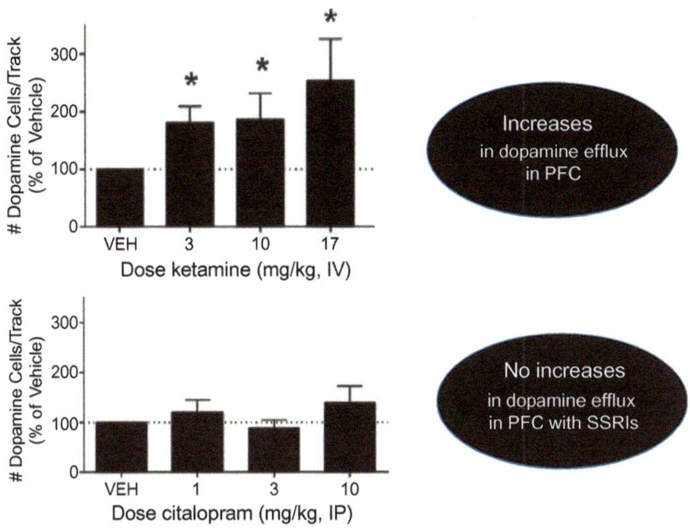

Fig. 11 Effects of ketamine or citalopram on the activity of dopamine neurons in the ventral tegmental area of anesthetized rats in comparison with the outflow of dopamine in the medial prefrontal cortex (PFC) of rats. $^*P < 0.05$ compared to vehicle control. *Data are from Witkin, J. M., Monn, J. A., Schoepp, D. D., Li, X., Overshiner, C., Mitchell, S. N., et al. (2016). The rapidly acting antidepressant ketamine rapidly engages dopaminergic mood circuits.* The Journal of Pharmacology and Experimental Therapeutics, 358, *71–82.*

receptor antagonists do not block the subjective effects of ketamine (Krystal et al., 1999) and antipsychotic drugs (dopamine antagonists) do not block the antidepressant effects of ketamine (C. Zarate, personal communication). Recent imaging studies in nonhuman primates suggested that (S)-ketamine but not (R)-ketamine increase dopamine release in the striatum and that this release might be associated with psychotomimetic effects (Hashimoto, Kakiuchi, Ohba, Nishiyama, & Tsukada, 2017).

Additional biochemical mediators of effects of rapid-acting antidepressants have recently been reported (Table 3). VGLUT1-mediated glutamate release and membrane GluA1 activation have been found to play a vital role in the rapid-acting effects of scopolamine (Chowdhury et al., 2017; Martin et al., 2017; Voleti et al., 2013; Yu, Li, Zhou, et al., 2018). Yu, Li, Shen, et al. (2018) also showed that, as with ketamine, L-type voltage-dependent calcium channels are required for the antidepressant-like effects of scopolamine. A role for TrkB-signaling through BDNF was shown to be a driver of bicaudal C homolog 1 gene expression for the antidepressant-like effects of the M_1-selective muscarinic antagonist, biperiden (Zhou et al., 2017). Protein kinase A is a mediator of the antidepressant-like effects of scopolamine with

Table 3 Some newly identified biological processes associated with the effects of rapid-acting antidepressants.

Biological effect	Drug	Reference
VEGF	Ketamine	Deyama et al. (2017)
VGLUT1	Scopolamine	Yu, Li, Zhou, et al. (2018)
L-type Ca^{++} channels	Scopolamine	Yu et al. (2018)
VGF and TLQP-62	Ketamine and GLYX-13	Jiang et al. (2018)
Bicaudal C homolog 1 gene	Biperiden	Zhou et al. (2017)
Protein kinase A	Scopolamine	Dong et al. (2018)
Hypocretin	GLYX-13	Liu et al. (2017)
Resolvin D1 and D2	–	Deyama et al. (2017)
Gut biome	Ketamine isomers	Yang, Qu, Abe, et al. (2017), Yang et al. (2017)
Peripheral IL-6 receptors	IL-6 antibody	Zhang et al. (2017)
Fibrinolytic system	Psilocybin	Idell et al. (2017)
Dopamine D_1 receptors	Brexpiprazole	Björkholm, Marcus, Konradsson-Geuken, Jardemark, and Svensson (2017)
GluN2D subunit of NMDA receptor	Ketamine	Ide, Ikekubo, Mishina, Hashimoto, and Ikeda (2017)
α7 nicotinic receptors	ANA-12	Zhang et al. (2016)
p11	Ketamine	Sun et al. (2016)
Insulin-like growth factor I (IGFI)	IGFI	Burgdorf et al. (2015)
$GABA_B$/Kir3/adaptor protein 14-3-3η	AP-5 and Ro 25-6891	Workman et al. (2015)

ANA-12, a TrkB antagonist, reversed depression-like phenotype in α7 deficient mice; *Kir3*, Potassium inwardly rectifying channel; *P11*, protein also known as S100A10; *TLQP-62*, VGF-derived C-terminal peptide (amino acids 556–617), *VGLUT1*, vesicular glutamate transporter.

AMPA receptor potentiation (GluA1 ser845 phosphorylation) as a provoker (Dong et al., 2018).

A role for VGF in the processing of rapid-antidepressant effects and their durability has been discussed. Jiang et al. (2018) identified an autoregulatory feedback loop that requires VGF and its C-terminal peptide (TLQP-62). These components are hypothesized to connect to pathways already discussed in this review: BDNF/TrkB signaling, mTOR activation, and AMPA receptor potentiation. The work of Deyama et al. (2017) disclosed that resolvin D1 and resolvin D2 produce antidepressant-like effects that are mTOR-dependent and involve the medial prefrontal cortex and dentate gyrus.

Bacteria in the gut have also been shown to play mechanistic roles (Table 3). For example, ketamine can alter the gut biome in mice subjected to chronic social defeat stress with the R-isomer being more efficacious overall (Qu et al., 2017; Yang, Qu, Fujita, et al., 2017). IL-6 receptors in the periphery may also be a target for rapid antidepressant response as an antibody produced antidepressant-like effects (Zhang et al., 2017). It has also been hypothesized that the activity of psychedelic drugs on depression also involves antiinflammatory and profibrinolytic actions that include blockade of TNF-α (Idell et al., 2017).

$GABA_B$ receptors have also been identified as biochemical mediators of rapid-acting antidepressant effects (Table 3). Workman et al. (2015) had shown that rapid-acting antidepressants induce $GABA_B$ receptors to increase resting dendritic calcium signaling and mTOR activity. Thus, $GABA_B$ receptor signaling through Kir3 (GIRK) channels decreases upon NMDA receptor blockade. The shift away from GIRK was shown to stabilize 14-3-3η, an adaptor protein, which decouples $GABA_B$ receptor signaling from Kir3.

Additional mechanisms have been gleaned from studies with antidepressant add-on therapies that might induce more rapid effects and impact treatment-resistant patients (Table 3). Brexpiprazole (Rexulti®) is a dopamine $D_{2/3}$ receptor partial agonist that is approved as an adjunct therapy for depression where more rapid onset of action has been reported. Induction of rapid antidepressant-like effects of brexpiprazole is dependent on BDNF-TrkB signaling (Ma et al., 2016). Brexpiprazole potentiated NMDA-induced currents and electrically evoked EPSPs; these excitatory effects in the medial prefrontal cortex were dependent upon dopamine D_1 receptors (Björkholm et al., 2017). In contrast, the neurite outgrowth facilitated by brexpiprazole was mediated by serotonin receptors (5-HT_{1A} agonism and 5-HT_{2A} antagonism) (Ishima et al., 2015).

Metabolomics, proteomics, and genetic analysis have also begun to be utilized as methods for defining mechanisms of action of rapid-acting antidepressants (Table 2). For example, data from a study with ketamine and the $mGlu_{2/3}$ receptor antagonist LY3020371 utilized network pathway analysis of metabolites found in cerebral spinal fluid of rats. In that study GRIA2, the gene associated with a principle subunit of AMPA receptors, showed predicted activation after both drugs (Witkin, Overshiner, et al., 2017) thus providing alternative substantiation for the AMPA potentiation hypothesis of rapid-acting antidepressants (Alt et al., 2006) and the predicted rapid-acting efficacy of the $mGlu_{2/3}$ receptor antagonist mechanism (Chaki, 2019; Witkin et al., 2018; Witkin, Overshiner, et al., 2017). A GWAS study evaluating SNPs in ketamine and scopolamine-treated patients was conducted (Guo et al., 2018). Although the sample size was too small to detect the robust changes needed for statistical significance, genetic analysis should provide valuable insight into mechanisms and to identify treatment-responsive patient populations.

Imaging, electroencephalography, and other methods have been used to identify brain circuits regulating effects of rapid-acting antidepressants. In general, it has been found that the circuits have marked overlap with those defined as relevant to major depressive disorder (Price & Drevets, 2010). Brain structures important to several of the antidepressant effects of ketamine are outline in Fig. 3. Global connectivity enhancements within the prefrontal cortex were identified for the first time by Abdallah, Sanacora, et al. (2018) after ketamine administration. Such findings should enable the use of imaging methods in the identification of new chemical entities proposed as rapid-acting antidepressants. Donegan and Lodge (2017) provided evidence for the necessity of parvalbumin interneuron function in the ventral hippocampus for the sustained antidepressant-like effects of ketamine in rats. Another recent study utilized the NMDA receptor antagonist nitrous oxide in human volunteers to generate data suggesting that rapid-acting antidepressants operate through the induction of a transient cortical excitability; TrkB and GSK3β signaling was implicated in the induction of a slow cortical oscillatory state (Kohtala et al., 2018).

High-density electroencephalogram (EEG) was utilized in healthy human volunteers to study brain areas involved in the effects of psilocybin (spiritual effects and insightfulness). Psilocybin decreased current density within brain circuits involving the anterior and posterior cingulate cortices and the parahippocampal regions. Behavioral effects of psilocybin were positively associated with the lagged phase synchronization of delta oscillations (1.5–4 Hz) between the retrosplenial cortex, the parahippocampus, and the lateral orbitofrontal area (Kometer, Pokorny, Seifritz, & Volleinweider, 2015). In treatment-resistant patients given psilocybin, decreases in blood flow in the amygdala were associated with decreased depression symptoms

(Carhart-Harris et al., 2017). In response to emotional faces, psilocybin increased fMRI responses in the amygdala in contrast to the decreases generally reported for biogenic-amine antidepressants (Roseman, Demetriou, et al., 2018). The later finding suggests that while conventional antidepressants dampen emotionality, psilocybin enhances cognitive review of these data. In a study with healthy human volunteers, LSD enhanced sensory-somatomotor brain-wide and thalamic connectivity as a result of 5-HT_{2A} receptor activation (Preller et al., 2018).

Preclinical studies that are designed to pin-point brain areas involved in the effects of rapid-acting antidepressants can also aid in the understanding of underlying mechanisms of action and to identify novel compounds exerting these effects (Pešić, Petrović, & Jukić, 2016). For example, Yang et al. (2018) have suggested that the decreases in bursting activity in the lateral habenula are necessary for the antidepressant effects of ketamine and that the astroglial potassium channel Kir4.1 is a controlling mechanism (Cui et al., 2018); however, the role of this channel is not without debate (Xiong et al., 2018, 2019).

$GABA_A$ receptors containing the α5 protein can selectively modulate cortical and hippocampal circuits involved in depression (Sur, Fresu, Howell, McKernan, & Atack, 1999). Negative allosteric modulators of α5-associated $GABA_A$ receptors encourage coherent neuronal activity that is associated with positive mood states (Hajós, Hoffmann, Orbán, Kiss, & Erdi, 2004; Towers et al., 2004: Zanos et al., 2017). Schulz, Knoflach, Hernandez, and Bischofberger (2018) have described how these receptors can control the GABA interneuron modulation of NMDA receptors.

For the compounds that have been most widely investigated for potential underlying mechanisms of action (ketamine, scopolamine, and mGlu2/3 receptor antagonists), there is substantial overlap in a host of biological processes (Table 2). Despite the absence of a complete understanding of mechanisms or a formal theory of rapid-antidepressant action, the biology that has been described might serve as a guide to the discovery of additional compounds or manipulations that have the antidepressant properties like those of the already described rapid-acting agents. Compounds currently in development will help confirm this idea; for example, if an mGlu2/3 receptor antagonist with biological mechanistic overlap with ketamine shows rapid antidepressant effects in patients. Serendipity will be another major driver of new drug discovery. Rational methods will also continue to help bring improved antidepressants to patients. Remember, the idea that ketamine might function as an antidepressant came from the brilliant connections in diverse data sets made by Ramon Trullas and Phil Skolnick 10 years prior to clinical proof of concept. They related the findings of inescapable stress inducing depressive-like behaviors to the effects of stress on hippocampal long-term potentiation (LTP) to the data connecting LTP to NMDA receptors: "A competitive NMDA antagonist (2-amino-7-phosphonoheptanoic acid [AP-7]), a non-competitive NMDA antagonist (Dizolcipine [MK-801]), and a partial agonist at strychnine-insensitive glycine receptors (1-aminocylopropanecarboxylic acid [ACPC]) mimicked the effects of clinically effective antidepressants in these models. These findings indicate that the NMDA receptor complex may be involved in the behavioral deficits induced by inescapable stress, and that substances capable of reducing neurotransmission at the NMDA receptor complex may represent a new class of antidepressants. Based on these findings, the hypothesis that pathways subserved by the NMDA subtype of glutamate receptors are involved in the pathophysiology of affective disorders may have heuristic value" (Trullas & Skolnick, 1990).

7. Conclusions

In contrast to standard of care, biogenic amine-based antidepressants, a new class of antidepressants has demonstrated rapid onset, large effect size, activity after only a single or few dose applications, and positive impact in treatment refractory patients and against some treatment-resistant symptoms. Rapid-acting antidepressant drug action has been demonstrated in controlled clinical studies for ketamine, a few other NMDA receptor antagonists, and scopolamine. Less clinical data are currently available for psychedelic drugs such as psilocybin, lysergic acid diethylamide, and ayahuasca. The U.S. FDA approved (S)-ketamine (esketamine) as an antidepressant in February 2019. In addition to rapid onset, these compounds have demonstrated effects not typically observed with standard of care antidepressants that include effects on anhedonia and sometimes long-lasting effects after one or few doses. Compounds currently in clinical development include the NMDA receptor antagonist (R)-ketamine (arketamine), and an NMDA receptor modulator, GLYX-13 (Rapastinel). There is also an AMPA receptor potentiator in clinical development (TAK-653). Preclinical development is ongoing with mGlu2/3 receptor antagonists, and negative allosteric modulators of $GABA_A(\alpha5)$ receptors. Understanding of the mechanisms underlying rapid antidepressant action has rapidly accumulated since 2006 for some of the drug classes but a universal field theory has yet to be established. Current understanding, primarily based upon the pharmacology of ketamine, implicates amplification of AMPA receptors as a trigger for downstream enhancement of cortical connectivity.

In addition to efficacy, two conditions need to be met to inaugurate new medicines as rapid-antidepressants—(1) tolerability and safety and (2) the ability of drug treatment to provide enduring antidepressant coverage. Given the rapid recruitment of rapid-acting antidepressants into high-level scientific inquiry at both the preclinical and clinical level, the likelihood of improved medicines being marketed for depression appears high. An ultimate goal for a new antidepressant called rapid-acting would be the production of remission within a few doses that could be maintained by that drug on a periodic basis or by transition to another maintenance drug. Additional benefits of this new medicine would be the large effect size produced and the impact upon otherwise drug-resistant symptoms.

Acknowledgments

We are grateful for the Henry and Nellie Pence family for supporting this work by a Pence foundation grant awarded to Jodi L. Smith. We are also grateful to John and Nancy Peterson for their support of this research. We thank the following granting agencies for support: MH-096463 and NS-076517. We also acknowledge the UW-Milwaukee Shimadzu Laboratory for Advanced and Applied Analytical Chemistry and support from the Milwaukee Institute of Drug Discovery and the University of Wisconsin-Milwaukee Research Foundation. We also thank Kenji Hashimoto and Shigeyuki Chaki for providing information pertinent to this manuscript.

Conflict of interest

The authors declare no conflicts of interest. All data reported in the present review are from the public scientific literature.

References

Abdallah, C., Averill, L. A., Gueorguieva, R., Goktas, S., Purohit, P., Ranganathan, M., et al. (2018). *Rapamycin, an immunosuppressant and mTORC1 inhibitor, triples the antidepressant response rate of ketamine at 2 weeks following treatment: A double-blind, placebo-controlled, cross-over, randomized clinical trial.* bioRxiv.

Abdallah, C. G., Sanacora, G., Duman, R. S., & Krystal, J. H. (2018). The neurobiology of depression, ketamine and rapid-acting antidepressants: Is it glutamate inhibition or activation? *Pharmacology and Therapeutics*, *190*, 148–158.

Adams, B. W., Bradberry, C. W., & Moghaddam, B. (2002). NMDA antagonist effects on striatal dopamine release: Microdialysis studies in awake monkeys. *Synapse*, *43*(1), 12–18.

Ago, Y., Yano, K., Araki, R., Hiramatsu, N., Kita, Y., Kawasaki, T., et al. (2013). Metabotropic glutamate 2/3 receptor antagonists improve behavioral and prefrontal dopaminergic alterations in the chronic corticosterone-induced depression model in mice. *Neuropharmacology*, *65*, 29–38.

Alt, A., Nisenbaum, E. S., Bleakman, D., & Witkin, J. M. (2006). A role for AMPA receptors in mood disorders. *Biochemical Pharmacology*, *71*, 1273–1288.

Anderson, T., Petranker, R., Rosenbaum, D., Weissman, C. R., Dinh-Williams, L. A., Hui, K., et al. (2019). Microdosing psychedelics: Personality, mental health, and creativity differences in microdosers. *Psychopharmacology (Berlin)*, *236*, 731–740.

Argyropoulos, S. V., & Nutt, D. J. (2013). Anhedonia revisited: Is there a role for dopamine-targeting drugs for depression? *Journal of Psychopharmacology*, *27*, 869–877.

Atack, J. R., Maubach, K. A., Wafford, K. A., et al. (2009). In vitro and in vivo properties of 3-tert-butyl-7-(5-methylisoxazol-3-yl)-2-(1-methyl-1H-1,2,4-triazol-5-ylmethoxy)-pyrazolo[1,5-d]-[1,2,4]triazine (MRK-016), a GABAA receptor alpha5 subtype-selective inverse agonist. *The Journal of Pharmacology and Experimental Therapeutics*, *331*, 470–484.

Autry, A. E., Adachi, M., Nosyreva, E., Na, E. S., Los, M. F., Cheng, P. F., et al. (2011). NMDA receptor blockade at rest triggers rapid behavioural antidepressant responses. *Nature*, *475*(7354), 91–95.

Belujon, P., & Grace, A. A. (2014). Restoring mood balance in depression: Ketamine reverses deficit in dopamine-dependent synaptic plasticity. *Biological Psychiatry*, *76*(12), 927–936.

Berman, R. M., Cappiello, A., Anand, A., Oren, D. A., Heninger, G. R., Charney, D. S., et al. (2000). Antidepressant effects of ketamine in depressed patients. *Biological Psychiatry*, *47*, 351–354.

Björkholm, C., Marcus, M. M., Konradsson-Geuken, Å., Jardemark, K., & Svensson, T. H. (2017). The novel antipsychotic drug brexpiprazole, alone and in combination with escitalopram, facilitates prefrontal glutamatergic transmission via a dopamine D1 receptor-dependent mechanism. *European Neuropsychopharmacology*, *27*(4), 411–417.

Bodkin, J. A., Zornberg, G. L., Lukas, S. E., & Cole, J. O. (1995). Buprenorphine treatment of refractory depression. *Journal of Clinical Psychopharmacology*, *15*(1), 49–57.

Brocks, D. R. (1999). Anticholinergic drugs used in Parkinson's disease: An overlooked class of drugs from a pharmacokinetic perspective. *Journal of Pharmacy & Pharmaceutical Sciences*, *2*(2), 39–46.

Burgdorf, J., Zhang, X. L., Nicholson, K. L., Balster, R. L., Leander, J. D., Stanton, P. K., et al. (2013). GLYX-13, a NMDA receptor glycine-site functional partial agonist, induces antidepressant-like effects without ketamine-like side effects. *Neuropsychopharmacology*, *38*(5), 729–742.

Burgdorf, J., Zhang, X. L., Weiss, C., Gross, A., Boikess, S. R., Kroes, R. A., et al. (2015). The long-lasting antidepressant effects of rapastinel (GLYX-13) are associated with a metaplasticity process in the medial prefrontal cortex and hippocampus. *Neuroscience*, *308*, 202–211.

Cadeddu, R., Jadzic, D., & Carboni, E. (2016). Ketamine modulates catecholamine transmission in the bed nucleus of stria terminalis: The possible role of this region in the antidepressant effects of ketamine. *European Neuropsychopharmacology*, *26*(10), 1678–1682.

Cannon, D. M., Carson, R. E., Nugent, A. C., Eckelman, W. C., Kiesewetter, D. O., Williams, J., et al. (2006). Reduced muscarinic type 2 receptor binding in subjects with bipolar disorder. *Archives of General Psychiatry*, *63*, 741–747.

Cao, B., Zhu, J., Zuckerman, H., Rosenblat, J. D., Brietzke, E., Pan, Z., et al. (2019). Pharmacological interventions targeting anhedonia in patients with major depressive disorder: A systematic review. *Progress in Neuro-Psychopharmacology & Biological Psychiatry*, *92*, 109–117.

Carhart-Harris, R. L., Bolstridge, M., Day, C. M. J., Rucker, J., Watts, R., Erritzoe, D. E., et al. (2018). Psilocybin with psychological support for treatment-resistant depression: Six-month follow-up. *Psychopharmacology*, *235*(2), 399–408.

Carhart-Harris, R. L., Bolstridge, M., Rucker, J., Day, C. M., Erritzoe, D., Kaelen, M., et al. (2016). Psilocybin with psychological support for treatment-resistant depression: An open-label feasibility study. *Lancet Psychiatry*, *3*(7), 619–627.

Carhart-Harris, R. L., Roseman, L., Bolstridge, M., Demetriou, L., Pannekoek, J. N., Wall, M. B., et al. (2017). Psilocybin for treatment-resistant depression: fMRI-measured brain mechanisms. *Scientific Reports*, 7(1), 13187.

Carreno, F. R., Collins, G. T., Frazer, A., & Lodge, D. J. (2017). Selective pharmacological augmentation of hippocampal activity produces a sustained antidepressant-like response without abuse-related or psychotomimetic effects. *The International Journal of Neuropsychopharmacology*, *20*(6), 504–509.

Carrillo, F., Sigman, M., Fernández Slezak, D., Ashton, P., Fitzgerald, L., Stroud, J., et al. (2018). Natural speech algorithm applied to baseline interview data can predict which patients will respond to psilocybin for treatment-resistant depression. *Journal of Affective Disorders*, *230*, 84–86.

Chaki, S. (2017). mGlu2/3 receptor antagonists as novel antidepressants. *Trends in Pharmacological Sciences*, *38*(6), 569–580.

Chaki, S. (2019). mGlu2/3 receptor antagonists. In J. M. Witkin (Ed.), *Neuropsychopharmacology, advances in pharmacology: Vol. 86*. Elsevier.

Chaki, S., & Yamaguchi, J. I. (2018). Is the history repeated? Can (2R,6R)-hydroxynorketamine be another antidepressant? *Journal of Experimental Neuroscience*, *12*. 1179069518815445.

Chiu, M., Vigod, S., Rahman, F., Wilton, A. S., Lebenbaum, M., & Kurdyak, P. (2018). Mortality risk associated with psychological distress and major depression: A population-based cohort study. *Journal of Affective Disorders*, *234*, 117–123.

Chowdhury, G. M. I., Zhang, J., Thomas, M., Banasr, M., Ma, X., Pittman, B., et al. (2017). Transiently increased glutamate cycling in rat PFC is associated with rapid onset of antidepressant-like effects. *Molecular Psychiatry*, *22*(1), 120–126.

Cui, Y., Yang, Y., Ni, Z., Dong, Y., Cai, G., Foncelle, A., et al. (2018). Astroglial Kir4.1 in the lateral habenula drives neuronal bursts in depression. *Nature*, *554*(7692), 323–327.

Dagyte, G., Den Boer, J. A., & Trentani, A. (2011). The cholinergic system and depression. *Behavioural Brain Research*, *221*, 574–582.

De Gregorio, D., Enns, J. P., Nuñez, N. A., Posa, L., & Gobbi, G. (2018). d-Lysergic acid diethylamide, psilocybin, and other classic hallucinogens: Mechanism of action and potential therapeutic applications in mood disorders. *Progress in Brain Research*, *242*, 69–96.

de la Vega, D., Piña, A., Peralta, F. J., Kelly, S. A., & Giner, L. A. (2018). Review on the general stability of mood disorder diagnoses along the lifetime. *Current Psychiatry Reports*, *20*, 29.

Deyama, S., Ishikawa, Y., Yoshikawa, K., Shimoda, K., Ide, S., Satoh, M., et al. (2017). Resolvin D1 and D2 reverse lipopolysaccharide-induced depression-like behaviors through the mTORC1 signaling pathway. *The International Journal of Neuropsychopharmacology*, *20*(7), 575–584.

Diazgranados, N., Ibrahim, L., Brutsche, N. E., Newberg, A., Kronstein, P., Khalife, S., et al. (2010). A randomized add-on trial of an N-methyl-D-aspartate antagonist in treatment-resistant bipolar depression. *Archives of General Psychiatry*, *67*(8), 793–802.

Donegan, J. J., & Lodge, D. J. (2017). Hippocampal perineuronal nets are required for the sustained antidepressant effect of ketamine. *The International Journal of Neuropsychopharmacology*, *20*(4), 354–358.

Donello, J. E., Banerjee, P., Li, Y. X., Guo, Y. X., Yoshitake, T., Zhang, X. L., et al. (2018). Positive N-methyl-D-aspartate receptor modulation by rapastinel promotes rapid and sustained antidepressant-like effects. *The International Journal of Neuropsychopharmacology*, *22*(3), 247–259.

Dong, J., Zhou, Q., Wei, Z., Yan, S., Sun, F., & Cai, X. (2018). Protein kinase A mediates scopolamine-induced mTOR activation and an antidepressant response. *Journal of Affective Disorders*, *227*, 633–642.

Doran, C. M., & Kinchin, I. (2017). A review of the economic impact of mental illness. *Australian Health Review*. https://doi.org/10.1071/AH16115.

Dos Santos, R. G., Bouso, J. C., Alcázar-Córcoles, M. Á., & Hallak, J. E. C. (2018). Efficacy, tolerability, and safety of serotonergic psychedelics for the management of mood, anxiety, and substance-use disorders: A systematic review of systematic reviews. *Expert Review of Clinical Pharmacology*, *11*(9), 889–902.

Drevets, W. C., Zarate, C. A., Jr., & Furey, M. L. (2013). Antidepressant effects of the muscarinic cholinergic receptor antagonist scopolamine: A review. *Biological Psychiatry*, *73*, 1156–1163.

Duman, R. S., Aghajanian, G. K., Sanacora, G., & Krystal, J. H. (2016). Synaptic plasticity and depression: New insights from stress and rapid-acting antidepressants. *Nature Medicine*, *22*(3), 238–249.

Duman, R. S., & Monteggia, L. M. (2006). A neurotrophic model for stress-related mood disorders. *Biological Psychiatry*, *59*(12), 1116–1127.

Duncan, W. C., Sarasso, S., Ferrarelli, F., Selter, J., Riedner, B. A., Hejazi, N. S., et al. (2013). Concomitant BDNF and sleep slow wave changes indicate ketamine-induced plasticity in major depressive disorder. *The International Journal of Neuropsychopharmacology*, *16*(2), 301–311.

Ehrich, E., Turncliff, R., Sellers, E., Jones, R., & Fava, M. (2012). Early clinical development of the opioid modulator ALKS 5461 in the treatment of depression. In *NCDEU, 2012*.

Feder, A., Parides, M. K., Murrough, J. W., Perez, A. M., Morgan, J. E., Saxena, S., et al. (2014). Efficacy of intravenous ketamine for treatment of chronic posttraumatic stress disorder: A randomized clinical trial. *JAMA Psychiatry*, *71*(6), 681–688.

Fischell, J., Van Dyke, A. M., Kvarta, M. D., LeGates, T. A., & Thompson, S. M. (2015). Rapid antidepressant action and restoration of excitatory synaptic strength after chronic stress by negative modulators of alpha5-containing $GABA_A$ receptors. *Neuropsychopharmacology*, *40*, 2499–2509.

Fukumoto, K., Iijima, M., & Chaki, S. (2016). The antidepressant effects of an mGlu2/3 receptor antagonist and ketamine require AMPA receptor stimulation in the mPFC and subsequent activation of the 5-HT neurons in the DRN. *Neuropsychopharmacology*, *41*(4), 1046–1056.

Fukumoto, K., Iijima, M., Funakoshi, T., & Chaki, S. (2018). $5\text{-}HT_{1A}$ receptor stimulation in the medial prefrontal cortex mediates the antidepressant effects of mGlu2/3 receptor antagonist in mice. *Neuropharmacology*, *137*, 96–103.

Fukumoto, K., Toki, H., Iijima, M., Hashihayata, T., Yamaguchi, J. I., Hashimoto, K., et al. (2017). Antidepressant potential of (R)-ketamine in rodent models: Comparison with (S)-ketamine. *The Journal of Pharmacology and Experimental Therapeutics*, *361*(1), 9–16.

Furey, M. L., & Drevets, W. C. (2006). Antidepressant efficacy of the antimuscarinic drug scopolamine: A randomized, placebo-controlled clinical trial. *Archives of General Psychiatry*, *63*(10), 1121–1129.

Gadient, R. A., Wedel, P., Frisbie, V., Leuchter, A. F., Targum, S. D., Truong, C., et al. (2012). Safety, pharmacokinetic and pharmacodynamic profile of BCI-632, a selective metabotropic glutamate 2/3 receptor antagonist, in healthy human subjects. Poster 841.20. In *Society for neuroscience meeting*.

Galvão, A. C. M., de Almeida, R. N., Silva, E. A. D. S., Freire, F. A. M., Palhano-Fontes, F., Onias, H., et al. (2018). Cortisol modulation by ayahuasca in patients with treatment resistant depression and healthy controls. *Frontiers in Psychiatry*, *9*, 185.

Garay, R. P., Zarate, C. A., Jr., Charpeaud, T., Citrome, L., Correll, C. U., Hameg, A., et al. (2017). Cortisol modulation by ayahuasca in patients with treatment resistant depression and healthy controls. *Expert Review of Neurotherapeutics*, *17*(6), 593–609.

Gasser, P., Holstein, D., Michel, Y., Doblin, R., Yazar-Klosinski, B., Passie, T., et al. (2014). Safety and efficacy of lysergic acid diethylamide-assisted psychotherapy for anxiety associated with life-threatening diseases. *The Journal of Nervous and Mental Disease, 202*(7), 513–520.

Gasser, P., Kirchner, K., & Passie, T. (2015). LSD-assisted psychotherapy for anxiety associated with a life-threatening disease: A qualitative study of acute and sustained subjective effects. *Journal of Psychopharmacology, 29*(1), 57–68.

Gerhard, D. M., & Duman, R. S. (2018). Rapid-acting antidepressants: Mechanistic insights and future directions. *Current Behavioral Neuroscience Reports, 5*(1), 36–47.

Ghoneim, M. M., Hinrichs, J. V., Mewaldt, S. P., & Petersen, R. C. (1985). Ketamine: Behavioral effects of subanesthetic doses. *Journal of Clinical Psychopharmacology, 5*(2), 70–77.

Ghosal, S., Bang, E., Yue, W., Hare, B. D., Lepack, A. E., Girgenti, M. J., et al. (2018). Activity-dependent brain-derived neurotrophic factor release is required for the rapid antidepressant actions of Scopolamine. *Biological Psychiatry, 83*(1), 29–37.

Gibbons, A. S., Scarr, E., McLean, C., Sundram, S., & Dean, B. (2009). Decreased muscarinic receptor binding in the frontal cortex of bipolar disorder and major depressive disorder subjects. *Journal of Affective Disorders, 116*, 184–191.

Gillin, J. C., Lauriello, J., Kelsoe, J. R., Rapaport, M., Golshan, S., Kenny, W. M., et al. (1995). No antidepressant effect of biperiden compared with placebo in depression: A double-blind 6-week clinical trial. *Psychiatry Research, 58*(2), 99–105.

Gould, T. D., Zarate, C. A., Jr., & Thompson, S. M. (2019). Molecular pharmacology and neurobiology of rapid-acting antidepressants. *Annual Review of Pharmacology and Toxicology, 59*, 213–236.

Griffiths, R. R., Johnson, M. W., Carducci, M. A., Umbricht, A., Richards, W. A., Richards, B. D., et al. (2016). Psilocybin produces substantial and sustained decreases in depression and anxiety in patients with life-threatening cancer: A randomized double-blind trial. *Journal of Psychopharmacology, 30*(12), 1181–1197.

Grob, C. S., Danforth, A. L., Chopra, G. S., Hagerty, M., McKay, C. R., Halberstadt, A. L., et al. (2011). Pilot study of psilocybin treatment for anxiety in patients with advanced-stage cancer. *Archives of General Psychiatry, 68*(1), 71–78.

Grof, S., Goodman, L. E., Richards, W. A., & Kurland, A. A. (1973). LSD-assisted psychotherapy in patients with terminal cancer. *International Pharmacopsychiatry, 8*(3), 129–144.

Guo, W., Machado-Vieira, R., Mathew, S., Murrough, J. W., Charney, D. S., Gruenbaum, M., et al. (2018). Exploratory genome-wide association analysis of response to ketamine and a polygenic analysis of response to scopolamine in depression. *Translational Psychiatry, 8*(1), 280.

Hajós, M., Hoffmann, W. E., Orbán, G., Kiss, T., & Erdi, P. (2004). Modulation of septo-hippocampal theta activity by $GABA_A$ receptors: An experimental and computational approach. *Neuroscience, 126*, 599–610.

Hamill, J., Hallak, J., Dursun, S. M., & Baker, G. (2018). Ayahuasca: Psychological and physiologic effects, pharmacology and potential uses in addiction and mental illness. *Current Neuropharmacology, 17*, 108–128.

Haridas, R. M., Parkar, S. R., Ghulam, R., Amin, G., Thombre, K. G., Srivastava, A., et al. (2003). Olanzapine and fluoxetine combination in severe or resistant depression. *Indian Journal of Psychiatry, 45*(4), 234–238.

Hashimoto, K. (2016). Ketamine's antidepressant action: Beyond NMDA receptor inhibition. *Expert Opinion on Therapeutic Targets, 20*(11), 1389–1392.

Hashimoto, K., Kakiuchi, T., Ohba, H., Nishiyama, S., & Tsukada, H. (2017). Reduction of dopamine $D_{2/3}$ receptor binding in the striatum after a single administration of esketamine, but not R-ketamine: A PET study in conscious monkeys. *European Archives of Psychiatry and Clinical Neuroscience, 267*(2), 173–176.

Hausrat, T. J., Muhia, M., Gerrow, K., Thomas, P., Hirdes, W., Tsukita, S., et al. (2015). Radixin regulates synaptic GABAA receptor density and is essential for reversal learning and short-term memory. *Nature Communications*, *6*, 6872.

Highland, J. N., Morris, P. J., Zanos, P., Lovett, J., Ghosh, S., Wang, A. Q., et al. (2018). Mouse, rat, and dog bioavailability and mouse oral antidepressant efficacy of (2R,6R)-hydroxynorketamine. *Journal of Psychopharmacology,* 269881118812095. https://doi.org/10.1177/0269881118812095 [Epub ahead of print].

Homayoun, H., & Moghaddam, B. (2007). NMDA receptor hypofunction produces opposite effects on prefrontal cortex interneurons and pyramidal neurons. *The Journal of Neuroscience*, *27*(43), 11496–11500.

Howland, R. H. (2009). The antidepressant effects of anticholinergic drugs. *Journal of Psychosocial Nursing and Mental Health Services*, *47*(6), 17–20.

Huang, C. C., & Hsu, K. S. (2010). Activation of muscarinic acetylcholine receptors induces a nitric oxide-dependent long-term depression in rat medial prefrontal cortex. *Cerebral Cortex*, *20*, 982–996.

Ide, S., Ikekubo, Y., Mishina, M., Hashimoto, K., & Ikeda, K. (2017). Role of NMDA receptor GluN2D subunit in the antidepressant effects of enantiomers of ketamine. *Journal of Pharmacological Sciences*, *135*(3), 138–140.

Idell, R. D., Florova, G., Komissarov, A. A., Shetty, S., Girard, R. B., & Idell, S. (2017). The fibrinolytic system: A new target for treatment of depression with psychedelics. *Medical Hypotheses*, *100*, 46–53.

Ishima, T., Futamura, T., Ohgi, Y., Yoshimi, N., Kikuchi, T., & Hashimoto, K. (2015). Potentiation of neurite outgrowth by brexpiprazole, a novel serotonin-dopamine activity modulator: A role for serotonin 5-HT1A and 5-HT2A receptors. *European Neuropsychopharmacology*, *25*(4), 505–511.

Iversen, L. (2005). The monoamine hypothesis of depression. In J. Licinio & M. L. Wong (Eds.), *Biology of depression* (pp. 71–86). Weinheim: Wiley-VCH.

Jaffe, R. J., Novakovic, V., & Peselow, E. D. (2013). Scopolamine as an antidepressant: A systematic review. *Clinical Neuropharmacology*, *36*, 24–26.

Janowsky, D. S. (2011). Serendipity strikes again: Scopolamine as an antidepressant agent in bipolar depressed patients. *Current Psychiatry Reports*, *13*, 443–445.

Janowsky, D. S., el-Yousef, M. K., Davis, J. M., & Sekerke, H. J. (1972). A cholinergic adrenergic hypothesis of mania and depression. *Lancet*, *2*, 632–635.

Jeon, W. J., Dean, B., Scarr, E., & Gibbons, A. (2015). The role of muscarinic receptors in the pathophysiology of mood disorders: A potential novel treatment? *Current Neuropharmacology*, *13*(6), 739–749.

Jiang, C., Lin, W. J., & Salton, S. R. (2018). Role of a VGF/BDNF/TrkB autoregulatory feedback loop in rapid-acting antidepressant efficacy. *Journal of Molecular Neuroscience*. https://doi.org/10.1007/s12031-018-1124-0.

Johnson, M. W., & Griffiths, R. R. (2017). Potential therapeutic effects of psilocybin. *Neurotherapeutics*, *14*(3), 734–740.

Johnson, M. W., Griffiths, R. R., Hendricks, P. S., & Henningfield, J. E. (2018). The abuse potential of medical psilocybin according to the 8 factors of the controlled substances act. *Neuropharmacology*, *142*, 143–166.

Johnson, M. W., Hendricks, P. S., Barrett, F. S., & Griffiths, R. R. (2018). Classic psychedelics: An integrative review of epidemiology, mystical experience, brain network function, and therapeutics. *Pharmacology & Therapeutics*. pii: S0163-7258(18)30215-8. https://doi.org/10.1016/j.pharmthera.2018.11.010.

Kadriu, B., Musazzi, L., Henter, I. D., Graves, M., Popoli, M., & Zarate, C. A., Jr. (2019). Glutamatergic neurotransmission: Pathway to developing novel rapid-acting antidepressant treatments. *The International Journal of Neuropsychopharmacology*, *22*, 119–135.

Karasawa, J., Kotani, M., Kambe, D., & Chaki, S. (2010). AMPA receptor mediates mGlu 2/3 receptor antagonist-induced dopamine release in the rat nucleus accumbens shell. *Neurochemistry International*, *57*(5), 615–619.
Karasawa, J., Shimazaki, T., Kawashima, N., & Chaki, S. (2005). AMPA receptor stimulation mediates the antidepressant-like effect of a group II metabotropic glutamate receptor antagonist. *Brain Research*, *1042*(1), 92–98.
Karasawa, J., Yoshimizu, T., & Chaki, S. (2006). A metabotropic glutamate 2/3 receptor antagonist, MGS0039, increases extracellular dopamine levels in the nucleus accumbens shell. *Neuroscience Letters*, *393*(2–3), 127–130.
Karp, J. F., Butters, M. A., Begley, A., Miller, M. D., Lenze, E. J., Blumberger, D., et al. (2014). Safety, tolerability, and clinical effect of low-dose buprenorphine for treatment-resistant depression in mid-life and older adults. *The Journal of Clinical Psychiatry*, *75*(8), e785–e793.
Kasper, S., Moises, H. W., & Beckmann, H. (1981). The anticholinergic biperiden in depressive disorders. *Pharmacopsychiatria*, *14*(6), 195–198.
Katz, M. M., Koslow, S. H., & Frazer, A. (1996-1997). Onset of antidepressant activity: Reexamining the structure of depression and multiple actions of drugs. *Depression and Anxiety*, *4*(6), 257–267.
Katz, M. M., Tekell, J. L., Bowden, C. L., Brannan, S., Houston, J. P., & Berman, N. (2004). Onset and early behavioral effects of pharmacologically different antidepressants and placebo in depression. *Neuropsychopharmacology*, *29*, 566–579.
Kawashima, N., Karasawa, J., Shimazaki, T., Chaki, S., Okuyama, S., Yasuhara, A., et al. (2005). Neuropharmacological profiles of antagonists of group II metabotropic glutamate receptors. *Neuroscience Letters*, *378*(3), 131–134.
Kelly, T. F., & Lieberman, D. Z. (2014). The utility of the combination of dextromethorphan and quinidine in the treatment of bipolar II and bipolar NOS. *Journal of Affective Disorders*, *167*, 333–335.
Kohtala, S., Theilmann, W., Rosenholm, M., Penna, L., Karabulut, G., Uusitalo, S., et al. (2018). Cortical excitability and activation of TrkB signaling during rebound slow oscillations are critical for rapid antidepressant responses. *Molecular Neurobiology*. https://doi.org/10.1007/s12035-018-1364-6.
Koike, H., & Chaki, S. (2014). Requirement of AMPA receptor stimulation for the sustained antidepressant activity of ketamine and LY341495 during the forced swim test in rats. *Behavioural Brain Research*, *271*, 111–115.
Koike, H., Iijima, M., & Chaki, S. (2011). Involvement of the mammalian target of rapamycin signaling in the antidepressant-like effect of group II metabotropic glutamate receptor antagonists. *Neuropharmacology*, *61*(8), 1419–1423.
Kometer, M., Pokorny, T., Seifritz, E., & Volleinweider, F. X. (2015). Psilocybin-induced spiritual experiences and insightfulness are associated with synchronization of neuronal oscillations. *Psychopharmacology*, *232*(19), 3663–3676.
Kroes, R. A., & Nilsson, C. L. (2017). Towards the molecular foundations of glutamatergic-targeted antidepressants. *Current Neuropharmacology*, *15*(1), 35–46.
Krystal, J. H., D'Souza, D. C., Karper, L. P., Bennett, A., Abi-Dargham, A., Abi-Saab, D., et al. (1999). Interactive effects of subanesthetic ketamine and haloperidol in healthy humans. *Psychopharmacology*, *145*, 193–204.
Kunugi, A., Tajima, Y., Kuno, H., Sogabe, S., & Kimura, H. (2018). HBT1, a novel AMPA receptor potentiator with lower agonistic effect, avoided bell-shaped response in in vitro BDNF production. *The Journal of Pharmacology and Experimental Therapeutics*, *364*(3), 377–389.
Kyzar, E. J., Nichols, C. D., Gainetdinov, R. R., Nichols, D. E., & Kalueff, A. V. (2017). Psychedelic drugs in biomedicine. *Trends in Pharmacological Sciences*, *38*(11), 992–1005.

Lally, N., Nugent, A. C., Luckenbaugh, D. A., Ameli, R., Roiser, J. P., & Zarate, C. A. (2014). Anti-anhedonic effect of ketamine and its neural correlates in treatment-resistant bipolar depression. *Translational Psychiatry*, *4*, e469.

Lally, N., Nugent, A. C., Luckenbaugh, D. A., Niciu, M. J., Roiser, J. P., & Zarate, C. A., Jr. (2015). Neural correlates of change in major depressive disorder anhedonia following open-label ketamine. *Journal of Psychopharmacology*, *29*(5), 596–607.

Lauterbach, E. C. (2016). Treatment resistant depression with loss of antidepressant response: Rapid-acting antidepressant action of dextromethorphan, a possible treatment bridging molecule. *Psychopharmacology Bulletin*, *46*(2), 53–58.

Lepack, A. E., Bang, E., Lee, B., Dwyer, J. M., & Duman, R. S. (2016). Fast-acting antidepressants rapidly stimulate ERK signaling and BDNF release in primary neuronal cultures. *Neuropharmacology*, *111*, 242–252.

Li, N., Lee, B., Liu, R. J., Banasr, M., Dwyer, J. M., Iwata, M., et al. (2010). mTOR-dependent synapse formation underlies the rapid antidepressant effects of NMDA antagonists. *Science*, *329*(5994), 959–964.

Lian, B., Xia, J., Yang, X., Zhou, C., Gong, X., Gui, S., et al. (2018). Mechanisms of ketamine on mice hippocampi shown by gas chromatography-mass spectrometry-based metabolomic analysis. *Neuroreport*, *29*(9), 704–711.

Liu, R. J., Duman, C., Kato, T., Hare, B., Lopresto, D., Bang, E., et al. (2017). GLYX-13 Produces rapid antidepressant responses with key synaptic and behavioral effects distinct from ketamine. *Neuropsychopharmacology*, *42*, 1231–1242.

Locher, C., Koechlin, H., Zion, S. R., Werner, C., Pine, D. S., Kirsch, I., et al. (2017). Efficacy and safety of selective serotonin reuptake inhibitors, serotonin-norepinephrine reuptake inhibitors, and placebo for common psychiatric disorders among children and adolescents: A systematic review and meta-analysis. *JAMA Psychiatry*, *74*(10), 1011–1020.

Lorrain, D. S., Baccei, C. S., Bristow, L. J., Anderson, J. J., & Varney, M. A. (2003). Effects of ketamine and N-methyl-D-aspartate on glutamate and dopamine release in the rat prefrontal cortex: Modulation by a group II selective metabotropic glutamate receptor agonist LY379268. *Neuroscience*, *117*(3), 697–706.

Lu, Y., Wang, C., Xue, Z., Li, C., Zhang, J., Zhao, X., et al. (2014). PI3K/AKT/mTOR signaling-mediated neuropeptide VGF in the hippocampus of mice is involved in the rapid onset antidepressant-like effects of GLYX-13. *The International Journal of Neuropsychopharmacology*, *18*(5), pii: pyu110, https://doi.org/10.1093/ijnp/pyu110.

Ly, C., Greb, A. C., Cameron, L. P., Wong, J. M., Barragan, E. V., Wilson, P. C., et al. (2018). Psychedelics promote structural and functional neural plasticity. *Cell Reports*, *23*(11), 3170–3182.

Ma, M., Ren, Q., Yang, C., Zhang, J. C., Yao, W., Dong, C., et al. (2016). Adjunctive treatment of brexpiprazole with fluoxetine shows a rapid antidepressant effect in social defeat stress model: Role of BDNF-TrkB signaling. *Scientific Reports*, *6*, 39209.

Machado-Vieira, R., Henter, I. D., & Zarate, C. A., Jr. (2017). New targets for rapid antidepressant action. *Progress in Neurobiology*, *152*, 21–37.

Martin, A. E., Schober, D. A., Nikolayev, A., Tolstikov, V. V., Anderson, W. H., Higgs, R. E., et al. (2017). Further evaluation of mechanisms associated with the antidepressant-like signature of scopolamine in mice. *CNS & Neurological Disorders: Drug Targets*, *16*, 492–500.

Meredith, G. E., Blank, B., & Groenewegen, H. J. (1989). The distribution and compartmental organization of the cholinergic neurons in nucleus accumbens of the rat. *Neuroscience*, *31*, 327–345.

Meyers, M. A. (2007). *Happy accidents: Serendipity in modern medical breakthroughs*. New York: Arcade Publishing.

Moaddel, R., Shardell, M., Khadeer, M., Lovett, J., Kadriu, B., Ravichandran, S., et al. (2018). Plasma metabolomic profiling of a ketamine and placebo crossover trial of major depressive disorder and healthy control subjects. *Psychopharmacology, 235*(10), 3017–3030.

Moghaddam, B., & Krystal, J. H. (2012). Capturing the angel in "angel dust": Twenty years of translational neuroscience studies of NMDA receptor antagonists in animals and humans. *Schizophrenia Bulletin, 38*, 942–949.

Molero, P., Ramos-Quiroga, J. A., Martin-Santos, R., Calvo-Sánchez, E., Gutiérrez-Rojas, L., & Meana, J. J. (2018). Antidepressant efficacy and tolerability of ketamine and esketamine: A critical review. *CNS Drugs, 32*, 411–420.

Monteggia, L. M., Gideons, E., & Kavalali, E. T. (2013). The role of eukaryotic elongation factor 2 kinase in rapid antidepressant action of ketamine. *Biological Psychiatry, 73*(12), 1199–1203.

Moskal, J. R., Burgdorf, J. S., Stanton, P. K., Kroes, R. A., Disterhoft, J. F., Burch, R. M., et al. (2017). The development of rapastinel (formerly GLYX-13); A rapid acting and long lasting antidepressant. *Current Neuropharmacology, 15*(1), 47–56.

Musazzi, L., Tornese, P., Sala, N., & Popoli, M. (2017). Acute or chronic? A stressful question. *Trends in Neurosciences, 40*(9), 525–535.

Navarria, A., Wohleb, E. S., Voleti, B., Ota, K. T., Dutheil, S., Lepack, A. E., et al. (2015). Rapid antidepressant actions of scopolamine: Role of medial prefrontal cortex and M1-subtype muscarinic acetylcholine receptors. *Neurobiology of Disease, 82*, 254–261.

Nichols, D. E. (1986). Differences between the mechanism of action of MDMA, MBDB, and the classic hallucinogens. Identification of a new therapeutic class: Entactogens. *Journal of Psychoactive Drugs, 18*(4), 305–313.

Nisenbaum, E. S., & Witkin, J. M. (2010). Positive allosteric modulation of AMPA receptors: A novel potential antidepressant therapy. In P. Skolnick (Ed.), *Glutamate-based therapies for psychiatric disorders* (pp. 39–56). Basel, Switzerland: Birkhäuser Verlag AG.

Novotný, V., & Faltus, F. (2003). First signs of improvement with tianeptine in the treatment of depression: An analysis of a double-blind study versus fluoxetine. *European Neuropsychopharmacology, 13*(13), S230.

Nugent, A. C., Wills, K. E., Gilbert, J. R., & Zarate, C. A., Jr. (2019). Synaptic potentiation and rapid antidepressant response to ketamine in treatment-resistant major depression: A replication study. *Psychiatry Research: Neuroimaging, 283*, 64–66.

Nyhuis, P. W., Gastpar, M., & Scherbaum, N. (2008). Opiate treatment in depression refractory to antidepressants and electroconvulsive therapy. *Journal of Clinical Psychopharmacology, 28*(5), 593–595.

Oertel, B. G., Felden, L., Tran, P. V., Bradshaw, M. H., Angst, M. S., Schmidt, H., et al. (2010). Selective antagonism of opioid-induced ventilatory depression by an ampakine molecule in humans without loss of opioid analgesia. *Clinical Pharmacology and Therapeutics, 87*(2), 204–211.

Orozco-Solis, R., Montellier, E., Aguilar-Arnal, L., Sato, S., Vawter, M. P., Bunney, B. G., et al. (2017). A circadian genomic signature common to ketamine and sleep deprivation in the anterior cingulate cortex. *Biological Psychiatry, 82*(5), 351–360.

Osório Fde, L., Sanches, R. F., Macedo, L. R., Santos, R. G., Maia-de-Oliveira, J. P., Wichert-Ana, L., et al. (2015). Antidepressant effects of a single dose of ayahuasca in patients with recurrent depression: A preliminary report. *Revista Brasileira de Psiquiatria, 37*(1), 13–20.

Pahnke, W. N., Kurland, A. A., Goodman, L. E., & Richards, W. A. (1969). LSD-assisted psychotherapy with terminal cancer patients. *Current Psychiatric Therapies, 9*, 144–152.

Palhano-Fontes, F., Barreto, D., Onias, H., Andrade, K. C., Novaes, M. M., Pessoa, J. A., et al. (2018). Rapid antidepressant effects of the psychedelic ayahuasca in treatment-resistant depression: A randomized placebo-controlled trial. *Psychological Medicine*, *15*, 1–9.

Pałucha-Poniewiera, A. (2018). The role of glutamatergic modulation in the mechanism of action of ketamine, a prototype rapid-acting antidepressant drug. *Pharmacological Reports*, *70*(5), 837–846.

Park, L., Furey, M., Nugent, A. C., Farmer, C., Ellis, J., Szczepanik, J., et al. (2019). Neurophysiological changes associated with antidepressant response to ketamine not observed in a negative trial of scopolamine in major depressive disorder. *The International Journal of Neuropsychopharmacology*, *22*(1), 10–18.

Pešić, V., Petrović, J., & Jukić, M. M. (2016). Molecular mechanism and clinical relevance of ketamine as rapid-acting antidepressant. *Drug Development Research*, *77*(7), 414–422.

Pham, T. H., Mendez-David, I., Defaix, C., Guiard, B. P., Tritschler, L., David, D. J., et al. (2017). Ketamine treatment involves medial prefrontal cortex serotonin to induce a rapid antidepressant-like activity in BALB/cJ mice. *Neuropharmacology*, *112*(Pt. A), 198–209.

Phillips, A. G., & Fibiger, H. C. (1976). Long-term deficits in stimulation-induced behaviors and self-stimulation after 6-hydroxydopamine administration in rats. *Behavioral Biology*, *16*, 127–143.

Podkowa, K., Pilc, A., Podkowa, A., Salat, K., Marciniak, M., & Palucha-Poniewiera, A. (2018). The potential antidepressant action and adverse effects profile of scopolamine co-administered with the mGlu7 receptor allosteric agonist AMN082 in mice. *Neuropharmacology*, *141*, 214–222.

Podkowa, A., Salat, K., Lenda, T., Pilc, A., & Palucha-Poniewiera, A. (2016). Antidepressant-like effects of scopolamine in mice are enhanced by the group II mGlu receptor antagonist LY341495. *Neuropharmacology*, *111*, 169–179.

Preller, K. H., Burt, J. B., Ji, J. L., Schleifer, C. H., Adkinson, B. D., Stämpfli, P., et al. (2018). Changes in global and thalamic brain connectivity in LSD-induced altered states of consciousness are attributable to the 5-HT2A receptor. *eLife*, 7. pii: e35082.

Preskorn, S. H., Baker, B., Kolluri, S., Menniti, F. S., Krams, M., & Landen, J. W. (2008). An innovative design to establish proof of concept of the antidepressant effects of the NR2B subunit selective N-methyl-D-aspartate antagonist, CP-101,606, in patients with treatment-refractory major depressive disorder. *Journal of Clinical Psychopharmacology*, *28*, 631–637.

Price, J. L., & Drevets, W. C. (2010). Neurocircuitry of mood disorders. *Neuropsychopharmacology*, *35*, 192–216.

Qiu, Y., Chen, D., Huang, X., Huang, L., Tang, L., Jiang, J., et al. (2016). Neuroprotective effects of HTR1A antagonist WAY-100635 on scopolamine-induced delirium in rats and underlying molecular mechanisms. *BMC Neuroscience*, *17*(1), 66.

Qu, Y., Yang, C., Ren, Q., Ma, M., Dong, C., & Hashimoto, K. (2017). Comparison of (R)-ketamine and lanicemine on depression-like phenotype and abnormal composition of gut microbiota in a social defeat stress model. *Scientific Reports*, 7(1), 15725.

Rantamäki, T., & Yalcin, I. (2016). Antidepressant drug action–From rapid changes on network function to network rewiring. *Progress in Neuro-Psychopharmacology & Biological Psychiatry*, *64*, 285–292.

Rawls, S. M., & Mcginty, J. F. (1998). Muscarinic receptors regulate extracellular glutamate levels in the rat striatum: An in vivo microdialysis study. *The Journal of Pharmacology and Experimental Therapeutics*, *286*(1), 91–98.

Romeo, B., Blecha, L., Locatelli, K., Benyamina, A., & Martelli, C. (2018). Meta-analysis and review of dopamine agonists in acute episodes of mood disorder: Efficacy and safety. *Journal of Psychopharmacology*, *32*(4), 385–396.

Roseman, L., Demetriou, L., Wall, M. B., Nutt, D. J., & Carhart-Harris, R. L. (2018). Increased amygdala responses to emotional faces after psilocybin for treatment-resistant depression. *Neuropharmacology*, *142*, 263–269.
Roseman, L., Nutt, D. J., & Carhart-Harris, R. L. (2018). Quality of acute psychedelic experience predicts therapeutic efficacy of psilocybin for treatment-resistant depression. *Frontiers in Pharmacology*, *8*, 974.
Ross, S., Bossis, A., Guss, J., Agin-Liebes, G., Malone, T., Cohen, B., et al. (2016). Rapid and sustained symptom reduction following psilocybin treatment for anxiety and depression in patients with life-threatening cancer: A randomized controlled trial. *Journal of Psychopharmacology*, *30*(12), 1165–1180.
Rotroff, D. M., Corum, D. G., Motsinger-Reif, A., Fiehn, O., Bottrel, N., Drevets, W. C., et al. (2016). Metabolomic signatures of drug response phenotypes for ketamine and esketamine in subjects with refractory major depressive disorder: New mechanistic insights for rapid acting antidepressants. *Translational Psychiatry*, *6*(9), e894.
Rucker, J. J. H., Iliff, J., & Nutt, D. J. (2018). Psychiatry & the psychedelic drugs. Past, present & future. *Neuropharmacology*, *142*, 200–218.
Rush, A. J., Trivedi, M. H., Wisniewski, S. R., Nierenberg, A. A., Stewart, J. W., Warden, D., et al. (2006). Acute and longer-term outcomes in depressed outpatients requiring one or several treatment steps: A STAR_D report. *The American Journal of Psychiatry*, *163*, 1905–1917.
Sakashita, Y., Abe, K., Katagiri, N., Kambe, T., Saitoh, T., Utsunomiya, I., et al. (2015). Effect of psilocin on extracellular dopamine and serotonin levels in the mesoaccumbens and mesocortical pathway in awake rats. *Biological & Pharmaceutical Bulletin*, *38*(1), 134–138.
Sakloth, F., Leggett, E., Moerke, M. J., Townsend, E. A., Banks, M. L., & Negus, S. S. (2019). Effects of acute and repeated treatment with serotonin 5-HT2A receptor agonist hallucinogens on intracranial self-stimulation in rats. *Experimental and Clinical Psychopharmacology*. https://doi.org/10.1037/pha0000253.
Sanacora, G., Johnson, M. R., Khan, A., Atkinson, S. D., Riesenberg, R. R., Schronen, J. P., et al. (2017). Adjunctive lanicemine (AZD6765) in patients with major depressive disorder and history of inadequate response to antidepressants: A randomized, placebo-controlled study. *Neuropsychopharmacology*, *42*(4), 844–853.
Sanacora, G., Smith, M. A., Pathak, S., Su, H. L., Boeijinga, P. H., McCarthy, D. J., et al. (2014). Lanicemine: A low-trapping NMDA channel blocker produces sustained antidepressant efficacy with minimal psychotomimetic adverse effects. *Molecular Psychiatry*, *19*(9), 978–985.
Sanches, R., Osório, F., dos Santos, R., Macedo, L., Maia-de-Oliveira, J., Wichert-Ana, L., et al. (2016). Antidepressant effects of a single dose of ayahuasca in patients with recurrent depression: A SPECT study. *Journal of Clinical Psychopharmacology*, *36*, 77–81.
Savage, C. (1952). Lysergic acid diethylamide; A clinical-psychological study. *Journal of Psychiatry*, *108*(12), 896–900.
Schulz, J. M., Knoflach, F., Hernandez, M. C., & Bischofberger, J. (2018). Dendrite-targeting interneurons control synaptic NMDA-receptor activation via nonlinear α5-$GABA_A$ receptors. *Nature Communications*, *9*(1), 3576.
Shaw, A. D., Saxena, N., E Jackson, L., Hall, J. E., Singh, K. D., & Muthukumaraswamy, S. D. (2015). Ketamine amplifies induced gamma frequency oscillations in the human cerebral cortex. *European Neuropsychopharmacology*, *25*(8), 1136–1146.
Shokry, I. M., Sinha, V., Da Silva, G., Park, S. B., Callanan, J. J., & Tao, R. (2018). Comparison of electroencephalogram (EEG) response to MDPV versus the hallucinogenic drugs MK-801 and ketamine in rats. *Experimental Neurology*, *313*, 26–36.

Siwek, M., Dudek, D., Paul, I. A., Sowa-Kućma, M., Zieba, A., Popik, P., et al. (2009). Zinc supplementation augments efficacy of imipramine in treatment resistant patients: A double blind, placebo-controlled study. *Journal of Affective Disorders*, *2009*(118), 187–195.

Skolnick, P. (2008). AMPA receptors: A target for novel antidepressants? *Biological Psychiatry*, *63*(4), 347–378.

Skolnick, P., Popik, P., & Trullas, R. (2009). Glutamate-based antidepressants: 20 years on. *Trends in Pharmacological Sciences*, *30*(11), 563–569.

Song, M., Martinowich, K., & Lee, F. S. (2017). BDNF at the synapse: Why location matters. *Molecular Psychiatry*, *22*(10), 1370–1375.

Strasburger, S. E., Bhimani, P. M., Kaabe, J. H., Krysiak, J. T., Nanchanatt, D. L., Nguyen, T. N., et al. (2017). What is the mechanism of ketamine's rapid-onset antidepressant effect? A concise overview of the surprisingly large number of possibilities. *Journal of Clinical Pharmacy and Therapeutics*, *42*(2), 147–154.

Stroud, J. B., Freeman, T. P., Leech, R., Hindocha, C., Lawn, W., Nutt, D. J., et al. (2018). Psilocybin with psychological support improves emotional face recognition in treatment-resistant depression. *Psychopharmacology*, *235*(2), 459–466.

Sun, H. L., Zhou, Z. Q., Zhang, G. F., Yang, C., Wang, X. M., Shen, J. C., et al. (2016). Role of hippocampal p11 in the sustained antidepressant effect of ketamine in the chronic unpredictable mild stress model. *Translational Psychiatry*, *6*, e741.

Sur, C., Fresu, L., Howell, O., McKernan, R. M., & Atack, J. R. (1999). Autoradiographic localization of alpha5 subunit-containing GABAA receptors in rat brain. *Brain Research*, *822*, 265–270.

Svenningsson, P., Tzavara, E. T., Witkin, J. M., Fienberg, A. A., Nomikos, G. G., & Greengard, P. (2002). Involvement of striatal and extrastriatal DARPP-32 in biochemical and behavioral effects of fluoxetine (Prozac). *Proceedings of the National Academy of Sciences of the United States of America*, *99*(5), 3182–3187.

Szczepanik, J., Drevets, W., Khanna, A., Zarate, C., & Furey, M. (2012). Amygdala response to implicit and explicit sad face stimuli at baseline predicts antidepressant treatment response to scopolamine in major depressive disorder. *Biological Psychiatry*, *71*(8), 293s.

Szewczyk, B., Poleszak, E., Sowa-Kućma, M., Wróbel, A., Słotwiński, S., Listos, J., et al. (2010). The involvement of NMDA and AMPA receptors in the mechanism of antidepressant-like action of zinc in the forced swim test. *Amino Acids*, *39*(1), 205–217.

Talbot, J. N., Geffert, L. M., Jorvig, J. E., Goldstein, R. I., Nielsen, C. L., Wolters, N. E., et al. (2016). Rapid and sustained antidepressant properties of an NMDA antagonist/monoamine reuptake inhibitor identified via transporter-based virtual screening. *Pharmacology, Biochemistry, and Behavior*, *150–151*, 22–30.

Thelen, C., Flaherty, E., Saurine, J., Sens, J., Mohamed, S., & Pitychoutis, P. M. (2019). Sex differences in the temporal neuromolecular and synaptogenic effects of the rapid-acting antidepressant drug ketamine in the mouse brain. *Neuroscience*, *398*, 182–192.

Thomas, A. M., & Duman, R. S. (2017). Novel rapid-acting antidepressants: Molecular and cellular signaling mechanisms. *Neuronal Signaling*, *1*(4), pii: NS20170010. https://doi.org/10.1042/NS20170010.

Tobe, E. H., & Rybakowski, J. K. (2013). Possible usefulness of tianeptine in treatment-resistant depression. *International Journal of Psychiatry in Clinical Practice*, *17*(4), 313–316.

Towers, S. K., Gloveli, T., Traub, R. D., Driver, J. E., Engel, D., Fradley, R., et al. (2004). Alpha 5 subunit-containing GABAA receptors affect the dynamic range of mouse hippocampal kainate-induced gamma frequency oscillations in vitro. *The Journal of Physiology*, *559*, 721–728.

Trullas, R., & Skolnick, P. (1990). Functional antagonists at the NMDA receptor complex exhibit antidepressant actions. *European Journal of Pharmacology*, *185*, 1–10.

Trzepacz, P. T., Cummings, J., Konechnik, T., Forrester, T. D., Chang, C., Dennehy, E. B., et al. (2013). Mibampator (LY451395) randomized clinical trial for agitation/aggression in Alzheimer's disease. *International Psychogeriatrics*, *25*(5), 707–719.

Tsukada, H., Harada, N., Nishiyama, S., Ohba, H., & Kakiuchi, T. (2000). Cholinergic neuronal modulation alters dopamine D2 receptor availability in vivo by regulating receptor affinity induced by facilitated synaptic dopamine turnover: Positron emission tomography studies with microdialysis in the conscious monkey brain. *The Journal of Neuroscience*, *20*(18), 7067.

Valentine, G. W., & Sanacora, G. (2009). Targeting glial physiology and glutamate cycling in the treatment of depression. *Biochemical Pharmacology*, *78*(5), 431–439.

Voleti, B., Navarria, A., Liu, R. J., Banasr, M., Li, N., Terwilliger, R., et al. (2013). Scopolamine rapidly increases mammalian target of rapamycin complex 1 signaling, synaptogenesis, and antidepressant behavioral responses. *Biological Psychiatry*, *74*(10), 742–749.

Wasko, M. J., Witt-Enderby, P. A., & Surratt, C. K. (2018). DARK classics in chemical neuroscience: Ibogaine. *ACS Chemical Neuroscience*, *9*(10), 2475–2483.

West, C. H., & Weiss, J. M. (2011). Effects of chronic antidepressant drug administration and electroconvulsive shock on activity of dopaminergic neurons in the ventral tegmentum. *The International Journal of Neuropsychopharmacology*, *14*, 201–210.

Wilkinson, S. T., Ballard, E. D., Bloch, M. H., Mathew, S. J., Murrough, J. W., Feder, A., et al. (2018). The effect of a single dose of intravenous ketamine on suicidal ideation: A systematic review and individual participant data meta-analysis. *The American Journal of Psychiatry*, *175*(2), 150–158.

Wilkinson, S. T., & Sanacora, G. (2018). A new generation of antidepressants: An update on the pharmaceutical pipeline for novel and rapid-acting therapeutics in mood disorders based on glutamate/GABA neurotransmitter systems. *Drug Discovery Today*, *24*, 606–615. pii: S1359-6446(18)30376-3.

Willner, P. (1997). The mesolimbic dopamine system as a target for rapid antidepressant action. *International Clinical Psychopharmacology*, *12*(Suppl. 3), S7–S14.

Witkin, J. M. (2011). The mood in the field of antidepressant drug discovery. *CNS & Neurological Disorders: Drug Targets*, *10*(7), 1–2.

Witkin, J. M. (2015). Obstacles to the discovery of medicines for psychiatric disorders in modern times. *CNS & Neurological Disorders: Drug Targets*, *14*(1), 4–6.

Witkin, J. M., Knutson, D. E., Rodriguez, G. J., & Shi, S. (2018). Rapid-acting antidepressants. *Current Pharmaceutical Design*, *24*, 1–8.

Witkin, J. M., Monn, J. A., Li, J., Johnson, B., McKinzie, D. L., Wang, X. S., et al. (2017). Preclinical predictors that the orthosteric mGlu2/3 receptor antagonist LY3020371 will not engender ketamine-associated neurotoxic, motor, cognitive, subjective, or abuse-liability-related effects. *Pharmacology Biochemistry and Behavior*, *155*, 43–55.

Witkin, J. M., Monn, J. A., Schoepp, D. D., Li, X., Overshiner, C., Mitchell, S. N., et al. (2016). The rapidly acting antidepressant ketamine rapidly engages dopaminergic mood circuits. *The Journal of Pharmacology and Experimental Therapeutics*, *358*, 71–82.

Witkin, J. M., Ornstein, P. L., Mitch, C. H., Li, R., Smith, S. C., Heinz, B. A., et al. (2017). In vitro pharmacological and rat pharmacokinetic characterization of LY3020371, a potent and selective $mGlu_{2/3}$ receptor antagonist. *Neuropharmacology*, *115*, 100–114.

Witkin, J. M., Overshiner, C., Li, X., Catlow, J. T., Schober, D. A., Heinz, B. A., et al. (2014). The M_1 and M_2 muscarinic receptor subtypes regulate antidepressant-like effects of the rapidly-acting antidepressant scopolamine. *The Journal of Pharmacology and Experimental Therapeutics*, *351*(2), 448–456.

Witkin, J. M., Overshiner, C., Li, X., Gilmour, G., Li, J., Rorick-Kehn, L., et al. (2017). Comparative effects of LY3020371, a potent and selective mGlu2/3 receptor antagonist, and ketamine, a non-competitive NMDA receptor antagonist, in rodents: Evidence supporting use for the treatment of depression. *The Journal of Pharmacology and Experimental Therapeutics*, *361*(1), 68–86.

Wohleb, E. S., Gerhard, D., Thomas, A., & Duman, R. S. (2017). Molecular and cellular mechanisms of rapid-acting antidepressants ketamine and scopolamine. *Current Neuropharmacology*, *15*(1), 11–20.

Wohleb, E. S., Wu, M., Gerhard, D. M., Taylor, S. R., Picciotto, M. R., Alreja, M., et al. (2016). GABA interneurons mediate the rapid antidepressant-like effects of scopolamine. *The Journal of Clinical Investigation*, *126*(7), 2482–2494.

Woo, Y. S., Bahk, W.-M., Jeong, J.-H., Lee, S.-H., Sung, H.-M., Pae, C.-U., et al. (2013). Tianeptine combination for partial or non-response to selective serotonin re-uptake inhibitor monotherapy. *Psychiatry and Clinical Neurosciences*, *67*(4), 219–227.

Workman, E. R., Haddick, P. C., Bush, K., Dilly, G. A., Niere, F., Zemelman, B. V., et al. (2015). Rapid antidepressants stimulate the decoupling of GABA(B) receptors from GIRK/Kir3 channels through increased protein stability of 14-3-3η. *Molecular Psychiatry*, *20*(3), 298–310.

Workman, E. R., Niere, F., & Raab-Graham, K. F. (2018). Engaging homeostatic plasticity to treat depression. *Molecular Psychiatry*, *23*(1), 26–35.

Wray, N. H., & Rasenick, M. M. (2019). NMDA-receptor independent actions of ketamine: A new chapter in a story that's not so old. *Neuropsychopharmacology*, *44*(1), 220–221.

Wray, N. H., Schappi, J. M., Singh, H., Senese, N. B., & Rasenick, M. M. (2018). NMDAR-independent, cAMP-dependent antidepressant actions of ketamine. *Molecular Psychiatry*. https://doi.org/10.1038/s41380-018-0083-8 [Epub ahead of print].

Xiong, Z., Zhang, K., Ishima, T., Ren, Q., Chang, L., Chen, J., et al. (2018). Comparison of rapid and long-lasting antidepressant effects of negative modulators of α5-containing $GABA_A$ receptors and (R)-ketamine in a chronic social defeat stress model. *Pharmacology, Biochemistry, and Behavior*, *175*, 139–145.

Xiong, Z., Zhang, K., Ishima, T., Ren, Q., Ma, M., Pu, Y., et al. (2019). Lack of rapid antidepressant effects of Kir4.1 channel inhibitors in a chronic social defeat stress model: Comparison with (R)-ketamine. *Pharmacology, Biochemistry, and Behavior*, *176*, 57–62.

Xiong, Z., Zhang, K., Ren, Q., Chang, L., Chen, J., & Hashimoto, K. (2018). Increased expression of inwardly rectifying Kir4.1 channel in the parietal cortex from patients with major depressive disorder. *Journal of Affective Disorders*, *245*, 265–269.

Xu, N. Z., Ernst, M., Treven, M., Cerne, R., Wakulchik, M., Li, X., et al. (2018). Negative allosteric modulation of alpha 5-containing $GABA_A$ receptors engenders antidepressant-like effects and selectively prevents age-associated hyperactivity in tau-depositing mice. *Psychopharmacology*, *235*(4), 1151–1161.

Xue, M., Liu, J. P., Yang, Y. H., Suo, Z. W., Yang, X., & Hu, X. D. (2017). Inhibition of α5 subunit-containing GABAA receptors facilitated spinal nociceptive transmission and plasticity. *European Journal of Pain*, *21*(6), 1061–1071.

Yamaguchi, J. I., Toki, H., Qu, Y., Yang, C., Koike, H., Hashimoto, K., et al. (2018). (2R,6R)-Hydroxynorketamine is not essential for the antidepressant actions of (R)-ketamine in mice. *Neuropsychopharmacology*, *43*(9), 1900–1907.

Yang, Y., Cui, Y., Sang, K., Dong, Y., Ni, Z., Ma, S., et al. (2018). Ketamine blocks bursting in the lateral habenula to rapidly relieve depression. *Nature*, *554*(7692), 317–322.

Yang, C., Kobayashi, S., Nakao, K., Dong, C., Han, M., Qu, Y., et al. (2018). AMPA receptor activation-independent antidepressant actions of ketamine metabolite (S)-norketamine. *Biological Psychiatry*, *84*(8), 591–600.

Yang, C., Qu, Y., Abe, M., Nozawa, D., Chaki, S., & Hashimoto, K. (2017). (R)-ketamine shows greater potency and longer lasting antidepressant effects than its metabolite (2R,6R)-hydroxynorketamine. *Biological Psychiatry*, *82*(5), e43–e44. https://doi.org/10.1016/j.biopsych.2016.12.020. Epub 2016 Dec 23.

Yang, C., Qu, Y., Fujita, Y., Ren, Q., Ma, M., Dong, C., et al. (2017). Possible role of the gut microbiota–brain axis in the antidepressant effects of (R)-ketamine in a social defeat stress model. *Translational Psychiatry*, *7*, 1294.

Yang, C., Ren, Q., Qu, Y., Zhang, J. C., Ma, M., Dong, C., et al. (2018). Mechanistic target of rapamycin-independent antidepressant effects of (r)-ketamine in a social defeat stress model. *Biological Psychiatry*, *83*(1), 18–28.

Yang, C., Shirayama, Y., Zhang, J. C., Ren, Q., Yao, W., Ma, M., et al. (2015). R-ketamine: A rapid-onset and sustained antidepressant without psychotomimetic side effects. *Translational Psychiatry*, *5*, e632.

Yellepeddi, V. K., Zhudeva, M. Y., Movahedi, F., Vo, A., Phan, J., Kirsh, R. D., et al. (2018). Biopharmaceutical characterization and oral efficacy of a new rapid acting antidepressant Ro 25-6981. *Journal of Pharmaceutical Sciences*, *107*(9), 2472–2478.

Yu, H., Li, M., Shen, X., Lv, D., Sun, X., Wang, J., et al. (2018). The requirement of L-type voltage-dependent calcium channel (L-VDCC) in the rapid-acting antidepressant-like effects of scopolamine in mice. *The International Journal of Neuropsychopharmacology*, *21*(2), 175–186.

Yu, H. J., Li, M. M., Zhou, D. S., Lv, D., Liao, Q., Lou, Z. Z., et al. (2018). Vesicular glutamate transporter 1 (VGLUT1)-mediated glutamate release and membrane GluA1 activation is involved in the rapid antidepressant-like effects of scopolamine in mice. *Neuropharmacology*, *131*, 209–222.

Yu, H., Lv, D., Shen, M., Zhang, Y., Zhou, D., Chen, Z., et al. (2018). BDNF mediates the protective effects of scopolamine in reserpine-induced depression-like behaviors via up-regulation of 5-HTT and TPH1. *Psychiatry Research*, *271*, 328–334.

Yuan, L. L., Wauson, E., & Duric, V. (2016). Kinase-mediated signaling cascades in mood disorders and antidepressant treatment. *Journal of Neurogenetics*, *30*(3-4), 178–184.

Zanos, P., & Gould, T. D. (2018). Mechanisms of ketamine action as an antidepressant. *Molecular Psychiatry*, *23*(4), 801–811.

Zanos, P., Moaddel, R., Morris, P. J., Georgiou, P., Fischell, J., Elmer, G. I., et al. (2016). NMDAR inhibition-independent antidepressant actions of ketamine metabolites. *Nature*, *533*(7604), 481–486.

Zanos, P., Moaddel, R., Morris, P. J., Riggs, L. M., Highland, J. N., Georgiou, P., et al. (2018). Ketamine and ketamine metabolite pharmacology: Insights into therapeutic mechanisms. *Pharmacological Reviews*, *70*(3), 621–660.

Zanos, P., Nelson, M. E., Highland, J. N., Krimmel, S. R., Georgiou, P., Gould, T. D., et al. (2017). A negative allosteric modulator for α5 subunit-containing GABA receptors exerts a rapid and persistent antidepressant-like action without the side effects of the NMDA receptor antagonist ketamine in mice. *eNeuro*, *4*(1). pii: ENEURO.0285-16.2017.

Zanos, P., Piantadosi, S. C., Wu, H. Q., Pribut, H. J., Dell, M. J., Can, A., et al. (2015). The prodrug 4-chlorokynurenine causes ketamine-like antidepressant effects, but not side effects, by NMDA/glycineB-site inhibition. *The Journal of Pharmacology and Experimental Therapeutics*, *355*(1), 76–85.

Zarate, C. A., Jr., Mathews, D., Ibrahim, L., Chaves, J. F., Marquardt, C., Ukoh, I., et al. (2013). A randomized trial of a low-trapping nonselective N-methyl-D-aspartate channel blocker in major depression. *Biological Psychiatry*, *74*(4), 257–264.

Zarate, C. A., Jr., Singh, J. B., Carlson, P. J., Brutsche, N. E., Ameli, R., & Luckenbaugh, D. A. (2006). A randomized trial of an N-methyl-D-aspartate antagonist in treatment-resistant major depression. *Archives of General Psychiatry*, *63*, 856–864.

Zhang, K., Dong, C., Fujita, Y., Fujita, A., & Hashimoto, K. (2018). 5-Hydroxytryptamine-independent antidepressant actions of (R)-ketamine in a chronic social defeat stress model. *The International Journal of Neuropsychopharmacology*, *21*(2), 157–163.

Zhang, K., & Hashimoto, K. (2018). An update on ketamine and its two enantiomers as rapid-acting antidepressants. *Expert Review of Neurotherapeutics*, *4*, 1–10.
Zhang, J., Li, S., & Hashimoto, K. (2014). R (−)-ketamine shows greater potency and longer lasting antidepressant effects than S (+)-ketamine. *Pharmacology Biochemistry and Behavior*, *116*, 137–141.
Zhang, K., Toki, H., Fujita, Y., Ma, M., Chang, L., Qu, Y., et al. (2018). Lack of deuterium isotope effects in the antidepressant effects of (R)-ketamine in a chronic social defeat stress model. *Psychopharmacology*, *235*(11), 3177–3185.
Zhang, J. C., Yao, W., Dong, C., Yang, C., Ren, Q., Ma, M., et al. (2017). Blockade of interleukin-6 receptor in the periphery promotes rapid and sustained antidepressant actions: A possible role of gut-microbiota-brain axis. *Translational Psychiatry*, 7(5), e1138.
Zhang, J. C., Yao, W., Ren, Q., Yang, C., Dong, C., Ma, M., et al. (2016). Depression-like phenotype by deletion of α7 nicotinic acetylcholine receptor: Role of BDNF-TrkB in nucleus accumbens. *Scientific Reports*, *6*, 36705.
Zhou, D., Zhang, Z., Liu, L., Li, C., Li, M., Yu, H., et al. (2017). The antidepressant-like effects of biperiden may involve BDNF/TrkB signaling-mediated BICC1 expression in the hippocampus and prefrontal cortex of mice. *Pharmacology, Biochemistry, and Behavior*, *157*, 47–57.

CHAPTER FOUR

mGlu2/3 receptor antagonists

Shigeyuki Chaki*
Research Headquarters, Taisho Pharmaceutical Co., Ltd., Yoshino-cho, Saitama, Japan
*Corresponding author: e-mail address: s-chaki@taisho.co.jp

Contents

1. Introduction 98
2. mGlu2/3 receptors—Localization and molecular properties 99
3. Pharmacology of mGlu2/3 receptor antagonists 101
4. Depression and role of mGlu2/3 receptors in depression 103
5. Antidepressant effects of mGlu2/3 receptor antagonists 104
6. Anxiolytic effects of mGlu2/3 receptor antagonists 110
7. Pro-cognitive effects of mGlu2/3 receptor antagonists 112
8. Conclusions 113
Acknowledgments 113
Conflict of interest statement 113
References 114

Abstract

Abnormalities of glutamatergic transmission are implicated in neuropsychiatric disorders. Among the glutamate receptors, metabotropic (mGlu) 2/3 receptors have recently gained much attention as molecular targets for the treatment of several neuropsychiatric disorders including depression and anxiety. Both orthosteric and allosteric antagonists of mGlu2/3 receptors have been synthesized, and their therapeutic potential has been examined. These research activities have demonstrated the promise of mGlu2/3 receptor antagonists as potential treatment agents for the above-mentioned neuropsychiatric disorders. In particular, it has been considered that the antidepressant effects of mGlu2/3 receptor antagonists are worthy of pursuing, since the antidepressant profiles as well as synaptic/neural mechanisms involved in the actions of mGlu2/3 receptor antagonists are similar to those of ketamine, which has been demonstrated to show potent, rapid and sustained efficacy in patients with depression, even those resistant to the conventionally prescribed antidepressants. In this chapter, the general pharmacology of mGlu2/3 receptor antagonists and their therapeutic potential are reviewed. In particular, I focus on the usefulness of mGlu2/3 receptor antagonists as novel antidepressants, in comparison with ketamine.

Advances in Pharmacology, Volume 86
ISSN 1054-3589
https://doi.org/10.1016/bs.apha.2019.03.004

Abbreviations

AD	Alzheimer's disease
AMPA	α-amino-3-hydroxy-5-methyl-isoxazole-4-propionate
BDNF	brain-derived neurotrophic factor
fEPSP	field excitatory postsynaptic potential
GABA	γ-aminobutyric acid
LAC	L-acetylcarnitine
MDD	major depressive disorder
mGlu receptor	metabotropic glutamate receptor
mPFC	medial prefrontal cortex
mTORC1	mammalian target of rapamycin complex 1
NAM	negative allosteric modulator
NMDA	*N*-methyl-D-aspartate
OCD	obsessive-convulsive disorder
PAM	positive allosteric modulator
TRD	treatment-resistant depression
TrkB	tropomyosin-related kinase B

1. Introduction

Glutamate is the major excitatory neurotransmitter in the brain, and is involved in a wide range of physiological functions of the central nervous system (CNS), including emotion, cognition, and motor functions. At present, glutamate receptors are classified into two major types: ionotropic glutamate (iGlu) receptors, represented by receptors having an ion channel structure, and metabotropic glutamate (mGlu) receptors, representing the receptors that are coupled to G-proteins (Nakanishi, 1992). mGlu receptors belong to class C G-protein-coupled receptors (GPCRs), and compared to other conventional GPCRs (class A and class B GPCRs), have a relatively larger N-terminal extracellular domain which confers them with the properties of glutamate binding, agonist activation of the glutamate receptor, and receptor subtype selectivity. The iGlu receptors are also classified into *N*-methyl-D-aspartate (NMDA), α-amino-3-hydroxy-5-methyl-isoxazole-4-propionate (AMPA), and kainate receptors (Nakanishi, 1992). In addition to the iGlu receptor subtypes, which facilitate fast synaptic transmission, mGlu receptors also have eight subtypes (mGlu1-mGlu8). The eight mGlu receptor subtypes are currently classified into three groups based on their sequence homology, second messenger coupling and pharmacological characteristics (Conn & Pin, 1997; Schoepp & Conn, 1993). The group I mGlu receptors include mGlu1 and mGlu5, which are coupled to phospholipase C, while both group II (mGlu2, mGlu3) and group III (mGlu4, mGlu6, mGlu7, mGlu8) mGlu receptors are negatively coupled to adenylyl cyclase activity. Among the mGlu receptors, a growing body of evidence suggests that the mGlu2/3 and mGlu5 receptors may serve as potential therapeutic targets for psychiatric disorders, including schizophrenia (Chaki, 2010; Stansley & Conn, 2018), depression (Chaki, Ago, Palucha-Paniewiera, Matrisciano, & Pilc, 2013; Pilc, Chaki, Nowak, & Witkin, 2008) and anxiety disorders (Palucha & Pilc, 2007). Localization, physiological functions and pharmacological properties of each receptor subtype are summarized in Table 1. In this chapter, I focus on the mGlu2 and mGlu3 receptors, and review mGlu2/3 receptor antagonists and their therapeutic potential, in particular, for the treatment of depression. In regard to the therapeutic potential of mGlu5 receptor antagonists for neuropsychiatric disorders, please refer to the cited review articles (Pałucha-Poniewiera et al., 2013; Stansley & Conn, 2018).

2. mGlu2/3 receptors—Localization and molecular properties

mGlu2 and mGlu3 receptors are coupled to Gi/Go to negatively regulate adenylyl cyclase activity, and are also well positioned, both anatomically and physiologically, to regulate the activities of glutamate and other neurotransmitters within the CNS in brain regions associated with the control of mood and cognition. High mRNA expression levels and immunoreactivity of mGlu2 receptor have been observed in the pyramidal neurons of the cerebral cortex, hippocampus (granule cells of the dentate gyrus) and olfactory bulb (Neki et al., 1996; Ohishi, Shigemoto, Nakanishi, & Mizuno, 1993a), while mGlu3 receptor mRNA is predominantly expressed in neurons of the thalamic nuclei, cerebral cortex, amygdaloid nuclei and granule cells of the dentate gyrus (Ohishi, Shigemoto, Nakanishi, & Mizuno, 1993b; Tanabe et al., 1993). Receptor mapping using selective radiolabeled ligands of mGlu2/3 receptors also revealed that the mGlu2/3 receptors are highly localized in the cortical and limbic regions (Schaffhauser, Richards, et al., 1998; Wright et al., 2013). In these brain regions, the mGlu2 receptor is mainly localized at the perisynaptic position, functioning as an autoreceptor or heteroreceptor (Shigemoto et al., 1997), while the mGlu3 receptor is localized at presynaptic/postsynaptic sites, as well as on glial cells (Ohishi et al., 1993b). The major function of the presynaptic mGlu2/3 receptors

Table 1 Signaling, localization and functions of mGlu receptor subtypes.

	Group I		Group II		Group III			
Receptor	**mGlu1**	**mGlu5**	**mGlu2**	**mGlu3**	**mGlu4**	**mGlu6**	**mGlu7**	**mGlu8**
Signaling	Gq/11 (PLC↑)	Gq/11 (PLC↑)	Gi/o (AC↓)	Gi/o (AC↓)	Gi/o (AC↓)	Gi/o (AC↓)	Gi/o (AC↓)	Gi/o (AC↓)
Distribution/ cell type	Cerebellum Olfactory bulb Hippocampus (neurons)	Cortex hippocampus Caudate-putamen (neurons, glial cells)	Cortex Hippocampus (neurons)	Cortex Hippocampus Amygdala (neurons, glial cells)	Cerebellum (neurons)	Retina (ON bipolar cells)	Cortex Hippocampus Amygdala (neurons)	Olfactory bulb Cortex (neurons)
Physiological functions	Primarily postsynaptic localization Positive modulation of glutamate and GABA transmission	Primarily postsynaptic localization Positive modulation of glutamate and GABA transmission	Perisynaptic and postsynaptic localization Negative modulation of glutamate and GABA transmission	Primary localization of postsynaptic to neurons and in glia	Presynaptic and postsynaptic localization Negative modulation of glutamate and GABA transmission	Regulation of visual sensory information processing	Presynaptic and postsynaptic localization Negative modulation of glutamate and GABA transmission	Presynaptic and postsynaptic localization Negative modulation of glutamate transmission
Pharmacological tools	DHPG (agonist) JNJ16567083 (NAM) LY367385 (NAM)	CHPG (agonist) ADX47273 (PAM) Basimglurant (NAM)	LY404039 (agonist) MGS0008 (agonist) Decoglurant (NAM) LY341495 (antagonist) MGS0039 (antagonist)	LY404039 (agonist) MGS0008 (agonist) Decoglurant (NAM) LY341495 (antagonist) MGS0039 (antagonist)	LSP4-2022 (agonist) ADX88178 (PAM) CPPG (antagonist)	HomoAMPA (agonist) CPPG (antagonist)	LSP4-2022 (agonist) AMN082 (allosteric agonist) MMPIP (NAM) ADX71743 (NAM)	LSP4-2022 (agonist) ADX88178 (PAM) LY341495 (antagonist)

is to inhibit the release of glutamate, as autoreceptors. Indeed, electrophysiological investigations on hippocampal slices have indicated that the mGlu2/3 receptor agonists, LY354740 and DCG-IV, presynaptically inhibited the field excitatory postsynaptic potential (fEPSP) in the dentate gyrus induced by the stimulation of perforant paths (Higgins et al., 2004; Hiyoshi et al., 2014) and reduced ketamine-induced cortical γ band oscillation in the rat cortical electroencephalogram (Hiyoshi et al., 2014). Notably, the inhibitory effect of LY354740 on the evoked fEPSP in the mid-molecular layer of the dentate gyrus or CA1 stratum lacunosum moleculare was attenuated in mGlu2 receptor-knockout mice (Higgins et al., 2004), suggesting that these inhibitory effects of the mGlu2/3 receptor agonists are mainly mediated through stimulation of the mGlu2 receptor. In addition to regulating glutamate release, mGlu2/3 receptor agonists also negatively regulate the release of other neurotransmitters, such as γ-aminobutyric acid (GABA) (Neale & Salt, 2006; Schaffhauser, Knoflach, et al., 1998), via a presynaptic mechanism. Conversely, blockade of the mGlu2/3 receptors causes a relative increase in the release of neurotransmitters, including glutamate, via blockade of their functions as auto- or hetero-receptors. Although the roles of the mGlu3 receptor expressed on the glial cells have not yet been fully elucidated, the mGlu3 receptor expressed on astrocytes may be involved in neuroprotective actions (Durand, Carniglia, Caruso, & Lasaga, 2013), while it also known to increase the release of the inflammatory cytokine interleukin-6 in the presence of interleukin-1β (Aronica, Gorter, Rozemuller, Yankaya, & Troost, 2005).

3. Pharmacology of mGlu2/3 receptor antagonists

There are two groups of mGlu2/3 receptor antagonists that interact with different sites of the mGlu2/3 receptors: the orthosteric mGlu2/3 receptor antagonists, which bind to the N-terminus of the receptors, and the negative allosteric modulators (NAMs) which bind to the allosteric sites on the receptor, where amino acid sequences are less highly conserved across the mGlu receptor subtypes (Fig. 1). Based on molecular pharmacological studies using site-directed mutated receptors, the binding sites for the mGlu2 positive allosteric modulators (PAMs) have been demonstrated to be localized in transmembrane (TM) regions, including TM3, TM5 and TM6 (Farinha et al., 2015). Because it is presumed that the binding sites of the mGlu2 PAMs and NAMs may possibly overlap (Farinha et al., 2015; Lundström et al., 2011; O'Brien et al., 2018), mGlu2/3 NAMs

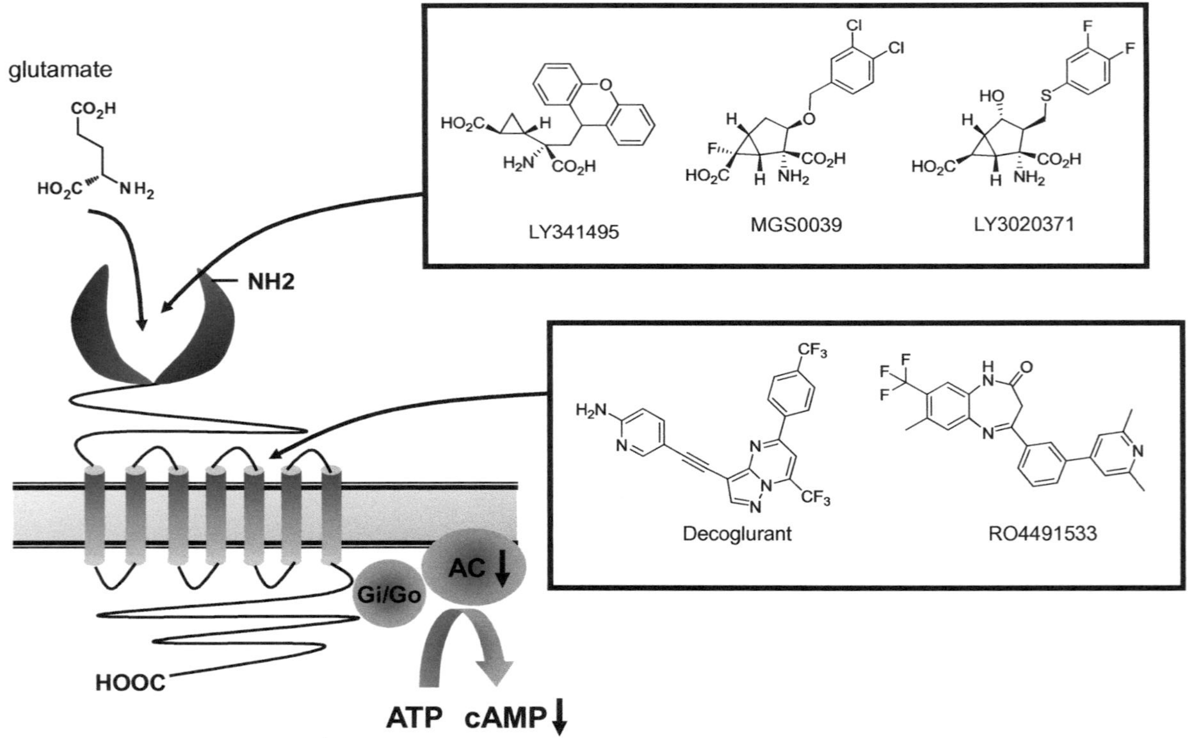

Fig. 1 Representative orthosteric and allosteric antagonists of mGlu2/3 receptor. Both mGlu2 and mGlu3 receptors belong to class C G-protein-coupled receptors, which have a relatively larger N-terminal extracellular domain to which an endogenous agonist glutamate bind. mGlu2 and mGlu3 receptors are coupled to Gi/Go to negatively regulate adenylyl cyclase activity. Orthosteric mGlu2/3 receptor antagonists, such as LY341495, MGS0039 and LY3020371, bind to the N-terminus of the receptors where they compete the binding of glutamate, while the negative allosteric modulators, such as decoglurant and RO4491533, bind to the allosteric sites on the receptor (transmembrane (TM) regions, presumably TM3, TM5 and TM6).

may bind to the same sites, although they may interact in a different manner with the sites (O'Brien et al., 2018). Among the mGlu2/3 receptor antagonists, three prototype mGlu2/3 receptor orthosteric antagonists have been widely utilized as pharmacological tools, MGS0039, LY341495 and LY3020371, all of which contain a glutamate moiety in their molecule. It should be noted that while LY341495 behaves as a pan-antagonist at multiple mGlu receptor subtypes (Kingston et al., 1998), MGS0039 and LY3020371 are more selective for the mGlu2/3 receptors (Chaki et al., 2004; Witkin, Ornstein, et al., 2017). Although most mGlu2/3 receptor NAMs exert practically equivalent antagonist activity on the mGlu2 receptor and mGlu3 receptor (Campo et al., 2011; Gleason et al., 2013), selective NAMs for the mGlu2 receptor and mGlu3 receptor have also recently been reported (Engers et al., 2017, 2015).

4. Depression and role of mGlu2/3 receptors in depression

Mood disorders, especially major depressive disorder (MDD), are among the most prevalent forms of mental illness. The economic burden of mood disorders is immense, amounting to about 100 billion USD in the United States and 105 billion Euros in the EU (Andlin-Sobocki, Jönsson, Wittchen, & Olesen, 2005; Greenberg et al., 2003), making this group of the disorders the most economically burdensome of all CNS diseases. All current antidepressant medications have stemmed from studies of the serendipitously discovered effects of the tricyclic antidepressants and the monoamine oxidase inhibitors, both of which exhibit their effects via modulation of monoamine neurotransmission. Indeed, the newer-generation antidepressants, such as the selective serotonin reuptake inhibitors (SSRIs) and serotonin- and noradrenaline reuptake inhibitors (SNRIs), have also been developed on the basis of these initial findings. Although the large majority of individuals with depression (about 70%) exhibit some improvement with antidepressant medication, remission is achieved in only about 50% of all patients (Rush et al., 2006). Moreover, it takes 3–6 weeks before the currently used antidepressant drugs begin to manifest any significant therapeutic effects. Therefore, novel targets, different from the monoaminergic system, have been sought for the development of newer antidepressants. Emerging evidence has suggested the role of the glutamatergic system in the development of depression (Sanacora, Treccani, & Popoli, 2012). Discovery of the antidepressant effect of ketamine, a non-competitive

N-methyl-D-aspartate (NMDA) receptor antagonist, highlights the importance of the glutamatergic system as a target for the treatment of depression. Indeed, ketamine has been reported to exert robust antidepressant activity in patients with MDD, including those who are resistant to treatment with conventional antidepressant agents, or so called treatment-resistant depression (TRD) (Berman et al., 2000; Newport et al., 2015; Zarate et al., 2006). In particular, ketamine is reported to exert rapid, sustained and robust antidepressant activity in patients with MDD, rapidly reducing suicidal ideation in these patients (Ionescu et al., 2016). Thus, modulation of glutamatergic transmission might be an effective approach for the treatment of depression, in particular, TRD.

Alterations of mGlu2/3 receptor expression have been demonstrated in depressed subjects and animal models of depression. Mice reared under isolated conditions, which displayed depressive-like behavior, were demonstrated to show increased mGlu2/3 receptor expression in the frontal cortex and hippocampus (Kawasaki et al., 2011). Consistent with this finding, postmortem investigations have also shown increased mGlu2/3 receptor expression levels in the prefrontal cortex of the brains of patients with MDD patients (Feyissa et al., 2010). In contrast, reduced mGlu2 receptor expression levels were found in the hippocampus in some rodent models of depression, such as models of Flinders sensitive line (Nasca et al., 2013), chronic unpredictable stress (CUS) (Nasca, Bigio, Zelli, Nicoletti, & McEwen, 2015), brain-derived neurotrophic factor (BDNF) (Val66Met) loss-of-function, and chronic restraint stress (Nasca, Zelli, et al., 2015). Interestingly, a subset of wild-type mice showing more depressive-like behavior after CUS showed lower brain mGlu2 expression levels as compared to other mice that were much less affected by CUS which showed higher brain mGlu2 expression (Nasca, Bigio, et al., 2015). Likewise, reduction of [^{3}H]LY341495 binding was demonstrated in the anterior cingulate cortex of the brain from MDD patients (McOmish et al., 2016).

5. Antidepressant effects of mGlu2/3 receptor antagonists

Antidepressant effects of mGlu2/3 receptor antagonists were reported for the first time in 2004 using MGS0039 and LY341495 (Chaki et al., 2004). Since then, a number of studies conducted in several animal models have demonstrated the antidepressant effects of mGlu2/3 receptor antagonists,

Table 2 Ketamine-like antidepressant profiles of mGlu2/3 receptor antagonists in rodent models.

Ketamine-like antidepressant profile	Model	mGlu2/3 receptor antagonist	Remarks
Rapid-acting, long-lasting	Chronic unpredictable stress model (rat, Sprague-Dawley)	LY341495	Onset of action (<1 day) lasted for >7 days
	Chronic social stress defeat model (mice, C57BL/6J)	MGS0039	Onset of action (<1 day) lasted for >7 days
	Tail suspension (mice, ICR)	MGS0039 LY341495	Lasted for >1 day
	Forced swimming test (rat, Sprague-Dawley)	LY341495	Lasted for >1 day
	Forced swimming test (mouse, C57BL/6J)	LY341495	Lasted for >1 day
Treatment-resistant	Learned helplessness (rat, Sprague-Dawley)	MGS0039	Effective
	Corticosterone-treatment (rat, Sprague-Dawley)	LY341495	Effective
	Corticosterone-treatment (mouse, ddY)	MGS0039	Effective
	Tail suspension test (Mouse, CD-1)	LY341495	Effective

using both mGlu2/3 receptor antagonists and mGlu2/3 receptor NAMs (Chaki, 2017). Importantly, the antidepressant profiles of mGlu2/3 receptor antagonists were similar to those of ketamine, as shown in Table 2. Indeed, MGS0039 and LY341495 were found to exert antidepressant effects within 24 h of administration in animal models (CUS model and chronic social defeat stress model), in which the effects of currently prescribed antidepressants have been shown to take a few weeks to manifest (Dong et al., 2017; Dwyer, Lepack, & Duman, 2013). Moreover, the antidepressant effects of these compounds lasted for at least a week after a single administration in these animal models. Therefore, mGlu2/3 receptor antagonists may also, like ketamine, have rapid-acting and long-lasting antidepressant effects. mGlu2/3 receptor antagonists have also been reported to exert antidepressant effects in animal models which are resistant to treatment with currently prescribed antidepressants, such as corticosterone-treated rodents (Ago et al., 2013; Koike, Iijima, & Chaki, 2013) and tail suspension test using CD-1 mice (Witkin et al., 2016). This characteristic of this class of drugs was also similar to that of ketamine. Of note, while mGlu2/3 receptor NAMs including RO4491533 have been reported to show antidepressant and anxiolytic effects in rodents (Campo et al., 2011), unlike orthosteric mGlu2/3 receptor antagonists, ketamine-like antidepressant profiles of mGlu2/3 receptor NAMs have not yet been demonstrated, and the potency of mGlu2/3 receptor NAMs is weaker than those of the orthosteric antagonists (Gleason et al., 2013). The discrepancy may be at least due to the different mechanism of antagonistic action against the mGlu2/3 receptor (orthosteric vs. allosteric). Indeed, different numbers of bindings of mGlu2/3 receptor radiolabeled ligands were reported between ligands bind to orthosteric site and allosteric site (Lavreysen et al., 2013).

The roles of the individual receptor subtype (mGlu2 or mGlu3 receptor) in the antidepressant actions of the mGlu2/3 receptor antagonists are still controversial. LY341495 no longer exerted antidepressant effect in knockout mice lacking mGlu2 receptor but still showed the effect in knockout mice lacking mGlu3 receptor (Gleason et al., 2013), suggesting that it is the mGlu2 receptor rather than the mGlu3 receptor that plays a critical role in the antidepressant actions of the mGlu2/3 receptor antagonists. In contrast, a selective mGlu3 receptor NAM was shown to exert both antidepressant (as assessed in the forced swimming test) and anxiolytic effects (as assessed from their marble-burying behavior) in rodent models (Engers et al., 2015). In another study, while a selective mGlu3 receptor NAM exerted an antidepressant effect comparable to that of ketamine (as assessed in the tail suspension test), a selective mGlu2 receptor NAM failed to show any significant effect at the appropriate exposure level (Engers et al., 2017), indicating a greater contribution of mGlu3 blockade in the antidepressant effects exerted by the mGlu2/3 receptor NAMs. Interestingly, functional interaction between postsynaptic mGlu3 receptor and mGlu5 receptor has been reported (Di Menna et al., 2018). Thus, mGlu3 receptor stimulation potentiated mGlu5 receptor-mediated signaling and mGlu3 and mGlu5 receptor synergized to induce long-term depression in the prefrontal cortex. Given that mGlu5 receptor antagonists have been shown to induce antidepressant effects in rodents (Chaki et al., 2013), functional blockade of mGlu5 receptor via mGlu3 receptor may contribute to the antidepressant effects.

A series of studies have revealed that the synaptic and neural mechanisms underlying the antidepressant effects of mGlu2/3 receptor antagonists are similar to those underlying the effect of ketamine. Both mGlu2/3 receptor antagonists and ketamine have been reported to normalize the reduced spine density through BDNF/tropomyosin-related kinase B (TrkB) signaling and subsequent activation of mechanistic target of rapamycin complex 1 (mTORC1) signaling, triggered by AMPA receptor stimulation (Dong et al., 2017; Dwyer, Lepack, & Duman, 2012; Koike, Fukumoto, Iijima, & Chaki, 2013; Koike, Iijima, & Chaki, 2011; Li et al., 2010, 2011) (Fig. 2). Because mGlu2/3 receptors expressed at the perisynaptic position of the glutamatergic nerve terminals negatively regulate the release of glutamate, the increase in glutamate release by mGlu2/3 receptor blockade may stimulate the postsynaptic AMPA receptor, while ketamine is presumed to increase glutamate release by disinhibition of pyramidal neurons (Krystal, Sanacora, & Duman, 2013). In addition to transient stimulation of the AMPA receptor, increased expression of the AMPA receptor may be required for mGlu2/3 receptor antagonists to exert their antidepressant effects (Koike & Chaki, 2014). In addition to sharing synaptic mechanisms involved in their antidepressant effects, it has been reported that mGlu2/3 receptor antagonists and ketamine also share their actions on the monoaminergic system (Fig. 2). It has been reported that mGlu2/3 receptor antagonists increased the number of spontaneously active dopamine neurons in the ventral tegmental area and increased the extracellular dopamine level in the medial prefrontal cortex (mPFC) and nucleus accumbens, and these effects were blocked by an AMPA receptor antagonist (Karasawa, Kotani, Kambe, & Chaki, 2010; Witkin, Mitchell, et al., 2017; Witkin et al., 2016). Thus, mGlu2/3 receptor antagonists positively regulate the mesolimbic and mesocortical dopaminergic systems, which are involved in reward and mood, through AMPA receptor stimulation. Consistent with this mechanism, mGlu2/3 receptor antagonists potentiated dopamine receptor agonist-increased locomotor activity (Witkin et al., 2016) and reversed depressive-like behavior induced by withdrawal from chronic administration of methamphetamine by acting in the nucleus accumbens (Iijima, Koike, & Chaki, 2013). In addition to acting on the dopaminergic system, mGlu2/3 receptor antagonists also increases the activity of the serotonergic system, which also has been proposed to have a critical role in its antidepressant actions. mGlu2/3 receptor antagonists have been shown to increase serotonergic neuronal activity in the dorsal raphe nucleus (Fukumoto, Iijima, & Chaki, 2016; Kawashima et al., 2005) and

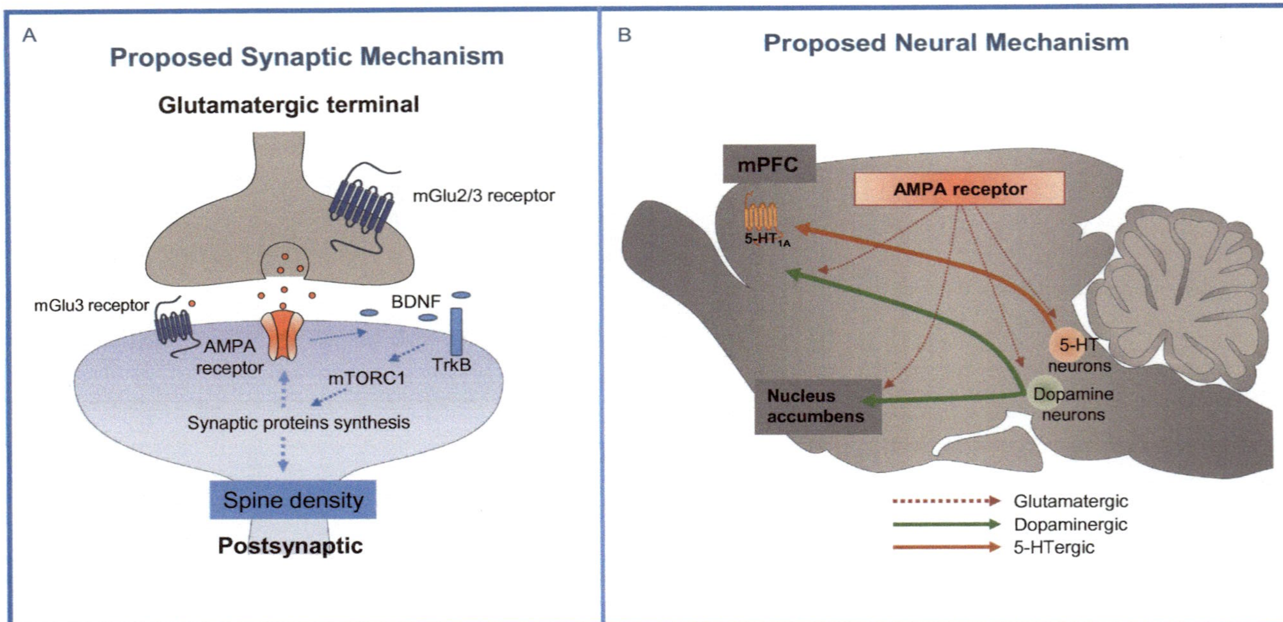

Fig. 2 Proposed synaptic (A) and neural (B) mechanisms of mGlu2/3 receptor antagonists. (A) mGlu2/3 receptor antagonist relatively increases synaptic glutamate release by blockade of presynaptic autoreceptor. Glutamate released, then, activates postsynaptic AMPA receptor to increase brain-derived neurotrophic factor secretion and/or synthesis, which stimulate tropomyosin-related kinase B (TrkB). Stimulation of TrkB signaling leads to activate mechanistic target of rapamycin complex 1 signaling to increase translation of synaptic proteins including GluR1, and subsequently to increase spine density. Additionally, mGlu3 receptors are localized in postsynapse where they interact with mGlu5 receptor. (B) mGlu2/3 receptor antagonist, via the AMPA receptor transmission, also activates dopamine neuronal activity in the ventral tegmental area and 5-HT neurons in the dorsal raphe nucleus. Consequently, dopamine release is increased in the medial prefrontal cortex (mPFC) and nucleus accumbens, and 5-HT release is increased in the mPFC. Stimulation of the mPFC 5-HT_{1A} receptor by increased 5-HT is also involved in the antidepressant actions of mGlu2/3 receptor antagonists.

extracellular serotonin levels in the medial prefrontal cortex (Karasawa, Shimazaki, Kawashima, & Chaki, 2005; Kawashima et al., 2005), both of which are mediated via AMPA receptor stimulation. It was further postulated that stimulation of the mPFC 5-HT_{1A} receptor, presumably stimulated by increased serotonin levels, mediates the actions of the mGlu2/3 receptor antagonist (Fukumoto, Iijima, Funakoshi, & Chaki, 2018a). All the above-mentioned actions on the monoaminergic systems have also been observed with ketamine. Notably, both depletion of serotonin and blockade of the 5-HT_{1A} receptor abrogated the antidepressant effects of both mGlu2/3 receptor antagonists and ketamine (Fukumoto, Iijima, & Chaki, 2014; Fukumoto, Iijima, Funakoshi, & Chaki, 2018b), indicating the involvement of the serotonergic system in the antidepressant effects of both mGlu2/3 receptor antagonists and ketamine. On the other hand, the mGlu2/3 receptor antagonist did not activate noradrenaline neurons in the locus coeruleus (Kawashima et al., 2005).

Because adverse effects and other limitations have limited the clinical usefulness of ketamine, development of an alternative treatment(s) that would act through similar biological mechanisms has been sought. Unlike ketamine, mGlu2/3 receptor antagonists do not increase locomotor activity or impair cognition, their use is not associated with abuse potential (Witkin, Monn, et al., 2017). Based on these findings, mGlu2/3 receptor antagonists could be developed as novel antidepressants with similar efficacy to ketamine, but without the unwanted side effects. Notably, combination of sub-effective doses of ketamine and LY341495 has been reported to induce significant antidepressant effects, both at 40 min and 24 h after administration (Podkowa, Pochwat, Brański, Pilc, & Pałucha-Poniewiera, 2016). Therefore, mGlu2/3 receptor antagonists can be used to reduce doses of ketamine, which mitigates side effects of ketamine.

To date, two mGlu2/3 receptor antagonists have been tested in clinical studies. Safety profiles of BCI-838, a prodrug of BCI-632 (MGS0039), was tested in Phase I study (Gadient et al., 2012). BCI-838 was well tolerated in both single ascending dose and multiple ascending dose studies. In addition, BCI-838 showed dose-dependent effects on EEG signal in the quantitative EEG study, indicating brain penetration. Efficacy data is not available for BCI-838. Moreover, a double-blinded, placebo-controlled study of decoglurant, an mGlu2/3 receptor NAM, was conducted in patients with MDD who were inadequately treated with antidepressants (Umbricht et al., 2015). Decoglurant demonstrated an insufficient efficacy on both primary (mean change in MADRS score) and secondary outcomes (proportion of patients exhibiting remission or response based on the MADRS score). However, because appropriateness of the trial has not been fully discussed, the results of this trial is not conclusive and other trials using different compounds are needed to prove whether mGlu2/3 receptor blockade would be beneficial for the treatment of depression.

Meanwhile, it should be noted that stimulation of the mGlu2/3 receptors could also be associated with antidepressant effects, while early findings revealed that LY354740, an mGlu2/3 receptor agonist, did not show antidepressant effects in the forced swimming test and tail suspension test (Kłodzińska et al., 1999). An mGlu2 receptor PAM, THIIC, has been shown to exert antidepressant effects in three animal models of depression (as assessed by the mouse forced swimming test, the rat differential reinforcement of low rate 72-s assay, and the rat dominant-submissive test) (Fell et al., 2011). The antidepressant effects of THIIC were no longer observed in knockout mice lacking mGlu2 receptor, suggesting that this effect is mediated through the mGlu2 receptor. Moreover, L-acetylcarnitine (LAC) exhibited an antidepressant effect in genetic (Flinders sensitive line) and environmental (CUS model) animal models much earlier than the currently medications (Nasca et al., 2013). LAC has been shown to increase mGlu2 receptor expression in the hippocampus and prefrontal cortex, and the antidepressant effect of LAC was partially attenuated in mGlu2 receptor-knockout mice and by an mGlu2/3 receptor antagonist, suggesting that LAC exerted its effect through increased mGlu2 receptor expression. Collectively, these findings suggest that stimulation of mGlu2 receptor signaling may be effective for the treatment of depression. However, it should also be noted that reports on the antidepressant effects of mGlu2 receptor agonists/PAMs are limited, and that the role of mGlu2 receptor stimulation in the antidepressant actions of some agents needs to be further investigated.

6. Anxiolytic effects of mGlu2/3 receptor antagonists

Several lines of evidence suggest that limbic glutamatergic neurotransmission also plays a pivotal role in the pathogenesis of anxiety disorders. To date, several lines of evidence have shown the anxiolytic effects of mGlu2/3 receptor agonists and mGlu2 receptor PAMs in numerous animal models of anxiety (Fell et al., 2011; Rorick-Kehn et al., 2007). In addition, LY544344 (a prodrug of LY354740) has been demonstrated to be effective for patients with generalized anxiety disorder (Dunayevich et al., 2008), although LY354740 failed to show efficacy in patients with panic disorder (Bergink & Westenberg, 2005). Thus, mGlu2/3 receptor activation has been proposed to be an effective strategy for the treatment of certain anxiety disorders. In contrast to these findings, mGlu2/3 receptor antagonists have also been reported to show anxiolytic effects in some animal models, such as in the marble-burying (Shimazaki, Iijima, & Chaki, 2004), fear-conditioning (Yoshimizu, Shimazaki, Ito, & Chaki, 2006), Vogel conflict (Stachowicz, Wierońska, Domin, Chaki, & Pilc, 2011), stress-induced hyperthermia (Iijima, Shimazaki, Ito, & Chaki, 2007) and novelty-suppressed feeding (Fukumoto et al., 2014). Interestingly, mGlu2/3 receptor antagonists are effective in models different from those in which mGlu2/3 receptor agonists have been shown to be effective. Therefore, both mGlu2/3 receptor agonists and antagonists may have potential roles in the treatment of different types of anxiety disorders. Experiments in some models suggest that the serotonergic system and 5-HT_{1A} receptor stimulation may have roles in the anxiolytic effects of mGlu2/3 receptor antagonists (Fukumoto et al., 2014; Iijima et al., 2007; Stachowicz et al., 2011). In addition, like in the case of the antidepressant effects of the mGlu2/3 receptor antagonists, AMPA receptor stimulation may also have an important role in the anxiolytic actions of mGlu2/3 receptor antagonists, as demonstrated in some models such as the marble-burying test (Shimazaki et al., 2004) and novelty-suppressed feeding test (Fukumoto et al., 2014). Notably, it has recently been reported that (*S*)-ketamine exerted an anxiolytic effect in mice showing marble-burying behavior via AMPA receptor stimulation (Tosta et al., 2018). Since the marble-burying behavior is considered as a characteristic of the animal model for obsessive-convulsive disorder (OCD), and glutamate-modulating drugs, including ketamine and rapastinel, both of which exert their activities via similar synaptic mechanisms to mGlu2/3 receptor antagonists, have been reported to be effective in patients with OCD (Marinova, Chuang, & Fineberg, 2017; Rodriguez et al., 2016), it would be of interest to identify the potential of mGlu2/3 receptor antagonists for the treatment of OCD. Moreover, recently, MGS0210, a pro-drug of MGS0039 (an mGlu2/3 receptor antagonist) has been reported to ameliorate post-traumatic stress disorder (PTSD)-like behavior in an animal model of blast-induced mild traumatic brain injury (Perez-Garcia et al., 2018). Given that an AMPA receptor potentiator may facilitate extinction of fear memory (Yamada, Wada, & Sekiguchi, 2011), it may be a reasonable strategy to use mGlu2/3 receptor antagonists for treatment of patients with PTSD.

7. Pro-cognitive effects of mGlu2/3 receptor antagonists

Pro-cognitive effects of mGlu2/3 receptor antagonists have been demonstrated in some animal models, such as the Morris water maze test (Higgins et al., 2004), social recognition test (Shimazaki, Kaku, & Chaki, 2007) and novel recognition test (Pitsikas, Kaffe, & Markou, 2012). Moreover, treatment with a selective mGlu2/3 receptor NAM, RO4432717, was shown to improve cognitive processes dependent upon effective functioning of the cortico-cortical and/or hippocampal regions (Goeldner et al., 2013). AMPA receptor stimulation may have a critical role in the pro-cognitive actions of mGlu2/3 receptor antagonists, because the pro-cognitive effects of MGS0039 in the social recognition test were reversed by an AMPA receptor antagonist (Shimazaki et al., 2007). Given that the AMPA receptor plays an important role in synaptic plasticity which is important for learning and memory, and there are several lines of evidence suggesting that AMPA receptor potentiators improved the cognitive performance in a variety of preclinical models (Black, 2005; Kunugi et al., 2019; Ward et al., 2017) and in patients with neuropsychiatric disorders (Koliaki, Messini, & Tsolaki, 2012; Marenco & Weinberger, 2006), it can be deduced that AMPA receptor stimulation is beneficial for pro-cognitive effects. Amelioration of amyloid β (Aβ)-associated abnormalities by mGlu2/3 receptor antagonists has also been suggested. Evidence suggests that aberrant accumulation of neurotoxic Aβ oligomers may underlie the cognitive dysfunctions in patients with Alzheimer's disease (AD). It has been reported that mGlu2/3 receptor stimulation triggered the production and release of Aβ42 peptides from isolated intact nerve terminals in TgCRND8 mice (expressing a human amyloid precursor protein with familial AD mutations), and that this event was counteracted by the mGlu2/3 receptor antagonist LY341495 (Kim et al., 2010). Moreover, the mGlu2 receptor PAM LY566332 has been reported to amplify Aβ-induced neurodegeneration, and this effect was prevented by LY341495 administration (Caraci et al., 2011). Consistent with these findings of vitro studies, chronic treatment with an mGlu2/3 receptor antagonist, MGS0210, for 3 months reversed transgene-related amnestic behavior, anxiety, as well as the brain Aβ monomer and oligomer levels in Dutch Aβ-oligomer-forming APP transgenic mice (APP E693Q) (Kim et al., 2014). Interestingly, 2-weeks treatment with MGS0039 significantly increased hippocampal neurogenesis in naïve mice (Yoshimizu & Chaki, 2004), and MGS0210 increased hippocampal neurogenesis more potently in Dutch APP mice than in wild-type (Kim et al., 2014). These findings are of particular interest, given the increased expression of the mGlu2 receptor in the regions and the cellular subtype of neural vulnerability to degeneration and neurofibrillary alterations in AD as compared to age-matched controls (Lee et al., 2004). Taken together, mGlu2/3 receptor antagonists have the potential to improve the cognitive dysfunctions observed in neuropsychiatric disorders, including AD.

8. Conclusions

Animal studies have shown that mGlu2/3 receptor antagonists have the potential to be developed as effective treatment agents for several neuropsychiatric disorders. In particular, recent studies have established that mGlu2/3 receptor antagonists possess antidepressant profiles similar to ketamine, which would satisfy the current unmet medical needs for depression therapy. Moreover, unlike ketamine, mGlu2/3 receptor antagonists do not appear to have any adverse effects, indicating their usefulness as an alternative to ketamine. Since anxiety and cognitive impairment are commonly encountered in patients with depression, and are associated with greater symptom severity and social functioning, the efficacy of these agents for these symptoms also is considered to be advantageous for the treatment of depression. Although one of mGlu2/3 receptor NAMs, decoglurant, failed to show efficacy in patients with MDD who did not show adequate response to treatment with SSRIs and SNRIs, this does not necessarily deny potential of mGlu2/3 receptor antagonists. The compound properties and study designs, including the dose-setting and patient stratification, should be carefully reviewed/set. Human proof-of-concept studies with appropriate compounds and study designs are expected to clarify the potential of mGlu2/3 receptor antagonists for clinical use in patients with neuropsychiatric disorders.

Acknowledgments

The author acknowledges Dr. Dai Nozawa for his artwork in Fig. 1.

Conflict of interest statement

S.C. is an employee of Taisho Pharmaceutical Co., Ltd.

References

Ago, Y., Yano, K., Araki, R., Hiramatsu, N., Kita, Y., Kawasaki, T., et al. (2013). Metabotropic glutamate 2/3 receptor antagonists improve behavioral and prefrontal dopaminergic alterations in the chronic corticosterone-induced depression model in mice. *Neuropharmacology, 65*, 29–38.

Andlin-Sobocki, P., Jönsson, B., Wittchen, H. U., & Olesen, J. (2005). Cost of disorders of the brain in Europe. *European Journal of Neurology, 12*, 1–27.

Aronica, E., Gorter, J. A., Rozemuller, A. J., Yankaya, B., & Troost, D. (2005). Activation of metabotropic glutamate receptor 3 enhances interleukin (IL)-1beta-stimulated release of IL-6 in cultured human astrocytes. *Neuroscience, 130*, 927–933.

Bergink, V., & Westenberg, H. G. (2005). Metabotropic glutamate II receptor agonists in panic disorder: A double blind clinical trial with LY354740. *International Clinical Psychopharmacology, 20*, 291–293.

Berman, R. M., Cappiello, A., Anand, A., Oren, D. A., Heninger, G. R., Charney, D. S., et al. (2000). Antidepressant effects of ketamine in depressed patients. *Biological Psychiatry, 47*, 351–354.

Black, M. D. (2005). Therapeutic potential of positive AMPA modulators and their relationship to AMPA receptor subunits. A review of preclinical data. *Psychopharmacology, 179*, 154–163.

Campo, B., Kalinichev, M., Lambeng, N., El Yacoubi, M., Royer-Urios, I., Schneider, M., et al. (2011). Characterization of an mGluR2/3 negative allosteric modulator in rodent models of depression. *Journal of Neurogenetics, 25*, 152–166.

Caraci, F., Molinaro, G., Battaglia, G., Giuffrida, M. L., Riozzi, B., Traficante, A., et al. (2011). Targeting group II metabotropic glutamate (mGlu) receptors for the treatment of psychosis associated with Alzheimer's disease: Selective activation of mGlu2 receptors amplifies beta-amyloid toxicity in cultured neurons, whereas dual activation of mGlu2 and mGlu3 receptors is neuroprotective. *Molecular Pharmacology, 79*, 618–626.

Chaki, S. (2010). Group II metabotropic glutamate receptor agonists as a potential drug for schizophrenia. *European Journal of Pharmacology, 639*, 59–66.

Chaki, S. (2017). mGlu2/3 receptor antagonists as novel antidepressants. *Trends in Pharmacological Sciences, 38*, 569–580.

Chaki, S., Ago, Y., Palucha-Paniewiera, A., Matrisciano, F., & Pilc, A. (2013). mGlu2/3 and mGlu5 receptors: Potential targets for novel antidepressants. *Neuropharmacology, 66*, 40–52.

Chaki, S., Yoshikawa, R., Hirota, S., Shimazaki, T., Maeda, M., Kawashima, N., et al. (2004). MGS0039: A potent and selective group II metabotropic glutamate receptor antagonist with antidepressant-like activity. *Neuropharmacology, 46*, 457–467.

Conn, P. J., & Pin, J. P. (1997). Pharmacology and functions of metabotropic glutamate receptors. *Annual Review of Pharmacology and Toxicology, 37*, 205–237.

Di Menna, L., Joffe, M. E., Iacovelli, L., Orlando, R., Lindsley, C. W., Mairesse, J., et al. (2018). Functional partnership between mGlu3 and mGlu5 metabotropic glutamate receptors in the central nervous system. *Neuropharmacology, 128*, 301–313.

Dong, C., Zhang, J. C., Yao, W., Ren, Q., Ma, M., Yang, C., et al. (2017). Rapid and sustained antidepressant action of the mGlu2/3 receptor antagonist MGS0039 in the social defeat stress model: Comparison with ketamine. *International Journal of Neuropsychopharmacology, 20*, 228–236.

Dunayevich, E., Erickson, J., Levine, L., Landbloom, R., Schoepp, D. D., & Tollefson, G. D. (2008). Efficacy and tolerability of an mGlu2/3 agonist in the treatment of generalized anxiety disorder. *Neuropsychopharmacology, 33*, 1603–1610.

Durand, D., Carniglia, L., Caruso, C., & Lasaga, M. (2013). mGlu3 receptor and astrocytes: Partners in neuroprotection. *Neuropharmacology, 66*, 1–11.

Dwyer, J. M., Lepack, A. E., & Duman, R. S. (2012). mTOR activation is required for the antidepressant effects of mGluR2/3 blockade. *International Journal of Neuropsychopharmacology*, *15*, 429–434.

Dwyer, J. M., Lepack, A. E., & Duman, R. S. (2013). mGluR2/3 blockade produces rapid and long-lasting reversal of anhedonia caused by chronic stress exposure. *Journal of Molecular Psychiatry*, *1*, 15.

Engers, J. L., Bollinger, K. A., Weiner, R. L., Rodriguez, A. L., Long, M. F., Breiner, M. M., et al. (2017). Design and synthesis of N-aryl phenoxyethoxy pyridinones as highly selective and CNS penetrant mGlu3 NAMs. *ACS Medicinal Chemistry Letters*, *8*, 925–930.

Engers, J. L., Rodriguez, A. L., Konkol, L. C., Morrison, R. D., Thompson, A. D., Byers, F. W., et al. (2015). Discovery of a selective and CNS penetrant negative allosteric modulator of metabotropic glutamate receptor subtype 3 with antidepressant and anxiolytic activity in rodents. *Journal of Medicinal Chemistry*, *58*, 7485–7500.

Farinha, A., Lavreysen, H., Peeters, L., Russo, B., Masure, S., Trabanco, A. A., et al. (2015). Molecular determinants of positive allosteric modulation of the human metabotropic glutamate receptor 2. *British Journal of Pharmacology*, *172*, 2383–2396.

Fell, M. J., Witkin, J. M., Falcone, J. F., Katner, J. S., Perry, K. W., Hart, J., et al. (2011). N-(4-((2-(Trifluoromethyl)-3-hydroxy-4-(isobutyryl)phenoxy)methyl)benzyl)-1-methyl-1H-imidazole-4-carboxamide (THIIC), a novel metabotropic glutamate 2 potentiator with potential anxiolytic/antidepressant properties: In vivo profiling suggests a link between behavioral and central nervous system neurochemical changes. *Journal of Pharmacology and Experimental Therapeutics*, *336*, 165–177.

Feyissa, A. M., Woolverton, W. L., Miguel-Hidalgo, J. J., Wang, Z., Kyle, P. B., Hasler, G., et al. (2010). Elevated level of metabotropic glutamate receptor 2/3 in the prefrontal cortex in major depression. *Progress in Neuro-Psychopharmacology & Biological Psychiatry*, *34*, 279–283.

Fukumoto, K., Iijima, M., & Chaki, S. (2014). Serotonin-1A receptor stimulation mediates effects of a metabotropic glutamate 2/3 receptor antagonist, 2S-2-amino-2-(1S,2S-2-carboxycycloprop-1-yl)-3-(xanth-9-yl)propanoic acid (LY341495), and an N-methyl-D-aspartate receptor antagonist, ketamine, in the novelty-suppressed feeding test. *Psychopharmacology*, *231*, 2291–2298.

Fukumoto, K., Iijima, M., & Chaki, S. (2016). The antidepressant effects of an mGlu2/3 receptor antagonist and ketamine require AMPA receptor stimulation in the mPFC and subsequent activation of the 5-HT neurons in the DRN. *Neuropsychopharmacology*, *41*, 1046–1056.

Fukumoto, K., Iijima, M., Funakoshi, T., & Chaki, S. (2018a). 5-HT1A receptor stimulation in the medial prefrontal cortex mediates the antidepressant effects of mGlu2/3 receptor antagonist in mice. *Neuropharmacology*, *137*, 96–103.

Fukumoto, K., Iijima, M., Funakoshi, T., & Chaki, S. (2018b). Role of 5-HT1A receptor stimulation in the medial prefrontal cortex in the sustained antidepressant effects of ketamine. *International Journal of Neuropsychopharmacology*, *21*, 371–381.

Gadient, R. A., Wedel, P. C., Frisbie, V. M., Leuchter, A. F., Targum, S. D., Truong, C. T., et al. (2012). Safety, pharmacokinetic and pharmacodynamics profile of BCI-632, a selective metabotropic glutamate 2/3 receptor antagonist, in healthy human subjects. In *Abstract of society for neuroscience*, 841.20.

Gleason, S. D., Li, X., Smith, I. A., Ephlin, J. D., Wang, X. S., Heinz, B. A., et al. (2013). mGlu2/3 agonist-induced hyperthermia: An in vivo assay for detection of mGlu2/3 receptor antagonism and its relation to antidepressant-like efficacy in mice. *CNS & Neurological Disorders—Drug Targets*, *12*, 554–566.

Goeldner, C., Ballard, T. M., Knoflach, F., Wichmann, J., Gatti, S., & Umbricht, D. (2013). Cognitive impairment in major depression and the mGlu2 receptor as a therapeutic target. *Neuropharmacology*, *64*, 337–346.

Greenberg, P. E., Kessler, R. C., Birnbaum, H. G., Leong, S. A., Lowe, S. W., Berglund, P. A., et al. (2003). The economic burden of depression in the United States: How did it change between 1990 and 2000? *Journal of Clinical Psychiatry*, *64*, 1465–1475.

Higgins, G. A., Ballard, T. M., Kew, J. N., Richards, J. G., Kemp, J. A., Adam, G., et al. (2004). Pharmacological manipulation of mGlu2 receptors influences cognitive performance in the rodent. *Neuropharmacology*, *46*, 907–917.

Hiyoshi, T., Marumo, T., Hikichi, H., Tomishima, Y., Urabe, H., Tamita, T., et al. (2014). Neurophysiologic and antipsychotic profiles of TASP0433864, a novel positive allosteric modulator of metabotropic glutamate 2 receptor. *Journal of Pharmacology and Experimental Therapeutics*, *351*, 642–653.

Iijima, M., Koike, H., & Chaki, S. (2013). Effect of an mGlu2/3 receptor antagonist on depressive behavior induced by withdrawal from chronic treatment with methamphetamine. *Behavioural Brain Research*, *246*, 24–28.

Iijima, M., Shimazaki, T., Ito, A., & Chaki, S. (2007). Effects of metabotropic glutamate 2/3 receptor antagonists in the stress-induced hyperthermia test in singly housed mice. *Psychopharmacology*, *190*, 233–239.

Ionescu, D. F., Swee, M. B., Pavone, K. J., Taylor, N., Akeju, O., Baer, L., et al. (2016). Rapid and sustained reductions in current suicidal ideation following repeated doses of intravenous ketamine: Secondary analysis of an open-label study. *Journal of Clinical Psychiatry*, *77*, 719–725.

Karasawa, J., Kotani, M., Kambe, D., & Chaki, S. (2010). AMPA receptor mediates mGlu 2/3 receptor antagonist-induced dopamine release in the rat nucleus accumbens shell. *Neurochemistry International*, *57*, 615–619.

Karasawa, J., Shimazaki, T., Kawashima, N., & Chaki, S. (2005). AMPA receptor stimulation mediates the antidepressant-like effect of a group II metabotropic glutamate receptor antagonist. *Brain Research*, *1042*, 92–98.

Kawasaki, T., Ago, Y., Yano, K., Araki, R., Washida, Y., Onoe, H., et al. (2011). Increased binding of cortical and hippocampal group II metabotropic glutamate receptors in isolation-reared mice. *Neuropharmacology*, *60*, 397–404.

Kawashima, N., Karasawa, J., Shimazaki, T., Chaki, S., Okuyama, S., Yasuhara, A., et al. (2005). Neuropharmacological profiles of antagonists of group II metabotropic glutamate receptors. *Neuroscience Letters*, *378*, 131–134.

Kim, S. H., Fraser, P. E., Westaway, D., St George-Hyslop, P. H., Ehrlich, M. E., & Gandy, S. (2010). Group II metabotropic glutamate receptor stimulation triggers production and release of Alzheimer's amyloid(beta)42 from isolated intact nerve terminals. *Journal of Neuroscience*, *30*, 3870–3875.

Kim, S. H., Steele, J. W., Lee, S. W., Clemenson, G. D., Carter, T. A., Treuner, K., et al. (2014). Proneurogenic group II mGluR antagonist improves learning and reduces anxiety in Alzheimer Aβ oligomer mouse. *Molecular Psychiatry*, *19*, 1235–1242.

Kingston, A. E., Ornstein, P. L., Wright, R. A., Johnson, B. G., Mayne, N. G., Burnett, J. P., et al. (1998). LY341495 is a nanomolar potent and selective antagonist of group II metabotropic glutamate receptors. *Neuropharmacology*, *37*, 1–12.

Kłodzińska, A., Chojnacka-Wójcik, E., Pałucha, A., Brański, P., Popik, P., & Pilc, A. (1999). Potential anti-anxiety, anti-addictive effects of LY 354740, a selective group II glutamate metabotropic receptors agonist in animal models. *Neuropharmacology*, *38*, 1831–1839.

Koike, H., & Chaki, S. (2014). Requirement of AMPA receptor stimulation for the sustained antidepressant activity of ketamine and LY341495 during the forced swim test in rats. *Behavioural Brain Research*, *271*, 111–115.

Koike, H., Fukumoto, K., Iijima, M., & Chaki, S. (2013). Role of BDNF/TrkB signaling in antidepressant-like effects of a group II metabotropic glutamate receptor antagonist in animal models of depression. *Behavioural Brain Research*, *238*, 48–52.

Koike, H., Iijima, M., & Chaki, S. (2011). Involvement of the mammalian target of rapamycin signaling in the antidepressant-like effect of group II metabotropic glutamate receptor antagonists. *Neuropharmacology, 61*, 1419–1423.
Koike, H., Iijima, M., & Chaki, S. (2013). Effects of ketamine and LY341495 on the depressive-like behavior of repeated corticosterone-injected rats. *Pharmacology, Biochemistry and Behavior, 107*, 20–23.
Koliaki, C. C., Messini, C., & Tsolaki, M. (2012). Clinical efficacy of aniracetam, either as monotherapy or combined with cholinesterase inhibitors, in patients with cognitive impairment: A comparative open study. *CNS Neuroscience & Therapeutics, 18*, 302–312.
Krystal, J. H., Sanacora, G., & Duman, R. S. (2013). Rapid-acting glutamatergic antidepressants: The path to ketamine and beyond. *Biological Psychiatry, 73*, 1133–1141.
Kunugi, A., Tanaka, M., Suzuki, A., Tajima, Y., Suzuki, N., Suzuki, M., et al. (2019). TAK-137, an AMPA-R potentiator with little agonistic effect, has a wide therapeutic window. *Neuropsychopharmacology, 44*, 961–970. https://doi.org/10.1038/s41386-018-0213-7.
Lavreysen, H., Langlois, X., Ahnaou, A., Drinkenburg, W., te Riele, P., Biesmans, I., et al. (2013). Pharmacological characterization of JNJ-40068782, a new potent, selective, and systemically active positive allosteric modulator of the mGlu2 receptor and its radioligand [3H]JNJ-40068782. *Journal of Pharmacology and Experimental Therapeutics, 346*, 514–527.
Lee, H. G., Ogawa, O., Zhu, X., O'Neill, M. J., Petersen, R. B., Castellani, R. J., et al. (2004). Aberrant expression of metabotropic glutamate receptor 2 in the vulnerable neurons of Alzheimer's disease. *Acta Neuropathologica, 107*, 365–371.
Li, N., Lee, B., Liu, R. J., Banasr, M., Dwyer, J. M., Iwata, M., et al. (2010). mTOR-dependent synapse formation underlies the rapid antidepressant effects of NMDA antagonists. *Science, 329*, 959–964.
Li, N., Liu, R. J., Dwyer, J. M., Banasr, M., Lee, B., Son, H., et al. (2011). Glutamate N-methyl-D-aspartate receptor antagonists rapidly reverse behavioral and synaptic deficits caused by chronic stress exposure. *Biological Psychiatry, 69*, 754–761.
Lundström, L., Bissantz, C., Beck, J., Wettstein, J. G., Woltering, T. J., Wichmann, J., et al. (2011). Structural determinants of allosteric antagonism at metabotropic glutamate receptor 2: Mechanistic studies with new potent negative allosteric modulators. *British Journal of Pharmacology, 164*, 521–537.
Marenco, S., & Weinberger, D. R. (2006). Therapeutic potential of positive AMPA receptor modulators in the treatment of neuropsychiatric disorders. *CNS Drugs, 20*, 173–185.
Marinova, Z., Chuang, D. M., & Fineberg, N. (2017). Glutamate-modulating drugs as a potential therapeutic strategy in obsessive-compulsive disorder. *Current Neuropharmacology, 15*, 977–995.
McOmish, C. E., Pavey, G., Gibbons, A., Hopper, S., Udawela, M., Scarr, E., et al. (2016). Lower [3H]LY341495 binding to mGlu2/3 receptors in the anterior cingulate of subjects with major depressive disorder but not bipolar disorder or schizophrenia. *Journal of Affective Disorders, 190*, 241–248.
Nakanishi, S. (1992). Molecular diversity of glutamate receptors and implications for brain function. *Science, 258*, 597–603.
Nasca, C., Bigio, B., Zelli, D., Nicoletti, F., & McEwen, B. S. (2015). Mind the gap: Glucocorticoids modulate hippocampal glutamate tone underlying individual differences in stress susceptibility. *Molecular Psychiatry, 20*, 755–763.
Nasca, C., Xenos, D., Barone, Y., Caruso, A., Scaccianoce, S., Matrisciano, F., et al. (2013). L-Acetylcarnitine causes rapid antidepressant effects through the epigenetic induction of mGlu2 receptors. *Proceedings of the National Academy of Sciences of the United States of America, 110*, 4804–4809.
Nasca, C., Zelli, D., Bigio, B., Piccinin, S., Scaccianoce, S., Nisticò, R., et al. (2015). Stress dynamically regulates behavior and glutamatergic gene expression in hippocampus by

opening a window of epigenetic plasticity. *Proceedings of the National Academy of Sciences of the United States of America*, *112*, 14960–14965.

Neale, S. A., & Salt, T. E. (2006). Modulation of GABAergic inhibition in the rat superior colliculus by a presynaptic group II metabotropic glutamate receptor. *Journal of Physiology*, *577*, 659–669.

Neki, A., Ohishi, H., Kaneko, T., Shigemoto, R., Nakanishi, S., & Mizuno, N. (1996). Pre- and postsynaptic localization of a metabotropic glutamate receptor, mGluR2, in the rat brain: An immunohistochemical study with a monoclonal antibody. *Neuroscience Letters*, *202*, 197–200.

Newport, D. J., Carpenter, L. L., McDonald, W. M., Potash, J. B., Tohen, M., Nemeroff, C. B., et al. (2015). Ketamine and other NMDA antagonists: Early clinical trials and possible mechanisms in depression. *American Journal of Psychiatry*, *172*, 950–966.

O'Brien, D. E., Shaw, D. M., Cho, H. P., Cross, A. J., Wesolowski, S. S., Felts, A. S., et al. (2018). Differential pharmacology and binding of mGlu2 receptor allosteric modulators. *Molecular Pharmacology*, *93*, 526–540.

Ohishi, H., Shigemoto, R., Nakanishi, S., & Mizuno, N. (1993a). Distribution of the messenger RNA for a metabotropic glutamate receptor, mGluR2, in the central nervous system of the rat. *Neuroscience*, *53*, 1009–1018.

Ohishi, H., Shigemoto, R., Nakanishi, S., & Mizuno, N. (1993b). Distribution of the mRNA for a metabotropic glutamate receptor (mGluR3) in the rat brain: An in situ hybridization study. *Journal of Comparative Neurology*, *335*, 252–266.

Palucha, A., & Pilc, A. (2007). Metabotropic glutamate receptor ligands as possible anxiolytic and antidepressant drugs. *Pharmacology & Therapeutics*, *115*, 116–147.

Pałucha-Poniewiera, A., Wierońska, J. M., Brański, P., Burnat, G., Chruścicka, B., & Pilc, A. (2013). Is the mGlu5 receptor a possible target for new antidepressant drugs? *Pharmacological Reports*, *65*, 1506–1511.

Perez-Garcia, G., De Gasperi, R., Gama Sosa, M. A., Perez, G. M., Otero-Pagan, A., Tschiffely, A., et al. (2018). PTSD-related behavioral traits in a rat model of blast-induced mTBI are reversed by the mGluR2/3 receptor antagonist BCI-838. *eNeuro*, *5*, 1–15. pii: ENEURO.0357-17.2018.

Pilc, A., Chaki, S., Nowak, G., & Witkin, J. M. (2008). Mood disorders: Regulation by metabotropic glutamate receptors. *Biochemical Pharmacology*, *75*, 997–1006.

Pitsikas, N., Kaffe, E., & Markou, A. (2012). The metabotropic glutamate 2/3 receptor antagonist LY341495 differentially affects recognition memory in rats. *Behavioural Brain Research*, *230*, 374–379.

Podkowa, K., Pochwat, B., Brański, P., Pilc, A., & Pałucha-Poniewiera, A. (2016). Group II mGlu receptor antagonist LY341495 enhances the antidepressant-like effects of ketamine in the forced swim test in rats. *Psychopharmacology*, *233*, 2901–2914.

Rodriguez, C. I., Zwerling, J., Kalanthroff, E., Shen, H., Filippou, M., Jo, B., et al. (2016). Effect of a novel NMDA receptor modulator, rapastinel (formerly GLYX-13), in OCD: Proof of concept. *American Journal of Psychiatry*, *173*, 1239–1241.

Rorick-Kehn, L. M., Johnson, B. G., Knitowski, K. M., Salhoff, C. R., Witkin, J. M., Perry, K. W., et al. (2007). In vivo pharmacological characterization of the structurally novel, potent, selective mGlu2/3 receptor agonist LY404039 in animal models of psychiatric disorders. *Psychopharmacology*, *193*, 121–136.

Rush, A. J., Trivedi, M. H., Wisniewski, S. R., Nierenberg, A. A., Stewart, J. W., Warden, D., et al. (2006). Acute and longer-term outcomes in depressed outpatients requiring one or several treatment steps: A STAR*D report. *American Journal of Psychiatry*, *163*, 1905–1917.

Sanacora, G., Treccani, G., & Popoli, M. (2012). Towards a glutamate hypothesis of depression: An emerging frontier of neuropsychopharmacology for mood disorders. *Neuropharmacology*, *62*, 63–77.

Schaffhauser, H., Knoflach, F., Pink, J. R., Bleuel, Z., Cartmell, J., Goepfert, F., et al. (1998). Multiple pathways for regulation of the KCl-induced [3H]-GABA release by metabotropic glutamate receptors, in primary rat cortical cultures. *Brain Research, 782*, 91–104.
Schaffhauser, H., Richards, J. G., Cartmell, J., Chaboz, S., Kemp, J. A., Klingelschmidt, A., et al. (1998). In vitro binding characteristics of a new selective group II metabotropic glutamate receptor radioligand, [3H]LY354740, in rat brain. *Molecular Pharmacology, 53*, 228–233.
Schoepp, D. D., & Conn, P. J. (1993). Metabotropic glutamate receptors in brain function and pathology. *Trends in Pharmacological Sciences, 14*, 13–20.
Shigemoto, R., Kinoshita, A., Wada, E., Nomura, S., Ohishi, H., Takada, M., et al. (1997). Differential presynaptic localization of metabotropic glutamate receptor subtypes in the rat hippocampus. *Journal of Neuroscience, 17*, 7503–7522.
Shimazaki, T., Iijima, M., & Chaki, S. (2004). Anxiolytic-like activity of MGS0039, a potent group II metabotropic glutamate receptor antagonist, in a marble-burying behavior test. *European Journal of Pharmacology, 501*, 121–125.
Shimazaki, T., Kaku, A., & Chaki, S. (2007). Blockade of the metabotropic glutamate 2/3 receptors enhances social memory via the AMPA receptor in rats. *European Journal of Pharmacology, 575*, 94–97.
Stachowicz, K., Wierońska, J., Domin, H., Chaki, S., & Pilc, A. (2011). Anxiolytic-like activity of MGS0039, a selective group II mGlu receptor antagonist, is serotonin- and GABA-dependent. *Pharmacological Reports, 63*, 880–887.
Stansley, B. J., & Conn, P. J. (2018). The therapeutic potential of metabotropic glutamate receptor modulation for schizophrenia. *Current Opinion in Pharmacology, 38*, 31–36.
Tanabe, Y., Nomura, A., Masu, M., Shigemoto, R., Mizuno, N., & Nakanishi, S. (1993). Signal transduction, pharmacological properties, and expression patterns of two rat metabotropic glutamate receptors, mGluR3 and mGluR4. *Journal of Neuroscience, 13*, 1372–1378.
Tosta, C. L., Silote, G. P., Fracalossi, M. P., Sartim, A. G., Andreatini, R., Joca, S. R. L., et al. (2018). S-ketamine reduces marble burying behaviour: Involvement of ventromedial orbitofrontal cortex and AMPA receptors. *Neuropharmacology, 144*, 233–243.
Umbricht, D., Niggli, M., Sanwald-Ducray, P., Deptula, D., Moore, R., Grunbauer, W., et al. (2015). A double-blind placebo-controlled study of the antidepressant effects of the mGlu2 negative allosteric modulator Rg1578 in patients with inadequate response to antidepressant therapy. *Biological Psychiatry*, 77(9 Suppl. 1), 305S–306S.
Ward, S. E., Beswick, P., Calcinaghi, N., Dawson, L. A., Gartlon, J., Graziani, F., et al. (2017). Pharmacological characterization of N-[(2S)-5-(6-fluoro-3-pyridinyl)-2, 3-dihydro-1H-inden-2-yl]-2-propanesulfonamide: A novel, clinical AMPA receptor positive allosteric modulator. *British Journal of Pharmacology, 174*, 370–385.
Witkin, J. M., Mitchell, S. N., Wafford, K. A., Carter, G., Gilmour, G., Li, J., et al. (2017). Comparative effects of LY3020371, a potent and selective metabotropic glutamate (mGlu) 2/3 receptor antagonist, and ketamine, a noncompetitive N-methyl-D-aspartate receptor antagonist in rodents: Evidence supporting the use of mGlu2/3 antagonists, for the treatment of depression. *Journal of Pharmacology and Experimental Therapeutics, 361*, 68–86.
Witkin, J. M., Monn, J. A., Li, J., Johnson, B., McKinzie, D. L., Wang, X. S., et al. (2017). Preclinical predictors that the orthosteric mGlu2/3 receptor antagonist LY3020371 will not engender ketamine-associated neurotoxic, motor, cognitive, subjective, or abuse-liability-related effects. *Pharmacology, Biochemistry and Behavior, 155*, 43–55.
Witkin, J. M., Monn, J. A., Schoepp, D. D., Li, X., Overshiner, C., Mitchell, S. N., et al. (2016). The rapidly acting antidepressant ketamine and the mGlu2/3 receptor antagonist LY341495 rapidly engage dopaminergic mood circuits. *Journal of Pharmacology and Experimental Therapeutics, 358*, 71–82.

Witkin, J. M., Ornstein, P. L., Mitch, C. H., Li, R., Smith, S. C., Heinz, B. A., et al. (2017). In vitro pharmacological and rat pharmacokinetic characterization of LY3020371, a potent and selective mGlu2/3 receptor antagonist. *Neuropharmacology*, *115*, 100–114.
Wright, R. A., Johnson, B. G., Zhang, C., Salhoff, C., Kingston, A. E., Calligaro, D. O., et al. (2013). CNS distribution of metabotropic glutamate 2 and 3 receptors: Transgenic mice and [^{3}H]LY459477 autoradiography. *Neuropharmacology*, *66*, 89–98.
Yamada, D., Wada, K., & Sekiguchi, M. (2011). Facilitating actions of an AMPA receptor potentiator upon extinction of contextually conditioned fear response in stressed mice. *Neuroscience Letters*, *488*, 242–246.
Yoshimizu, T., & Chaki, S. (2004). Increased cell proliferation in the adult mouse hippocampus following chronic administration of group II metabotropic glutamate receptor antagonist, MGS0039. *Biochemical and Biophysical Research Communications*, *315*, 493–496.
Yoshimizu, T., Shimazaki, T., Ito, A., & Chaki, S. (2006). An mGluR2/3 antagonist, MGS0039, exerts antidepressant and anxiolytic effects in behavioral models in rats. *Psychopharmacology*, *186*, 587–593.
Zarate, C. A., Jr., Singh, J. B., Carlson, P. J., Brutsche, N. E., Ameli, R., Luckenbaugh, D. A., et al. (2006). A randomized trial of an N-methyl-D-aspartate antagonist in treatment-resistant major depression. *Archives of General Psychiatry*, *63*, 856–864.

CHAPTER FIVE

Nitric oxide: Antidepressant mechanisms and inflammation

Mehdi Ghasemi*
Department of Neurology, University of Massachusetts Medical School, Worcester, MA, United States
Department of Neurology, Massachusetts and General Hospital, Boston, MA, United States
*Corresponding author: e-mail address: m82.ghasemi@gmail.com

Contents

1. Introduction 122
2. Nitrergic neurotransmission in the central nervous system 123
3. A role for NO signaling in MDD 124
4. Animal behavioral studies 125
5. Effects of antidepressants on nitrergic transmission 127
6. NO signaling and inflammatory processes in MDD 134
7. Conclusion 137
Acknowledgment 138
Conflict of interest 139
References 139

Abstract

Millions of individuals worldwide suffers from mood disorders, especially major depressive disorder (MDD), which has a high rate of disease burden in society. Although targeting the biogenic amines including serotonin, and norepinephrine have provided invaluable links with the pharmacological treatment of MDD over the last four decades, a growing body of evidence suggest that other biologic systems could contribute to the pathophysiology and treatment of MDD. In this chapter, we highlight the potential role of nitric oxide (NO) signaling in the pathophysiology and thereby treatment of MDD. This has been investigated over the last four decades by showing that (i) levels of NO are altered in patients with major depression; (ii) modulators of NO signaling exert antidepressant effects in patients with MDD or in the animal studies; (iii) NO signaling could be targeted by a variety of antidepressants in animal models of depression; and (iv) NO signaling can potentially modulate the inflammatory pathways that underlie the pathophysiology of MDD. These findings, which hypothesize an NO involvement in MDD, can provide a new insight into novel therapeutic approaches for patients with MDD in the future.

Advances in Pharmacology, Volume 86
ISSN 1054-3589
https://doi.org/10.1016/bs.apha.2019.04.004

Abbreviations

5-HT 5-hydroxytryptamine
7-NI 7-nitroindazole
BCG Bacillus Calmette-Guerin
BH_4 tetrahydrobiopterin
Ca^{2+} calcium
cGMP cyclic guanosine monophosphate
CNS central nervous system
COX-2 cyclooxygenase-2
eNOS endothelial nitric oxide synthase
FST forced swimming test
GABA γ-amino butyric acid
IDO indoleamine-2,3-dioxygenase
IFN interferon
IL interleukin
iNOS inducible nitric oxide synthase
L-NA N^G-nitro-L-arginine
L-NAME N^G-nitro-L-arginine methyl ester
L-NMMA *N*-monomethyl-L-arginine
LPS lipopolysaccharide
MDD major depressive disorder
NADPH α-nicotinamide adenine dinucleotide phosphate
NMDA *N*-methyl-D-aspartate
nNOS neuronal nitric oxide synthase
NO nitric oxide
NO^- nitroxyl anion
NOS NO synthase
NOx nitric oxide metabolites
O_2^- superoxide anion
ODQ 1H-163 [1,2,4]oxadiazole[4,3-*a*]quinoxalin-1-one
$ONOO^-$ peroxynitrite anion
RNS reactive nitrogen species
sGC soluble guanylyl cyclase
TNF tumor necrosis factor
TRIM 1-(2-trifluoromethylphenyl)imidazole
TST tail suspension test

1. Introduction

Reports of norepinephrine, serotonin, and dopamine levels correlating with depressive symptoms and mood expression were published in the 1960s (Bunney & Davis, 1965; Coppen, Shaw, & Malleson, 1965; Lapin & Oxenkrug, 1969; Schildkraut, 1965; Sloane, Hughes, & Haust, 1966) and have provided a critical insight into the therapeutic approaches for depressive disorders over the last five decades. However, accumulating evidence has suggested that other chemical systems also contribute to mood and behavior (Berman, Krystal, & Charney, 1996; Delgado, 2000). Among these systems, nitric oxide (NO) signaling pathway has been proposed as an important pathway in the pathophysiology of mood disorders, especially major depressive disorders (MDD) (Ghasemi, Claunch, & Niu, 2019). The first evidence of the role of NO in MDD was reported in the 1980s when it was found that the NO signaling inhibitor methylene blue had antidepressant effects in patients with MDD (Narsapur & Naylor, 1983; Naylor, Smith, & Connelly, 1987). A decade later it was found that brain-derived NO plays a pivotal role in the MDD pathogenesis (Harvey, 1996; Karatinos, Rosse, & Deutsch, 1995; van Amsterdam & Opperhuisen, 1999). In this chapter, the role of nitrergic neurotransmission in MDD is reviewed and the potential therapeutic targets in this system are explored.

2. Nitrergic neurotransmission in the central nervous system

NO plays a critical role as a neurotransmitter in the central nervous system (CNS). It is produced by the activity of NO synthase (NOS) enzymes which include three isoforms:

(i) Neuronal NOS (nNOS), a main NOS isoform in the CNS. nNOS-containing neurons are present in many CNS regions, but primarily in the hippocampus and cerebellum (Bredt, Hwang, & Snyder, 1990; Bredt & Snyder, 1989). Although nNOS producing neurons represent only roughly 1% of cell bodies in the cerebral cortex, every neuron in the cortex is exposed to nNOS nerve terminals (Ghasemi et al., 2019).

(ii) Endothelial NOS (eNOS), a main NOS isoform in the vascular system.

(iii) Inducible NOS (iNOS), a main NOS isoform in the inflammatory cells including glial cells (Galea, Feinstein, & Reis, 1992). These cells express the enzyme in neuropathological conditions (e.g., ischemia, trauma, neurotoxicity, and inflammation) (Ghasemi & Fatemi, 2014) including in mood disorders (Peng et al., 2012). Compared to other NOS isoforms, iNOS is capable of producing higher levels of NO, resulting in a variety of signaling and immunotoxicological effects (Stuehr, 1999).

Although both eNOS and iNOS are present in the CNS, nNOS is the primary enzyme that accounts for the neuronal NO production. Postsynaptic Ca^{2+} influx through the activation of NMDA (*N*-methyl-D-aspartate) receptors is the first step that regulates the nNOS-mediated central NO synthesis (Bredt & Snyder, 1989; Garthwaite, Garthwaite, Palmer, & Moncada, 1989; Ghasemi, Phillips, Fahimi, McNerney, & Salehi, 2017; Ghasemi et al., 2014). Activity of these enzymes result in the production of NO from the amino acid L-arginine. NO can act as a retrograde messenger in the presynaptic terminal (Shibuki & Okada, 1991), where it activates soluble guanylyl cyclase (sGC), thereby increasing cyclic guanosine monophosphate (cGMP) levels (Hara & Snyder, 2007). NO can also react with cysteine thiol, *S*-nitrosylation, and transition metal centers for numerous downstream effects (Drapier & Bouton, 1996; Stamler et al., 1992).

3. A role for NO signaling in MDD

In the late 1990s and early 2000s, it was hypothesized that central NO has a role in the pathogenesis of depression (Harvey, 1996; Karatinos et al., 1995; van Amsterdam & Opperhuisen, 1999). This hypothesis derived from reports demonstrating a significant reduction in the activity of both eNOS and nNOS in prefrontal cortex (Xing, Chavko, Zhang, Yang, & Post, 2002), platelet eNOS activity or levels of plasma NO metabolites (NOx) (Chrapko et al., 2004; Ozcan, Gulec, Ozerol, Polat, & Akyol, 2004; Selley, 2004), density of NOS immunoreactive neurons in the paraventricular nucleus (Bernstein et al., 1998), nNOS immunoreactivity in the locus coeruleus (Karolewicz et al., 2004) and polymorphonuclear leukocytes NOx levels (Srivastava, Barthwal, Dalal, et al., 2002) in patients with MDD. However, other reports indicated that MDD patients have higher plasma levels of nitrate and nitrite levels (Herken et al., 2007; Suzuki, Yagi, Nakaki, Kanba, & Asai, 2001; Wei et al., 2009) which were normalized after recovery over a 12-month period (Suzuki et al., 2001) or after 8 weeks treatment with antidepressants such as sertraline, citalopram, fluoxetine and fluvoxamine (Herken et al., 2007). Moreover, there was evidence that total serum nitrite/nitrate concentrations in depressed patients with ischemic heart disease were decreased after paroxetine treatment (Finkel, Laghrissi-Thode, Pollock, & Rong, 1996). Next, studies found that serum NOx levels were associated with indecisiveness, psychomotor retardation, sexual dysfunction, weight loss, fatigue, and irritability (Papageorgiou et al., 2001). Compared to non-suicidal depressed patients or normal control subjects, suicidal depressed patients had higher plasma NOx levels (Kim et al., 2006; Lee et al., 2006). Later, it was found that both nNOS and eNOS gene variants were associated with suicidal behavior (Rujescu et al., 2008). Even more recent studies have demonstrated a reduced mobilization of airway NO in depressed patients (Ritz, Trueba, Liu, Auchus, & Rosenfield, 2015; Ritz, Trueba, Simon, & Auchus, 2014; Trueba, Smith, Auchus, & Ritz, 2013). Together, these data implicate NO dysregulation in the presence and/or severity of MDD as well as various behavioral manifestations of the disease.

4. Animal behavioral studies

There is no doubt that use of animal models have helped scientists gain significant progress in therapeutic approaches in medical diseases. Objective modeling of psychiatric disorders in animals seems inherently problematic. However, several models associated with MDD have been established over the last several decades (Cryan, Markou, & Lucki, 2002). Some of the more commonly used models of depression include mild unpredicted stress, maternal separation and various chronic stress paradigms, learned helplessness model, and restraint/immobilization stress. The forced swimming test (FST) is the most commonly used behavioral method used to help identify antidepressant drugs (Yuen, Swanson, & Witkin, 2017).

Exposure to chronic mild stress in mice causes both hippocampal nNOS overexpression and depressive behaviors (Zhou et al., 2007) which are prevented or reversed in *nNOS* gene knockout ($nNOS^{-/-}$) mice or in the wild type mice treated with the nNOS inhibitor 7-NI (7-nitroindazole) (Zhou et al., 2007). $nNOS^{-/-}$ mice also demonstrated less depression-related behavior in the FST compared to wild-type mice (Tanda et al., 2009).

Accumulating lines of evidence using these models also indicate that various inhibitors of NOS or sGC can exert antidepressant-like effects. These include

(i) Non-selective NOS inhibitors: L-NA (N^G-nitro-L-arginine) (da Silva, Matteussi, dos Santos, Calixto, & Rodrigues, 2000; Gigliucci et al., 2014; Sherwin, Gigliucci, & Harkin, 2017); L-NAME (N^G-nitro-L-arginine methyl ester) (Ghasemi et al., 2008; Harkin, Bruce, Craft, & Paul, 1999; Heydarpour et al., 2016; Inan, Yalcin, & Aksu, 2004; Jefferys & Funder, 1996; Lian & An, 2010; Tomaz et al., 2014);

L-NMMA (N^G-monomethyl-L-arginine) (Harkin et al., 1999); agmatine (1-amino-4-guanidinobutane) (Li et al., 2003; Zomkowski et al., 2002); myricitrin (Meyer et al., 2017).

(ii) Selective nNOS inhibitors: L-NPA (N^ω-propyl-L-arginine) (Ghasemi et al., 2008; Pereira, Romano, Wegener, & Joca, 2015); 7-NI (7-nitroindazole) (Almeida, Duarte, Oliveira, & Crestani, 2015; Neis et al., 2014; Zhou et al., 2007).

(iii) Selective nNOS and iNOS inhibitor: TRIM (1-[2-(trifluoromethyl) phenyl]imidazole) (Ulak et al., 2008; Volke, Wegener, Bourin, & Vasar, 2003).

(iv) Selective iNOS inhibitors: aminoguanidine (Heydarpour et al., 2016; Wang, An, & Zhang, 2008); 1400W (da Silva Leal, Bonassoli, Soares, Milani, & de Oliveira, 2017).

(v) Non-selective NOS and sGC inhibitor: Methylene blue (Eroğlu & Çaglayan, 1997; Patil, Singh, & Kulkarni, 2005).

(vi) Selective sGC inhibitor: ODQ ([1H-163 [1,2,4]oxadiazole[4,3-*a*] quinoxalin-1-one]) (Heiberg, Wegener, & Rosenberg, 2002; Pereira et al., 2015; Sales, Hiroaki-Sato, & Joca, 2017).

The antidepressant-like effects of NO/cGMP pathway inhibitors were also prevented by treatment with L-arginine (Dhir & Kulkarni, 2008; Harkin et al., 1999; Inan et al., 2004; Joca & Guimarães, 2006; Yildiz, Erden, Ulak, Utkan, & Gacar, 2000) and sildenafil (Almeida, Felisbino, Lopez, Rodrigues, & Gabilan, 2006; Dhir & Kulkarni, 2008). Moreover, co-administration of non-effective doses of NMDA receptor inhibitors with NOS/cGMP inhibitors exerted synergistic antidepressant-like effects in these behavioral tests (Dhir & Kulkarni, 2008; Rosa, Lin, Calixto, Santos, & Rodrigues, 2003; Szewczyk et al., 2010).

It is noteworthy that some studies have shown that the profile of the effects achieved by NOS inhibitors in different doses was not identical but instead consisted of two paradoxical components, which was described as a U-shape effect (Ergun & Ergun, 2007; Ergun, Ergun, Orhan, & Kucuk, 2006; Harkin et al., 1999). While antidepressant-like effects were observed with low doses of NOS inhibitors (e.g., L-NA) exerted, higher doses exerted depressant effects. Additionally, L-arginine at lower doses had antidepressant effects, whereas at higher doses had pro-depressant effects (da Silva et al., 2000; Ergun & Ergun, 2007). Although these paradoxical effects could be related to distinct experimental conditions or animal strains used, it may suggest that a critical level of NO concentration in the brain above which NO may exert depressive behavior and below that level NO presents its antidepressant effects.

Overall, inhibitors of L-arginine/NO/cGMP pathway augment the antidepressant-like effects of various antidepressant medications including bupropion (Dhir & Kulkarni, 2007), citalopram (Harkin, Connor, Burns, & Kelly, 2004), duloxetine (Zomkowski, Engel, Cunha, Gabilan, & Rodrigues, 2012), escitalopram (Zomkowski, Engel, Gabilan, & Rodrigues, 2010), fluoxetine (Gigliucci, Buckley, Nunan, O'Shea, & Harkin, 2010; Harkin et al., 2004), imipramine (Harkin et al., 2004), lamotrigine (Ostadhadi et al., 2016), lithium (Ghasemi et al., 2008; Ghasemi, Sadeghipour, Poorheidari, & Dehpour, 2009), paroxetine (Ghasemi et al., 2009), reboxetine (Ulak et al., 2008), sertraline (Harkin et al., 2004), tianeptine (Ulak et al., 2008), trazodone (Kumar, Garg, & Kumar, 2008), and venlafaxine (Kumar, Garg, Gaur, & Kumar, 2010). Similar results were also reported when other agents were used including adenosine (Kaster, Rosa, Santos, & Rodrigues, 2005), agmatine (Zomkowski et al., 2002), berberine (Kulkarni & Dhir, 2007), bis selenide (Jesse, Wilhelm, Bortolatto, Rocha, & Nogueira, 2010), diphenyl diselenide (Savegnago et al., 2008), folic acid (Brocardo Pde, Budni, Lobato, Kaster, & Rodrigues, 2008), melatonin (Ergun et al., 2006; Mantovani, Pertile, Calixto, Santos, & Rodrigues, 2003), tramadol (Jesse, Bortolatto, Savegnago, Rocha, & Nogueira, 2008), and tropisetron (Haj-Mirzaian et al., 2016).

5. Effects of antidepressants on nitrergic transmission

In addition to behavioral evidence of interaction between antidepressants or mood stabilizers with NO modulators to exert antidepressant-like effects in a variety of animal models, biochemical studies over the last three decades have also demonstrated that various conventional antidepressants (e.g., fluoxetine, venlafaxine, paroxetine, and citalopram) or mood stabilizers (e.g., lithium, carbamazepine, lamotrigine, olanzapine, and valproic acid), especially after chronic administration, affect NOS enzymes activity and NO signaling (Table 1). These results support the hypothesis that chronic treatment with conventional antidepressants or even mood stabilizers lead to the same functional endpoints as administration of NOS inhibitors (Skolnick, 1999). All in all, both human and animal data provide a new insight into the treatment of mood disorders using inhibitors of NO signaling alone or combined with standard treatments.

Table 1 Effect of antidepressants or mood stabilizers on nitric oxide synthase (NOS) and NO levels.

Substance	Treatment duration	Measurement	Targeted tissue/cell	Result	Reference
Amitriptyline	3 d	Nitrite and nitrate levels	Human synovial cells	↓	Yaron et al. (1999)
Carbamazepine	–	Muscarine-induced cGMP production	Bovine cultured adrenal medullary cells	↓	Yoshimura et al. (1995)
	24 and 48 h	LPS-induced NO production	Rat glial cells	↓	Matoth, Pinto, Sicsic, and Brenner (2000)
	2 w	iNOS mRNA expression	Rat hypothalamus, hippocampus, frontal cortex, brain stem, cerebellum	↑	Suzuki, Nakaki, Shintani, Kanba, and Miyaoka (2002)
	15 min	LPS-induced iNOS and NO production	Mouse microglial BV-2 cells	↓	Wang et al. (2014)
Citalopram	12 w	Total NO level	MDD patients' plasma	↑	van Zyl et al. (2009)
	2 w	L-[^{3}H]arginine to L-[^{3}H]citrulline conversion	Rat cortex, hippocampus, cerebellum	↔	Jopek, Kata, and Nowak (1999)
	15 min	NMDA receptor-induced cGMP production	Rat cerebellar slices	↓	Raiteri, Maura, and Barzizza (1991)
	3 h	L-[^{3}H]arginine to L-[^{3}H]citrulline conversion	Rat hippocampus	↓	Wegener, Volke, Harvey, and Rosenberg (2003)

Clomipramine	24 h	Nitrite levels after LPS stimulation, iNOS mRNA expression	Mouse glial cultures	↓	Hwang et al. (2008)
Desipramine	4 h	Absorbance at wavelength of 530 nm resulting from the conversion of L-arginine to NO	PC12 cells	↓	Li et al. (2006)
Escitalopram	3 w	Immunohistochemical NOS staining	Rat hippocampus, cortex, striatum	↓	Saglam et al. (2008)
Fluoxetine	0.5–6 h	iNOS mRNA expression, nitrite level	Mouse microglial cells	↑	Ha et al. (2006)
	1 h	eNOS mRNA	Rat cerebellum, hippocampus, midbrain, pons, striatum, thalamus	↑	Yoshino et al. (2015)
		nNOS or iNOS mRNA		↔	
	72 h	Nitrite and nitrate level	Human synovial cells	↓	Yaron et al. (1999)
	3 w	NADPH-diaphorase staining	Rat hippocampus (CA1/CA2–3)	↓	Luo and Tan (2001)
	90 min	Differential pulse voltammetry and amperometry	Rat striatum	↓	Crespi (2010)
	3 and 7 d	nNOS immunoblotting	Mouse hippocampus	↓	Zhang et al. (2010)
	5 d prior BCG and 2 w	NO level in BCG-induced depression	Mouse whole brain	↓	Saleh et al. (2014)
Fluvoxamine	2 w	iNOS mRNA expression	Rat hypothalamus, hippocampus, frontal cortex, brain stem, cerebellum	↑	Suzuki et al. (2002)

Continued

Table 1 Effect of antidepressants or mood stabilizers on nitric oxide synthase (NOS) and NO levels.—cont'd

Substance	Treatment duration	Measurement	Targeted tissue/cell	Result	Reference
Imipramine	24 h	Nitrite levels after LPS stimulation, iNOS mRNA expression	Mouse glial cultures	↓	Hwang et al. (2008)
	3 w or 3 h 3 h	L-[^{3}H]arginine to L-[^{3}H]citrulline conversion	Rat hippocampus	↓	Harvey, Retief, Korff, and Wegener (2006); Wegener et al. (2003)
	30 min prior 6 h acute immobilization stress	Nitrite level	Mouse brain	↓	Kumar, Garg, Gaur, and Kumar (2009)
	20–60 min	NOx level	Rat amygdala	↑	Maruta et al. (2005)
	4 w	Nitrate level, iNOS mRNA expression	Rat hypothalamus, hippocampus, cerebral cortex, brain stem, cerebellum	↑	Suzuki, Nakaki, Kanba, Shintani, and Miyaoka (2003)
	2 w	L-[^{3}H]arginine to L-[^{3}H]citrulline conversion	Rat cortex, ↔ hippocampus, cerebellum	↔	Jopek et al. (1999)
Lamotrigine	30 min	cGMP level, L-[U—^{14}C]arginine to [U-^{14}C]citrulline conversion	Rat forebrain slices	↓	Lizasoain, Knowles, and Moncada (1995)
	30 min	Focal cerebral ischemia-induced increase in nitrite and cGMP levels	Rat cortex and cerebellum	↓	Balkan et al. (1997)
Lithium	24 h	nNOS mRNA expression	Rat hippocampus	↑	Bagetta et al. (1993)
	3 w	cGMP and NO_2^- levels	Rat cortex	↑	Harvey, Carstens, and Taljaard (1994)
	–	Muscarinic-induced increase in nitrite/nitrate levels	Mouse neuroblastoma clone, N1E-115	↔	Shintani et al. (1994)
		Muscarinic- or SNP-induced increase in cGMP levels		↓	

	24 h	L-Citrulline level	Rat brain	↑	Bagetta et al. (1995)
	24 h	LPS plus IFN-γ-induced increase in nitrite levels	C6 glioma cells	↑	Feinstein (1998)
	24 h	LPS plus CM-induced nitrite accumulation, conversion of L-arginine to L-citrulline, and iNOS mRNA expression	Rat primary astrocytes	↑	
	4 w	NADPH-diaphorase staining and nNOS mRNA expression	Rat paraventricular and supraoptic nuclei	↑	Anai et al. (2001)
	5 d	L-Citrulline level	Rat frontal cortex, hippocampus and cerebellum	↔	Wegener et al. (2004)
	2–4 h		hippocampus	↓	
	60 and 90 min	NO_3^- and NOx levels	Rat amygdala	↓	Maruta et al. (2005)
	24 h	LPS-induced accumulation of NO_2^-	Murine microglial 6-3 cells	↓	Hashioka et al. (2007)
	30 min	LPS-induced accumulation of NO_2^- and iNOS mRNA expression	BV-2 microglia	↓	Yuskaitis and Jope (2009)
	8 w	Aluminum-induced conversion of L-arginine to L-citrulline and nitrite accumulation	Rat cerebrum and cerebellum	↓	Bhalla, Singla, and Dhawan (2009)
	30 min	Nitrite level	Murine prefrontal cortex, hippocampus	↓	Haj-Mirzaian et al. (2016)

Continued

Table 1 Effect of antidepressants or mood stabilizers on nitric oxide synthase (NOS) and NO levels.—cont'd

Substance	Treatment duration	Measurement	Targeted tissue/cell	Result	Reference
Maprotiline	2 w	iNOS mRNA expression	Rat hypothalamus, hippocampus, frontal cortex, brain stem, cerebellum	↑	Suzuki et al. (2002)
Mirtazapine	1 h	Serum NO level	Rat plasma	↑	Yoshino et al. (2015)
Milnacipran	2 w	L-[^{3}H]arginine to L-[^{3}H]citrulline conversion, nitrite level	Mouse cerebral cortex, hippocampus	↓	Ikenouchi-Sugita et al. (2009)
Moclobemide or fluoxetine	4 h	Absorbance at wavelength of 530 nm resulting from the conversion of L-arginine to NO	PC12 cells	↓	Li et al. (2006)
Olanzapine	28 d	nNOS levels using computed autoradiography	Rat cortical, limbic, and extrapyramidal brain	↔	Tarazi, Zhang, and Baldessarini (2002)
	24 h	NO production	Mouse microglial cell line N9	↓	Hou et al. (2006)
Paroxetine	30 min	Nitrate level	Mouse brain	↓	Umathe et al. (2009)
	Acute or 2 w	Nitrite and nitrate level, nNOS protein expression	Rat serum, corpus cavernosum	↓	Angulo et al. (2001)
	3 h	L-[^{3}H]arginine to L-[^{3}H]citrulline conversion	Rat hippocampus	↓	Wegener et al. (2003)
	8 w	Chemiluminescence of NO metabolite	Human serum	↑	Chrapko et al. (2006)
	11 w	Nitric oxide metabolites	Rat hippocampus	↑	Khedr, Nassar, El-Denshary, and Abdel-Tawab (2015)

Tianeptine	3h	L-[^{3}H]arginine to L-[^{3}H]citrulline conversion	Rat hippocampus	↓	Wegener et al. (2003)
Valproic acid	72h	eNOS protein level	Human umbilical vein endothelial cells	↓	Michaelis et al. (2004)
	12–24h	IFN-γ-mediated increase in nitrite, iNOS protein level and mRNA expression	Murine RAW 264.7 macrophages	↓	Guo et al. (2007)
Venlafaxine	4 w	Nitrite level	Rat cortex	↓	Eren et al. (2007)
	5 d	Nitrite level	Rat brain	↓	Kumar and Garg (2008)
	30min prior 6h acute immobilization stress	Nitrite level	Mouse brain	↓	Kumar et al. (2009)
	7 d	Nitrite level	Mouse brain	↓	Kumar et al. (2010)
Venlafaxine plus Ginkgo biloba	2–3 w	Immunohistochemistry for nNOS protein, nitrite level	Rat Hippocampus (CA3), serum	↓	Qin, Jin, Ding, Xie, and Ma (2005)

BCG, Bacillus Calmette-Guerin; IFN, interferon; LPS, lipopolysaccharide; NO, nitric oxide; NOS, nitric oxide synthase; iNOS, inducible NOS; nNOS, neuronal NOS.

6. NO signaling and inflammatory processes in MDD

It has been well established that diseases in which inflammatory process are involved in their pathophysiology (including coronary artery disease, diabetes, rheumatoid arthritis, Crohn's disease, cancers, human immunodeficiency virus, and multiple sclerosis) confer an increased relative risk of developing a major mood disorder (Benton, Staab, & Evans, 2007; Elenkov, 2008). Consistently, social stressors have been shown to play a pivotal role in increasing CNS and systemic inflammation (Amini-Khoei et al., 2017; Calcia et al., 2016; Rohleder, 2014). These data have additionally suggested a potential role of inflammatory processes in the pathophysiology of MDD. Accordingly, mounting lines of evidence have shown elevation of inflammatory markers in the MDD and other mood disorders (Inserra, Mastronardi, Rogers, Licinio, & Wong, 2018; Strawbridge, Young, & Cleare, 2017). Plasma of patients with MDD or other mood disorders have higher levels of pro-inflammatory mediators (i.e., interleukin (IL)-1, IL-2, IL-6, tumor necrosis factor (TNF), and C-reactive protein) (Bremmer et al., 2008; Cepeda, Stang, & Makadia, 2016; Guloksuz et al., 2010; Irwin & Miller, 2007; Penninx et al., 2003; Soczynska et al., 2009; Zorrilla et al., 2001) compared to controls. The increased ratio of IFN-γ to IL-4 was normalized with antidepressant treatment in these patients (Myint, Leonard, Steinbusch, & Kim, 2005). Patients with hepatitis C or other conditions receiving IFN-α treatment develop or experience exacerbation of depressive symptoms in about 50% of cases with hepatitis C (Asnis & De La Garza, 2006; Dieperink, Willenbring, & Ho, 2000; Suzuki, Yoshida, Shibuya, & Miyaoka, 2003). Low doses of endotoxin (0.8 ng/kg) can also induce depressive symptoms (Reichenberg et al., 2001). On the other hand, medications with anti-inflammatory properties including inhibitors of cyclooxygenase-2 (COX-2, celecoxib) or TNF (infliximab, etanercept, and adalimumab) can improve depression in patients with MDD or other psychiatric disorders (Krishnan et al., 2007; Menter et al., 2010; Muller et al., 2006; Persoons et al., 2005; Soczynska et al., 2009). It is noteworthy that celecoxib or other COX-2 inhibitors may not directly affect NOS activity or NO production; however, they can indirectly reduce the expression of NO and its downstream pathway (Wang et al., 2018).

Administration of endotoxin to rodents (which decreases sucrose preference (akin to human anhedonia), reduces exploratory and social behaviors, reduces food intake and hypersomnia (Dantzer, O'Connor, Freund, Johnson, & Kelley, 2008)) has made it a good animal model for investigating depression and depression-related behaviors. Additionally, administration of IFN-α, IL-1β and LPS have provided similar results in animal behavioral studies including the FST and TST (tail suspension test) (Dunn & Swiergiel, 2005; Frenois et al., 2007; Orsal, Blois, Bermpohl, Schaefer, & Coquery, 2008). However, investigators need to be cautious when interpreting the data from these studies as LPS administration may also produce systemic effects both in the periphery and CNS (e.g., hypotension, septic shock, and fever) (Fraifeld & Kaplanski, 1998), which can reduce motor activity (i.e., increase immobility time in FST) or food consumption (sucrose intake) (Dunn & Swiergiel, 2005). These abnormalities may also involve mood, but are more likely to affect the animal behavior regardless of mood. Mood stabilizers such as lithium also decrease the generation of INF-γ and TNF-α, and increase IL-10 levels (an anti-inflammatory cytokine) in both human and animal studies (Ballanger, Tenaud, Volteau, Khammari, & Dreno, 2008; Kim, Jung, Myint, Kim, & Park, 2007; Knijff et al., 2007).

Interference with serotonin synthesis, glutamate metabolism and NMDA receptor/NO signaling as well as glial function has been proposed as an underlying mechanism in the inflammatory/depression link. Excess glutamate levels have been shown to increase the release of inflammatory cytokines (e.g., TNF-α) from endotoxin-activated microglia (Hagino et al., 2004). NMDA receptor antagonists (e.g., ketamine and memantine) decrease endotoxin-induced microglial activation (Chang et al., 2009; Rosi et al., 2006) and inhibit LPS-induced NO, IL-1β and TNF-α release in primary cultured microglia (Chang et al., 2009; Shibakawa et al., 2005). Additionally, inflammatory cytokines (e.g., INF) evoke iNOS gene expression (McDonald, Mann, & Thomas, 1987). INF-induced NO overproduction in the murine microglial 6-3 cells is found to be attenuated by both antidepressants and mood stabilizers (Hashioka et al., 2007). Inhibitors of iNOS (e.g., aminoguanidine and 1400W) also exert antidepressant-like effects in animal models of depression (da Silva Leal et al., 2017; Heydarpour et al., 2016; Wang et al., 2008; Zhou et al., 2017). On the other hand, NOS inhibitors (e.g., L-NAME and aminoguanidine) prevent LPS-induced depressive behavior in several models in mice including the FST, sucrose preference, and prepulse inhibition of the startle reflex (Tomaz et al., 2014). It has been hypothesized that excess NO may incite a low-grade, but persistent, inflammatory state, which ultimately leads to a disruption in neurogenesis and reduction in hippocampal volume as observed in MDD patients (Dowlati et al., 2010). Other investigators also demonstrated that iNOS-mediated excess NO production mediates neuroinflammatory actions, is neurotoxic, and may have negative impacts on mood (Dhir & Kulkarni, 2011). Accordingly, polymorphisms in the genes encoding iNOS and nNOS are associated with depression (Galecki et al., 2010, 2011).

One major mechanism underlying the iNOS-mediated NO neurotoxicity is production of reactive nitrogen species (RNS) and reactive oxygen species (ROS) (Ghasemi & Fatemi, 2014). This induces inflammatory processes associated with MDD (Dowlati et al., 2010) which include elevation of inflammatory cytokines and inhibition of mitochondrial respiration (Dowlati et al., 2010; Howren, Lamkin, & Suls, 2009; Kudlow, Cha, Carvalho, & McIntyre, 2016). One of the adverse effects of a NO-induced pro-inflammatory state is the change in the production of precursors that are essentials for the biosynthesis of those neurotransmitters that are critical for mood regulation. IL-6 has been found to activate indoleamine-2,3-dioxygenase (IDO) enzyme. This enzyme catalyzes tryptophan degradation and thereby kynurenine synthesis (Sperner-Unterweger, Kohl, & Fuchs, 2014); the latter per se causes depressive behaviors (Maes, Leonard, Myint, Kubera, & Verkerk, 2011). Moreover, a decrease in the availability of the precursor for 5-HT synthesis (i.e., tryptophan) is involved in depression (Anderson & Maes, 2015).

Excess NO and chronic inflammatory conditions lead to a reduction in tetrahydrobiopterin (BH_4) (Kudlow et al., 2016; Loftis, Huckans, & Morasco, 2010; Sperner-Unterweger et al., 2014) which is a pivotal cofactor of aromatic amino acid hydroxylase enzymes and NOS for biosynthesis of biogenic amines (serotonin, noradrenaline, dopamine, adrenaline, and melatonin) and NO, respectively. Moreover, when the BH_4 supply is insufficient, the NOS enzyme generates RNS and ROS (Sperner-Unterweger et al., 2014). Either BH4 or L-arginine deficient cells inadequately catalyze oxidation of L-arginine into L-citrulline, increasing the conversion reaction of O_2 to superoxide (O_2^-) and thereby increasing free radicals and peroxynitrite ($ONOO^-$, a potent neurotoxic agent) (Steinert, Chernova, & Forsythe, 2010). Taken together, these data suggest that BH_4 deficiency (due to the increased utilization and/or the oxidative stress/inflammatory state) may lead to attenuation of monoamines biosynthesis, contributing to the pathophysiology of MDD.

Therefore, the above mentioned evidence suggests an important role for NMDA receptor/NO signaling in the inflammatory processes involved in the MDD pathophysiology. These inflammatory mediators can (A) enhance excess glutamate release and thereby NMDA receptor/NO-mediated neurotoxicity, (B) inhibit the glutamate removal by astroglia; and (C) induce iNOS overexpression and NO overproduction which leads to decreased neurogenesis in some brain regions (i.e., hippocampus) and related alteration in the level of neurotrophic factors (Tomaz et al., 2014). Additionally, attenuated levels of the NOS cofactor BH_4 may also contribute to MDD pathogenesis through (i) increasing RNS and ROS generation by disrupted NOS signaling and (ii) reducing monoamine biosynthesis. In addition to directly targeting iNOS, anti-inflammatory drugs (i.e., COX-2 inhibitors) seems to be promising in MDD treatment (Na, Lee, Lee, Cho, & Jung, 2014). Celecoxib has shown its efficacy in the improvement of depressive symptoms when it was used as an adjunctive therapy to antidepressants (sertraline, reboxetine, or fluoxetine) (Kohler et al., 2014; Na et al., 2014). Celecoxib also decreases microglial cell release of pro-inflammatory cytokines, which was associated with excess NO generation (Miller, Maletic, & Raison, 2009; Najjar, Pearlman, Alper, Najjar, & Devinsky, 2013). Although recent systematic review and meta-analysis study (Husain, Strawbridge, Stokes, & Young, 2017) as well as others (Kopschina Feltes et al., 2017) have demonstrated efficacy of anti-inflammatory medications as mono or adjuvant therapy in depressive symptoms, further high quality trials are still needed in this regard. Even though accumulating evidence supports the immunological hypothesis of depression, the current therapeutic approaches are still mainly targeting the monoaminergic system. It is possibly because the evidence for effective treatment of MDD with anti-inflammatory drugs is still insufficient to adapt treatment guidelines for the subgroup of MDD patients with elevated levels of inflammatory markers (i.e., cytokines).

7. Conclusion

It has become increasingly pivotal for physicians to understand the role of NO signaling as a part of a comprehensive model of MDD, integrating the monoamine model, the NMDA/glutamate model, and the neuroinflammation model. Alterations in serum NOx are found in MDD patients. Changes in NOx are also observed in patients that exhibit specific symptoms associated with depressive episodes including weight loss, fatigue, sexual dysfunction, psychomotor retardation, indecisiveness and irritability. An integrated understanding of NO signaling in these contexts should help with the discovery and implementation of new medications that primarily target the nitrergic neurotransmission. Although these studies have raised the NO hypothesis in MDD, the exact mechanisms that initially trigger nitrergic system aberration in these models are still elusive and further studies are clearly needed to understand how NO changes are generated in mood states.

Consistently, inhibition of NO signaling has been found to be involved in the antidepressant effects of various agents including conventional antidepressants and mood stabilizers (Ghasemi et al., 2019; Ghasemi & Dehpour, 2011). As our growing knowledge of mechanisms of these medications gets more closely linked to specific symptoms or disease states, personalization of treatment options can be foreseen in future clinical practice. As discussed earlier, various NMDA receptor blockers (e.g., ketamine), non-selective NOS inhibitors (e.g., agmatine, L-NA, L-NAME, L-NMMA, and myricitrin), selective nNOS inhibitors (e.g., L-NPA and 7-NI), iNOS inhibitors (e.g., TRIM, aminoguanidine, and 1400W), and NOS/sGC inhibitors (e.g., methylene blue and ODQ) are currently being tested extensively in animal models, showing antidepressant-like effects as well as modulation of monoaminergic transmission, NMDA/glutamatergic transmission, and neurotrophic amplification (Ghasemi, 2013; Ghasemi et al., 2019, 2017). Taken as a whole, several lines of evidence over the last four decades have demonstrated a role for NO signaling in mood disorders as found by (A) changes in the levels of NO or its metabolites in MDD patients; (B) antidepressant effects of NO blockers in MDD patients; (C) antidepressant-like effects of NO inhibitors in animal behavioral studies; (D) interaction between conventional antidepressants or mood stabilizers with NO modulators in several biochemical and behavioral studies; and finally (E) an essential role for nitrergic transmission in the inflammatory processes likely involved in the MDD pathophysiology. Adding to the monoamine hypothesis of depression, these findings have provided new insights into the discovery of multimodal therapies that comprehensively target depressive symptoms.

Acknowledgment

There was no financial support for preparation of this work.

Conflict of interest

The author declares no conflict of interest.

References

Almeida, J., Duarte, J. O., Oliveira, L. A., & Crestani, C. C. (2015). Effects of nitric oxide synthesis inhibitor or fluoxetine treatment on depression-like state and cardiovascular changes induced by chronic variable stress in rats. *Stress (Amsterdam, Netherlands)*, *18*(4), 462–474. https://doi.org/10.3109/10253890.2015.1038993.

Almeida, R. C., Felisbino, C. S., Lopez, M. G., Rodrigues, A. L., & Gabilan, N. H. (2006). Evidence for the involvement of L-arginine-nitric oxide-cyclic guanosine monophosphate pathway in the antidepressant-like effect of memantine in mice. *Behavioural Brain Research*, *168*(2), 318–322. https://doi.org/10.1016/j.bbr.2005.11.023.

Amini-Khoei, H., Mohammadi-Asl, A., Amiri, S., Hosseini, M. J., Momeny, M., Hassanipour, M., et al. (2017). Oxytocin mitigated the depressive-like behaviors of maternal separation stress through modulating mitochondrial function and neuroinflammation. *Progress in Neuro-Psychopharmacology & Biological Psychiatry*, *76*, 169–178. https://doi.org/10.1016/j.pnpbp.2017.02.022.

Anai, H., Ueta, Y., Serino, R., Nomura, M., Nakashima, Y., & Yamashita, H. (2001). Activation of hypothalamic neuronal nitric oxide synthase in lithium-induced diabetes insipidus rats. *Psychoneuroendocrinology*, *26*(2), 1009–1020.

Anderson, G., & Maes, M. (2015). Bipolar disorder: Role of immune-inflammatory cytokines, oxidative and nitrosative stress and tryptophan catabolites. *Current Psychiatry Reports*, *17*(2), 8. https://doi.org/10.1007/s11920-014-0541-1.

Angulo, J., Peiro, C., Sanchez-Ferrer, C. F., Gabancho, S., Cuevas, P., Gupta, S., et al. (2001). Differential effects of serotonin reuptake inhibitors on erectile responses, NO-production, and neuronal NO synthase expression in rat corpus cavernosum tissue. *British Journal of Pharmacology*, *134*(6), 1190–1194. https://doi.org/10.1038/sj.bjp.0704351.

Asnis, G. M., & De La Garza, R., 2nd. (2006). Interferon-induced depression in chronic hepatitis C: A review of its prevalence, risk factors, biology, and treatment approaches. *Journal of Clinical Gastroenterology*, *40*, 322–335.

Bagetta, G., Corasaniti, M. T., Melino, G., Paoletti, A. M., Finazzi-Agro, A., & Nistico, G. (1993). Lithium and tacrine increase the expression of nitric oxide synthase mRNA in the hippocampus of rat. *Biochemical and Biophysical Research Communications*, *197*(3), 1132–1139.

Bagetta, G., Rodino, P., Paoletti, A. M., Arabia, A., Massoud, R., & Nistico, G. (1995). Systemic administration of lithium chloride and tacrine but not kainic acid augments citrulline content of rat brain. *European Journal of Pharmacology*, *294*(1), 341–344.

Balkan, S., Ozben, T., Balkan, E., Oguz, N., Serteser, M., & Gumuslu, S. (1997). Effects of Lamotrigine on brain nitrite and cGMP levels during focal cerebral ischemia in rats. *Acta Neurologica Scandinavica*, *95*(3), 140–146.

Ballanger, F., Tenaud, I., Volteau, C., Khammari, A., & Dreno, B. (2008). Anti-inflammatory effects of lithium gluconate on keratinocytes: A possible explanation for efficiency in seborrhoeic dermatitis. *Archives of Dermatological Research*, *300*(5), 215–223. https://doi.org/10.1007/s00403-007-0824-z.

Benton, T., Staab, J., & Evans, D. L. (2007). Medical co-morbidity in depressive disorders. *Annals of Clinical Psychiatry*, *19*, 289–303.

Berman, R. M., Krystal, J. H., & Charney, D. S. (1996). Mechanism of action of antidepressants: Monoamine hypotheses and beyond. In S. J. Watson (Ed.), *Biology of schizophrenia and affective disease* (pp. 295–368). Washington, DC: American Psychiatric Press.

Bernstein, H.-G., Stanarius, A., Baumann, B., Henning, H., Krell, D., Danos, P., et al. (1998). Nitric oxide synthase-containing neurons in human hypothalamus: Reduced number of immunoreactive cells in the paraventricular nucleus of depressive patients and schizophrenics. *Neuroscience*, *83*, 867–875.

Bhalla, P., Singla, N., & Dhawan, D. K. (2009). Potential of lithium to reduce aluminium-induced cytotoxic effects in rat brain. *Biometals*, *23*, 197–206. https://doi.org/10.1007/s10534-009-9278-4.

Bredt, D. S., Hwang, P. M., & Snyder, S. H. (1990). Localization of nitric oxide synthase indicating a neural role for nitric oxide. *Nature*, *347*(6295), 768–770. https://doi.org/10.1038/347768a0.

Bredt, D. S., & Snyder, S. H. (1989). Nitric oxide mediates glutamate-linked enhancement of cGMP levels in the cerebellum. *Proceedings of the National Academy of Sciences of the United States of America*, *86*(22), 9030–9033.

Bremmer, M. A., Beekman, A. T., Deeg, D. J., Pennix, B. W., Dik, M. G., Hack, C. E., et al. (2008). Inflammatory markers in late-life depression: Results from a population-based study. *Journal of Affective Disorders*, *106*, 249–255.

Brocardo Pde, S., Budni, J., Lobato, K. R., Kaster, M. P., & Rodrigues, A. L. (2008). Antidepressant-like effect of folic acid: Involvement of NMDA receptors and L-arginine-nitric oxide-cyclic guanosine monophosphate pathway. *European Journal of Pharmacology*, *598*(1-3), 37–42. https://doi.org/10.1016/j.ejphar.2008.08.033.

Bunney, W. E., Jr., & Davis, J. M. (1965). Norepinephrine in depressive reactions. A review. *Archives of General Psychiatry*, *13*(6), 483–494.

Calcia, M. A., Bonsall, D. R., Bloomfield, P. S., Selvaraj, S., Barichello, T., & Howes, O. D. (2016). Stress and neuroinflammation: A systematic review of the effects of stress on microglia and the implications for mental illness. *Psychopharmacology*, *233*(9), 1637–1650. https://doi.org/10.1007/s00213-016-4218-9.

Cepeda, M. S., Stang, P., & Makadia, R. (2016). Depression is associated with high levels of C-reactive protein and low levels of fractional exhaled nitric oxide: Results from the 2007-2012 national health and nutrition examination surveys. *The Journal of Clinical Psychiatry*, 77(12), 1666–1671. https://doi.org/10.4088/JCP.15m10267.

Chang, Y., Lee, J. J., Hsieh, C. Y., Hsiao, G., Chou, D. S., & Sheu, J. R. (2009). Inhibitory effects of ketamine on lipopolysaccharide-induced microglial activation. *Mediators of Inflammation*, *2009*, 705379. https://doi.org/10.1155/2009/705379.

Chrapko, W., Jurasz, P., Radomski, M. W., Archer, S. L., Newman, S. C., Baker, G., et al. (2006). Alteration of decreased plasma NO metabolites and platelet NO synthase activity by paroxetine in depressed patients. *Neuropsychopharmacology*, *31*(6), 1286–1293. https://doi.org/10.1038/sj.npp.1300961.

Chrapko, W. E., Jurasz, P., Radomski, M. W., Lara, N., Archer, S. L., & Le Mellédo, J.-M. (2004). Decreased platelet nitric oxide synthase activity and plasma nitric oxide metabolites in major depressive disorder. *Biological Psychiatry*, *56*, 129–134.

Coppen, A., Shaw, D. M., & Malleson, A. (1965). Changes in 5-hydroxytryptophan metabolism in depression. *The British Journal of Psychiatry*, *111*, 105–107.

Crespi, F. (2010). The selective serotonin reuptake inhibitor fluoxetine reduces striatal in vivo levels of voltammetric nitric oxide (NO): A feature of its antidepressant activity? *Neuroscience Letters*, *470*(2), 95–99. https://doi.org/10.1016/j.neulet.2009.12.049.

Cryan, J. F., Markou, A., & Lucki, I. (2002). Assessing antidepressant activity in rodents: Recent developments and future needs. *Trends in Pharmacological Sciences*, *23*(5), 238–245.

da Silva Leal, V. M., Bonassoli, V. T., Soares, L. M., Milani, H., & de Oliveira, R. M. W. (2017). Depletion of 5 hydroxy-triptamine (5-HT) affects the antidepressant-like effect of neuronal nitric oxide synthase inhibitor in mice. *Neuroscience Letters*, *656*, 131–137. https://doi.org/10.1016/j.neulet.2017.07.035.

da Silva, G. D., Matteussi, A. S., dos Santos, A. R., Calixto, J. B., & Rodrigues, A. L. (2000). Evidence for dual effects of nitric oxide in the forced swimming test and in the tail suspension test in mice. *Neuroreport*, *11*(17), 3699–3702.

Dantzer, R., O'Connor, J. C., Freund, G. G., Johnson, R. W., & Kelley, K. W. (2008). From inflammation to sickness and depression: When the immune system subjugates the brain. *Nature Reviews. Neuroscience*, *9*, 45–46.

Delgado, P. L. (2000). Depression: The case for a monoamine deficiency. *The Journal of Clinical Psychiatry*, *61*(Suppl. 6), 7–11.

Dhir, A., & Kulkarni, S. K. (2007). Involvement of nitric oxide (NO) signaling pathway in the antidepressant action of bupropion, a dopamine reuptake inhibitor. *European Journal of Pharmacology*, *568*(1-3), 177–185. https://doi.org/10.1016/j.ejphar.2007.04.028.

Dhir, A., & Kulkarni, S. K. (2008). Possible involvement of nitric oxide (NO) signaling pathway in the antidepressant-like effect of MK-801(dizocilpine), a NMDA receptor antagonist in mouse forced swim test. *Indian Journal of Experimental Biology*, *46*(3), 164–170.

Dhir, A., & Kulkarni, S. K. (2011). Nitric oxide and major depression. *Nitric Oxide*, *24*(3), 125–131. https://doi.org/10.1016/j.niox.2011.02.002.

Dieperink, E., Willenbring, M., & Ho, S. B. (2000). Neuropsychiatric symptoms associated with hepatitis C and interferon alpha: A review. *The American Journal of Psychiatry*, *157*(6), 867–876.

Dowlati, Y., Herrmann, N., Swardfager, W., Liu, H., Sham, L., Reim, E. K., et al. (2010). A meta-analysis of cytokines in major depression. *Biological Psychiatry*, *67*(5), 446–457. https://doi.org/10.1016/j.biopsych.2009.09.033.

Drapier, J. C., & Bouton, C. (1996). Modulation by nitric oxide of metalloprotein regulatory activities. *BioEssays*, *18*(7), 549–556. https://doi.org/10.1002/bies.950180706.

Dunn, A. J., & Swiergiel, A. H. (2005). Effects of interleukin-1 and endotoxin in the forced swim and tail suspension tests in mice. *Pharmacology, Biochemistry, and Behavior*, *81*(3), 688–693. https://doi.org/10.1016/j.pbb.2005.04.019.

Elenkov, I. J. (2008). Neurohormonal-cytokine interactions: Implications for inflammation common human diseases and well-being. *Neurochemistry International*, *52*, 40–51.

Eren, I., Naziroglu, M., Demirdas, A., Celik, O., Uguz, A. C., Altunbasak, A., et al. (2007). Venlafaxine modulates depression-induced oxidative stress in brain and medulla of rat. *Neurochemical Research*, *32*(3), 497–505. https://doi.org/10.1007/s11064-006-9258-9.

Ergun, Y., & Ergun, U. G. (2007). Prevention of pro-depressant effect of L-arginine in the forced swim test by NG-nitro-L-arginine and [1H-[1,2,4]oxadiazole[4,3-a] quinoxalin-1-one]. *European Journal of Pharmacology*, *554*(2-3), 150–154. https://doi.org/10.1016/j.ejphar.2006.09.067.

Ergun, Y., Ergun, U. G., Orhan, F. O., & Kucuk, E. (2006). Co-administration of a nitric oxide synthase inhibitor and melatonin exerts an additive antidepressant-like effect in the mouse forced swim test. *Medical Science Monitor*, *12*(9), BR307–312.

Eroğlu, L., & Çaglayan, B. (1997). Anxiolytic and antidepressant properties of methylene blue in animal models. *Pharmacological Research*, *36*, 381–385.

Feinstein, D. L. (1998). Potentiation of astroglial nitric oxide synthase type-2 expression by lithium chloride. *Journal of Neurochemistry*, *71*, 883–886.

Finkel, M. S., Laghrissi-Thode, F., Pollock, B. G., & Rong, J. (1996). Paroxetine is a novel nitric oxide synthase inhibitor. *Psychopharmacology Bulletin*, *32*(4), 653–658.

Fraifeld, V., & Kaplanski, J. (1998). Brain eicosanoids and LPS fever: Species and age differences. *Progress in Brain Research*, *115*, 141–157.

Frenois, F., Moreau, M., O'Connor, J., Lawson, M., Micon, C., Lestage, J., et al. (2007). Lipopolysaccharide induces delayed FosB/DeltaFosB immunostaining within the mouse extended amygdala, hippocampus and hypothalamus, that parallel the expression of depressive-like behavior. *Psychoneuroendocrinology*, *32*(5), 516–531. https://doi.org/10.1016/j.psyneuen.2007.03.005.

Galea, E., Feinstein, D. L., & Reis, D. J. (1992). Induction of calcium-independent nitric oxide synthase activity in primary rat glial cultures. *Proceedings of the National Academy of Sciences of the United States of America*, *89*(22), 10945–10949.

Galecki, P., Maes, M., Florkowski, A., Lewinski, A., Galecka, E., Bienkiewicz, M., et al. (2010). An inducible nitric oxide synthase polymorphism is associated with the risk of recurrent depressive disorder. *Neuroscience Letters*, *486*(3), 184–187. https://doi.org/10.1016/j.neulet.2010.09.048.

Galecki, P., Maes, M., Florkowski, A., Lewinski, A., Galecka, E., Bienkiewicz, M., et al. (2011). Association between inducible and neuronal nitric oxide synthase polymorphisms and recurrent depressive disorder. *Journal of Affective Disorders*, *129*(1-3), 175–182. https://doi.org/10.1016/j.jad.2010.09.005.

Garthwaite, J., Garthwaite, G., Palmer, R. M., & Moncada, S. (1989). NMDA receptor activation induces nitric oxide synthesis from arginine in rat brain slices. *European Journal of Pharmacology*, *172*(4-5), 413–416.

Ghasemi, M. (2013). Ketamine as a promising drug for rapid treatment of major depression. In A. Costa & E. Villalba (Eds.), *Vol. 10. Horizons in neuroscience research* (pp. 75–102). New York, USA: Nova Science Publisher.

Ghasemi, M., Claunch, J., & Niu, K. (2019). Pathologic role of nitrergic neurotransmission in mood disorders. *Progress in Neurobiology*, *173*, 54–87. https://doi.org/10.1016/j.pneurobio.2018.06.002.

Ghasemi, M., & Dehpour, A. R. (2011). The NMDA receptor/nitric oxide pathway: A target for the therapeutic and toxic effects of lithium. *Trends in Pharmacological Sciences*, *32*, 420–434. Epub ahead of print.

Ghasemi, M., & Fatemi, A. (2014). Pathologic role of glial nitric oxide in adult and pediatric neuroinflammatory diseases. *Neuroscience and Biobehavioral Reviews*, *45*, 168–182. https://doi.org/10.1016/j.neubiorev.2014.06.002.

Ghasemi, M., Montaser-Kouhsari, L., Shafaroodi, H., Nezami, B. G., Ebrahimi, F., & Dehpour, A. R. (2009). NMDA receptor/nitrergic system blockage augments antidepressant-like effects of paroxetine in the mouse forced swimming test. *Psychopharmacology*, *206*(2), 325–333. https://doi.org/10.1007/s00213-009-1609-1.

Ghasemi, M., Phillips, C., Fahimi, A., McNerney, M. W., & Salehi, A. (2017). Mechanisms of action and clinical efficacy of NMDA receptor modulators in mood disorders. *Neuroscience and Biobehavioral Reviews*, *80*, 555–572. https://doi.org/10.1016/j.neubiorev.2017.07.002.

Ghasemi, M., Phillips, C., Trillo, L., De Miguel, Z., Das, D., & Salehi, A. (2014). The role of NMDA receptors in the pathophysiology and treatment of mood disorders. *Neuroscience and Biobehavioral Reviews*, *47*, 336–358. https://doi.org/10.1016/j.neubiorev.2014.08.017.

Ghasemi, M., Sadeghipour, H., Mosleh, A., Sadeghipour, H. R., Mani, A. R., & Dehpour, A. R. (2008). Nitric oxide involvement in the antidepressant-like effects of acute lithium administration in the mouse forced swimming test. *European Neuropsychopharmacology*, *18*(5), 323–332.

Ghasemi, M., Sadeghipour, H., Poorheidari, G., & Dehpour, A. R. (2009). A role for nitrergic system in the antidepressant-like effects of chronic lithium treatment in the mouse forced swimming test. *Behavioural Brain Research*, *200*, 76–82.

Gigliucci, V., Buckley, K. N., Nunan, J., O'Shea, K., & Harkin, A. (2010). A role for serotonin in the antidepressant activity of N(G)-nitro-L-arginine, in the rat forced swimming test. *Pharmacology, Biochemistry, and Behavior*, *94*(4), 524–533. https://doi.org/10.1016/j.pbb.2009.11.007.

Gigliucci, V., Gormley, S., Gibney, S., Rouine, J., Kerskens, C., Connor, T. J., et al. (2014). Characterisation of the antidepressant properties of nitric oxide synthase inhibitors in the olfactory bulbectomised rat model of depression. *European Neuropsychopharmacology*, *24*(8), 1349–1361. https://doi.org/10.1016/j.euroneuro.2014.05.003.

Guloksuz, S., Aktas Cetin, E., Cetin, T., Deniz, G., Oral, E. T., & Nutt, D. J. (2010). Cytokine levels in euthymic bipolar patients. *Journal of Affective Disorders*, *126*(3), 458–462. https://doi.org/10.1016/j.jad.2010.04.027.

Guo, L., Guo, H., Gao, C., Mi, Z., Russell, W. B., & Kuo, P. C. (2007). Stat1 acetylation inhibits inducible nitric oxide synthase expression in interferon-gamma-treated RAW264.7 murine macrophages. *Surgery*, *142*(2), 156–162. https://doi.org/10.1016/j.surg.2007.02.016.

Ha, E., Jung, K. H., Choe, B. K., Bae, J. H., Shin, D. H., Yim, S. V., et al. (2006). Fluoxetine increases the nitric oxide production via nuclear factor kappa B-mediated pathway in BV2 murine microglial cells. *Neuroscience Letters*, *397*(3), 185–189. https://doi.org/10.1016/j.neulet.2005.12.022.

Hagino, Y., Kariura, Y., Manago, Y., Amano, T., Wang, B., Sekiguchi, M., et al. (2004). Heterogeneity and potentiation of AMPA type of glutamate receptors in rat cultured microglia. *Glia*, *47*(1), 68–77. https://doi.org/10.1002/glia.20034.

Haj-Mirzaian, A., Amiri, S., Kordjazy, N., Momeny, M., Razmi, A., Rahimi-Balaei, M., et al. (2016). Lithium attenuated the depressant and anxiogenic effect of juvenile social stress through mitigating the negative impact of interlukin-1beta and nitric oxide on hypothalamic-pituitary-adrenal axis function. *Neuroscience*, *315*, 271–285. https://doi.org/10.1016/j.neuroscience.2015.12.024.

Hara, M. R., & Snyder, S. H. (2007). Cell signaling and neuronal death. *Annual Review of Pharmacology and Toxicology*, *47*, 117–141.

Harkin, A. J., Bruce, K. H., Craft, B., & Paul, I. A. (1999). Nitric oxide synthase inhibitors have antidepressant-like properties in mice. 1. Acute treatments are active in the forced swim test. *European Journal of Pharmacology*, *372*(3), 207–213.

Harkin, A., Connor, T. J., Burns, M. P., & Kelly, J. P. (2004). Nitric oxide synthase inhibitors augment the effects of serotonin re-uptake inhibitors in the forced swimming test. *European Neuropsychopharmacology*, *14*(4), 274–281. https://doi.org/10.1016/j.euroneuro.2003.08.010.

Harvey, B. H. (1996). Affective disorders and nitric oxide: A role in pathways to relapse and refractoriness? *Human Psychopharmacology*, *11*, 309–319.

Harvey, B. H., Carstens, M. E., & Taljaard, J. J. (1994). Evidence that lithium induces a glutamatergic: Nitric oxide-mediated response in rat brain. *Neurochemical Research*, *19*(4), 469–474.

Harvey, B. H., Retief, R., Korff, A., & Wegener, G. (2006). Increased hippocampal nitric oxide synthase activity and stress responsiveness after imipramine discontinuation: Role of 5HT 2A/C-receptors. *Metabolic Brain Disease*, *21*(2-3), 211–220. https://doi.org/10.1007/s11011-006-9018-1.

Hashioka, S., Klegeris, A., Monji, A., Kato, T., Sawada, M., McGeer, P. L., et al. (2007). Antidepressants inhibit interferon-gamma-induced microglial production of IL-6 and nitric oxide. *Experimental Neurology*, *206*(1), 33–42.

Heiberg, I. L., Wegener, G., & Rosenberg, R. (2002). Reduction of cGMP and nitric oxide has antidepressant-like effects in the forced swimming test in rats. *Behavioural Brain Research*, *134*, 479–484.

Herken, H., Gurel, A., Selek, S., Armutcu, F., Ozen, M. E., Bulut, M., et al. (2007). Adenosine deaminase, nitric oxide, superoxide dismutase, and xanthine oxidase in patients with major depression: Impact of antidepressant treatment. *Archives of Medical Research*, *38*, 247–252.

Heydarpour, P., Rahimian, R., Fakhfouri, G., Khoshkish, S., Fakhraei, N., Salehi-Sadaghiani, M., et al. (2016). Behavioral despair associated with a mouse model of Crohn's disease: Role of nitric oxide pathway. *Progress in Neuro-Psychopharmacology & Biological Psychiatry*, *64*, 131–141. https://doi.org/10.1016/j.pnpbp.2015.08.004.

Hou, Y., Wu, C. F., Yang, J. Y., He, X., Bi, X. L., Yu, L., et al. (2006). Effects of clozapine, olanzapine and haloperidol on nitric oxide production by lipopolysaccharide-activated N9 cells. *Progress in Neuro-Psychopharmacology & Biological Psychiatry*, *30*(8), 1523–1528. https://doi.org/10.1016/j.pnpbp.2006.05.006.

Howren, M. B., Lamkin, D. M., & Suls, J. (2009). Associations of depression with C-reactive protein, IL-1, and IL-6: A meta-analysis. *Psychosomatic Medicine*, *71*(2), 171–186. https://doi.org/10.1097/PSY.0b013e3181907c1b.

Husain, M. I., Strawbridge, R., Stokes, P. R., & Young, A. H. (2017). Anti-inflammatory treatments for mood disorders: Systematic review and meta-analysis. *Journal of Psychopharmacology*, *31*(9), 1137–1148. https://doi.org/10.1177/0269881117725711.

Hwang, J., Zheng, L. T., Ock, J., Lee, M. G., Kim, S. H., Lee, H. W., et al. (2008). Inhibition of glial inflammatory activation and neurotoxicity by tricyclic antidepressants. *Neuropharmacology*, *55*(5), 826–834. https://doi.org/10.1016/j.neuropharm.2008.06.045.

Ikenouchi-Sugita, A., Toyohira, Y., Yoshimura, R., Ueno, S., Tsutsui, M., Nakamura, J., et al. (2009). Opposite effects of milnacipran, a serotonin norepinephrine reuptake inhibitor, on the levels of nitric oxide and brain-derived neurotrophic factor in mouse brain cortex. *Naunyn-Schmiedeberg's Archives of Pharmacology*, *380*(6), 479–486. https://doi.org/10.1007/s00210-009-0467-z.

Inan, S. Y., Yalcin, I., & Aksu, F. (2004). Dual effects of nitric oxide in the mouse forced swimming test: Possible contribution of nitric oxide-mediated serotonin release and potassium channel modulation. *Pharmacology, Biochemistry, and Behavior*, 77(3), 457–464.

Inserra, A., Mastronardi, C. A., Rogers, G., Licinio, J., & Wong, M. L. (2018). Neuroimmunomodulation in major depressive disorder: Focus on caspase 1, inducible nitric oxide synthase, and interferon-gamma. *Molecular Neurobiology*, *56*, 4288–4305. https://doi.org/10.1007/s12035-018-1359-3.

Irwin, M. R., & Miller, A. H. (2007). Depressive disorders and immunity: 20 years of progress and discovery. *Brain, Behavior, and Immunity*, *21*, 374–383.

Jefferys, D., & Funder, J. (1996). Nitric oxide modulates retention of immobility in the forced swimming test in rats. *European Journal of Pharmacology*, *295*(2-3), 131–135.

Jesse, C. R., Bortolatto, C. F., Savegnago, L., Rocha, J. B., & Nogueira, C. W. (2008). Involvement of L-arginine-nitric oxide-cyclic guanosine monophosphate pathway in the antidepressant-like effect of tramadol in the rat forced swimming test. *Progress in Neuro-Psychopharmacology & Biological Psychiatry*, *32*(8), 1838–1843. https://doi.org/10.1016/j.pnpbp.2008.08.010.

Jesse, C. R., Wilhelm, E. A., Bortolatto, C. F., Rocha, J. B., & Nogueira, C. W. (2010). Involvement of L-arginine-nitric oxide-cyclic guanosine monophosphate pathway in the antidepressant-like effect of bis selenide in the mouse tail suspension test. *European Journal of Pharmacology*, *635*(1-3), 135–141. https://doi.org/10.1016/j.ejphar.2010.03.019.

Joca, S. R., & Guimarães, F. S. (2006). Inhibition of neuronal nitric oxide synthase in the rat hippocampus induces antidepressant-like effects. *Psychopharmacology*, *185*, 298–305.

Jopek, R., Kata, M., & Nowak, G. (1999). The activity of rat brain nitric oxide synthase following chronic antidepressant treatment. *Acta Poloniae Pharmaceutica*, *56*(4), 307–310.

Karatinos, J., Rosse, R. B., & Deutsch, S. I. (1995). The nitric oxide pathway: Potential implications for treatment of neuropsychiatric disorders. *Clinical Neuropharmacology*, *18*(6), 482–499.

Karolewicz, B., Szebeni, K., Stockmeier, C. A., Konick, L., Overholser, J. C., Jurjus, G., et al. (2004). Low nNOS protein in the locus coeruleus in major depression. *Journal of Neurochemistry*, *91*, 1057–1066.

Kaster, M. P., Rosa, A. O., Santos, A. R., & Rodrigues, A. L. (2005). Involvement of nitric oxide-cGMP pathway in the antidepressant-like effects of adenosine in the forced swimming test. *The International Journal of Neuropsychopharmacology*, *8*(4), 601–606. https://doi.org/10.1017/S1461145705005316.

Khedr, L. H., Nassar, N. N., El-Denshary, E. S., & Abdel-Tawab, A. M. (2015). Paroxetine ameliorates changes in hippocampal energy metabolism in chronic mild stress-exposed rats. *Neuropsychiatric Disease and Treatment, 11*, 2887–2901. https://doi.org/10.2147/ndt.s87089.

Kim, Y. K., Jung, H. G., Myint, A. M., Kim, H., & Park, S. H. (2007). Imbalance between pro-inflammatory and anti-inflammatory cytokines in bipolar disorder. *Journal of Affective Disorders, 104*(1-3), 91–95. https://doi.org/10.1016/j.jad.2007.02.018.

Kim, Y.-K., Paik, J.-W., Lee, S.-W., Yoon, D., Han, C., & Lee, B.-H. (2006). Increased plasma nitric oxide level associated with suicide attempt in depressive patients. *Progress in Neuro-Psychopharmacology and Biological Psychiatry, 30*, 1091–1096.

Knijff, E. M., Breunis, M. N., Kupka, R. W., de Wit, H. J., Ruwhof, C., Akkerhuis, G. W., et al. (2007). An imbalance in the production of IL-1beta and IL-6 by monocytes of bipolar patients: Restoration by lithium treatment. *Bipolar Disorders, 9*(7), 743–753. https://doi.org/10.1111/j.1399-5618.2007.00444.x.

Kohler, O., Benros, M. E., Nordentoft, M., Farkouh, M. E., Iyengar, R. L., Mors, O., et al. (2014). Effect of anti-inflammatory treatment on depression, depressive symptoms, and adverse effects: A systematic review and meta-analysis of randomized clinical trials. *JAMA Psychiatry, 71*(12), 1381–1391. https://doi.org/10.1001/jamapsychiatry.2014.1611.

Kopschina Feltes, P., Doorduin, J., Klein, H. C., Juarez-Orozco, L. E., Dierckx, R. A., Moriguchi-Jeckel, C. M., et al. (2017). Anti-inflammatory treatment for major depressive disorder: Implications for patients with an elevated immune profile and non-responders to standard antidepressant therapy. *Journal of Psychopharmacology, 31*(9), 1149–1165. https://doi.org/10.1177/0269881117711708.

Krishnan, R., Cella, D., Leonardi, C., Papp, K., Gottlieb, A. B., Dunn, M., et al. (2007). Effects of etanercept therapy on fatigue and symptoms of depression in subjects treated for moderate to severe plaque psoriasis for up to 96 weeks. *The British Journal of Dermatology, 157*(6), 1275–1277. https://doi.org/10.1111/j.1365-2133.2007.08205.x.

Kudlow, P., Cha, D. S., Carvalho, A. F., & McIntyre, R. S. (2016). Nitric oxide and major depressive disorder: Pathophysiology and treatment implications. *Current Molecular Medicine, 16*(2), 206–215.

Kulkarni, S. K., & Dhir, A. (2007). Possible involvement of L-arginine-nitric oxide (NO)-cyclic guanosine monophosphate (cGMP) signaling pathway in the antidepressant activity of berberine chloride. *European Journal of Pharmacology, 569*(1-2), 77–83. https://doi.org/10.1016/j.ejphar.2007.05.002.

Kumar, A., & Garg, R. (2008). A role of nitric oxide mechanism involved in the protective effects of venlafaxine in sleep deprivation. *Behavioural Brain Research, 194*(2), 169–173. https://doi.org/10.1016/j.bbr.2008.07.003.

Kumar, A., Garg, R., Gaur, V., & Kumar, P. (2009). Nitric oxide mechanism in protective effect of imipramine and venlafaxine against acute immobilization stress-induced behavioral and biochemical alteration in mice. *Neuroscience Letters, 467*(2), 72–75. https://doi.org/10.1016/j.neulet.2009.10.004.

Kumar, A., Garg, R., Gaur, V., & Kumar, P. (2010). Venlafaxine involves nitric oxide modulatory mechanism in experimental model of chronic behavior despair in mice. *Brain Research, 1311*, 73–80. https://doi.org/10.1016/j.brainres.2009.11.050.

Kumar, A., Garg, R., & Kumar, P. (2008). Nitric oxide modulation mediates the protective effect of trazodone in a mouse model of chronic fatigue syndrome. *Pharmacological Reports, 60*(5), 664–672.

Lapin, I. P., & Oxenkrug, G. F. (1969). Intensification of the central serotoninergic processes as a possible determinant of the thymoleptic effect. *Lancet, 1*(7586), 132–136.

Lee, B. H., Lee, S. W., Yoon, D., Lee, H. J., Yang, J. C., Shim, S. H., et al. (2006). Increased plasma nitric oxide metabolites in suicide attempters. *Neuropsychobiology, 53*(3), 127–132. https://doi.org/10.1159/000092542.

Li, Y. F., Gong, Z. H., Cao, J. B., Wang, H. L., Luo, Z. P., & Li, J. (2003). Antidepressant-like effect of agmatine and its possible mechanism. *European Journal of Pharmacology, 469*(1–3), 81–88.

Li, Y. F., Zhang, Y. Z., Liu, Y. Q., Wang, H. L., Cao, J. B., Guan, T. T., et al. (2006). Inhibition of N-methyl-D-aspartate receptor function appears to be one of the common actions for antidepressants. *Journal of Psychopharmacology, 20*(5), 629–635. https://doi.org/10.1177/0269881106059692.

Lian, T., & An, S. C. (2010). Antidepressant effect of microinjection of neuropeptide Y into the hippocampus is mediated by decreased expression of nitric oxide synthase. *Sheng Li Xue Bao, 62*(3), 237–246.

Lizasoain, I., Knowles, R. G., & Moncada, S. (1995). Inhibition by lamotrigine of the generation of nitric oxide in rat forebrain slices. *Journal of Neurochemistry, 64*(2), 636–642.

Loftis, J. M., Huckans, M., & Morasco, B. J. (2010). Neuroimmune mechanisms of cytokine-induced depression: Current theories and novel treatment strategies. *Neurobiology of Disease, 37*(3), 519–533. https://doi.org/10.1016/j.nbd.2009.11.015.

Luo, L., & Tan, R. X. (2001). Fluoxetine inhibits dendrite atrophy of hippocampal neurons by decreasing nitric oxide synthase expression in rat depression model. *Acta Pharmacologica Sinica, 22*(10), 865–870.

Maes, M., Leonard, B. E., Myint, A. M., Kubera, M., & Verkerk, R. (2011). The new '5-HT' hypothesis of depression: Cell-mediated immune activation induces indoleamine 2,3-dioxygenase, which leads to lower plasma tryptophan and an increased synthesis of detrimental tryptophan catabolites (TRYCATs), both of which contribute to the onset of depression. *Progress in Neuro-Psychopharmacology & Biological Psychiatry, 35*(3), 702–721. https://doi.org/10.1016/j.pnpbp.2010.12.017.

Mantovani, M., Pertile, R., Calixto, J. B., Santos, A. R., & Rodrigues, A. L. (2003). Melatonin exerts an antidepressant-like effect in the tail suspension test in mice: Evidence for involvement of N-methyl-D-aspartate receptors and the L-arginine-nitric oxide pathway. *Neuroscience Letters, 343*(1), 1–4.

Maruta, S., Suzuki, E., Yokoyama, M., Sato, T., Inada, K., Watanabe, S., et al. (2005). Effects of intraperitoneally injected lithium, imipramine and diazepam on nitrate levels in rat amygdala. *Psychiatry and Clinical Neurosciences, 59*(3), 358–361.

Matoth, I., Pinto, F., Sicsic, C., & Brenner, T. (2000). Inhibitory effect of carbamazepine on inflammatory mediators produced by stimulated glial cells. *Neuroscience Research, 38*(2), 209–212.

McDonald, E. M., Mann, A. H., & Thomas, H. C. (1987). Interferons as mediators of psychiatric morbidity: An investigation in a trial of recombinant α-interferon in hepatitis-B carriers. *Lancet, ii*, 1175–1178.

Menter, A., Augustin, M., Signorovitch, J., Yu, A. P., Wu, E. Q., Gupta, S. R., et al. (2010). The effect of adalimumab on reducing depression symptoms in patients with moderate to severe psoriasis: A randomized clinical trial. *Journal of the American Academy of Dermatology, 62*(5), 812–818. https://doi.org/10.1016/j.jaad.2009.07.022.

Meyer, E., Mori, M. A., Campos, A. C., Andreatini, R., Guimaraes, F. S., Milani, H., et al. (2017). Myricitrin induces antidepressant-like effects and facilitates adult neurogenesis in mice. *Behavioural Brain Research, 316*, 59–65. https://doi.org/10.1016/j.bbr.2016.08.048.

Michaelis, M., Michaelis, U. R., Fleming, I., Suhan, T., Cinatl, J., Blaheta, R. A., et al. (2004). Valproic acid inhibits angiogenesis in vitro and in vivo. *Molecular Pharmacology, 65*(3), 520–527. https://doi.org/10.1124/mol.65.3.520.

Miller, A. H., Maletic, V., & Raison, C. L. (2009). Inflammation and its discontents: The role of cytokines in the pathophysiology of major depression. *Biological Psychiatry, 65*(9), 732–741. https://doi.org/10.1016/j.biopsych.2008.11.029.

Muller, N., Schwarz, M. J., Dehning, S., Douhe, A., Cerovecki, A., Goldstein-Muller, B., et al. (2006). The cyclooxygenase-2 inhibitor celecoxib has therapeutic effects in major depression: Results of a double-blind, randomized, placebo controlled, add-on pilot study to reboxetine. *Molecular Psychiatry, 11*(7), 680–684. https://doi.org/10.1038/sj.mp.4001805.

Myint, A. M., Leonard, B. E., Steinbusch, H. W., & Kim, Y. K. (2005). Th1, Th2, and Th3 cytokine alterations in major depression. *Journal of Affective Disorders, 88*, 167–173.

Na, K. S., Lee, K. J., Lee, J. S., Cho, Y. S., & Jung, H. Y. (2014). Efficacy of adjunctive celecoxib treatment for patients with major depressive disorder: A meta-analysis. *Progress in Neuro-Psychopharmacology & Biological Psychiatry, 48*, 79–85. https://doi.org/10.1016/j.pnpbp.2013.09.006.

Najjar, S., Pearlman, D. M., Alper, K., Najjar, A., & Devinsky, O. (2013). Neuroinflammation and psychiatric illness. *Journal of Neuroinflammation, 10*. 43. https://doi.org/10.1186/1742-2094-10-43.

Narsapur, S. L., & Naylor, G. J. (1983). Methylene blue. A possible treatment for manic depressive psychosis. *Journal of Affective Disorders, 5*(2), 155–161.

Naylor, G. J., Smith, A. H. W., & Connelly, P. (1987). A controlled trial of methylene blue in severe depressive illness. *Biological Psychiatry, 22*, 657–659.

Neis, V. B., Manosso, L. M., Moretti, M., Freitas, A. E., Daufenbach, J., & Rodrigues, A. L. (2014). Depressive-like behavior induced by tumor necrosis factor-alpha is abolished by agmatine administration. *Behavioural Brain Research, 261*, 336–344. https://doi.org/10.1016/j.bbr.2013.12.038.

Orsal, A. S., Blois, S. M., Bermpohl, D., Schaefer, M., & Coquery, N. (2008). Administration of interferon-alpha in mice provokes peripheral and central modulation of immune cells, accompanied by behavioral effects. *Neuropsychobiology, 58*(3-4), 211–222. https://doi.org/10.1159/000201718.

Ostadhadi, S., Ahangari, M., Nikoui, V., Norouzi-Javidan, A., Zolfaghari, S., Jazaeri, F., et al. (2016). Pharmacological evidence for the involvement of the NMDA receptor and nitric oxide pathway in the antidepressant-like effect of lamotrigine in the mouse forced swimming test. *Biomedicine & Pharmacotherapy, 82*, 713–721. https://doi.org/10.1016/j.biopha.2016.05.035.

Ozcan, M. E., Gulec, M., Ozerol, E., Polat, R., & Akyol, O. (2004). Antioxidant enzyme activities and oxidative stress in affective disorders. *International Clinical Psychopharmacology, 19*(2), 89–95.

Papageorgiou, C., Graspa, E., Chirstodoulou, N. G., Zerefos, N., Stamatellopouols, S., & Chirstodoulou, G. N. (2001). Association of serum nitric oxide levels with depressive symptoms: A study with end-stage renal failure patients. *Psychotherapy and Psychosomatics, 70*, 216–220.

Patil, C. S., Singh, V. P., & Kulkarni, S. K. (2005). Peripheral and central activation of nitric oxide-cyclic GMP pathway by sildenafil. *Inflammopharmacology, 13*, 467–478.

Peng, Y. L., Liu, Y. N., Liu, L., Wang, X., Jiang, C. L., & Wang, Y. X. (2012). Inducible nitric oxide synthase is involved in the modulation of depressive behaviors induced by unpredictable chronic mild stress. *Journal of Neuroinflammation, 9*, 75. https://doi.org/10.1186/1742-2094-9-75.

Penninx, B. W., Kritchevsky, S. B., Yaffe, K., Newman, A. B., Simonsick, E. M., Rubin, S., et al. (2003). Inflammatory markers and depressed mood in older persons: Results from the Health, Aging and Body Composition Study. *Biological Psychiatry, 54*, 566–572.

Pereira, V. S., Romano, A., Wegener, G., & Joca, S. R. (2015). Antidepressant-like effects induced by NMDA receptor blockade and NO synthesis inhibition in the ventral medial prefrontal cortex of rats exposed to the forced swim test. *Psychopharmacology, 232*(13), 2263–2273. https://doi.org/10.1007/s00213-014-3853-2.

Persoons, P., Vermeire, S., Demyttenaere, K., Fischler, B., Vandenberghe, J., Van Oudenhove, L., et al. (2005). The impact of major depressive disorder on the short- and long-term outcome of Crohn's disease treatment with infliximab. *Alimentary Pharmacology & Therapeutics*, *22*(2), 101–110. https://doi.org/10.1111/j.1365-2036.2005.02535.x.

Qin, X. S., Jin, K. H., Ding, B. K., Xie, S. F., & Ma, H. (2005). Effects of extract of Ginkgo biloba with venlafaxine on brain injury in a rat model of depression. *Chinese Medical Journal*, *118*(5), 391–397.

Raiteri, M., Maura, G., & Barzizza, A. (1991). Activation of presynaptic 5-hydroxytryptamine1-like receptors on glutamatergic terminals inhibits N-methyl-D-aspartate-induced cyclic GMP production in rat cerebellar slices. *The Journal of Pharmacology and Experimental Therapeutics*, *257*(3), 1184–1188.

Reichenberg, A., Yirmiya, R., Schuld, A., Kraus, T., Haack, M., Morag, A., et al. (2001). Cytokine-associated emotional and cognitive disturbances in humans. *Archives of General Psychiatry*, *58*(5), 445–452.

Ritz, T., Trueba, A. F., Liu, J., Auchus, R. J., & Rosenfield, D. (2015). Exhaled nitric oxide decreases during academic examination stress in asthma. *Annals of the American Thoracic Society*, *12*(11), 1638–1645. https://doi.org/10.1513/AnnalsATS.201504-213OC.

Ritz, T., Trueba, A. F., Simon, E., & Auchus, R. J. (2014). Increases in exhaled nitric oxide after acute stress: Association with measures of negative affect and depressive mood. *Psychosomatic Medicine*, *76*(9), 716–725. https://doi.org/10.1097/psy.0000000000000118.

Rohleder, N. (2014). Stimulation of systemic low-grade inflammation by psychosocial stress. *Psychosomatic Medicine*, *76*(3), 181–189. https://doi.org/10.1097/psy.0000000000000049.

Rosa, A. O., Lin, J., Calixto, J. B., Santos, A. R., & Rodrigues, A. L. (2003). Involvement of NMDA receptors and L-arginine-nitric oxide pathway in the antidepressant-like effects of zinc in mice. *Behavioural Brain Research*, *144*(1-2), 87–93.

Rosi, S., Vazdarjanova, A., Ramirez-Amaya, V., Worley, P. F., Barnes, C. A., & Wenk, G. L. (2006). Memantine protects against LPS-induced neuroinflammation, restores behaviorally-induced gene expression and spatial learning in the rat. *Neuroscience*, *142*(4), 1303–1315. https://doi.org/10.1016/j.neuroscience.2006.08.017.

Rujescu, D., Giegling, I., Mandelli, L., Schneider, B., Hartmann, A. M., Schnabel, A., et al. (2008). NOS-I and -III gene variants are differentially associated with facets of suicidal behavior and aggression-related traits. *American Journal of Medical Genetics. Part B, Neuropsychiatric Genetics*, *147B*(1), 42–48. https://doi.org/10.1002/ajmg.b.30569 [doi].

Saglam, E., Ates, L. E., Kayir, H., Celik, T., Terzioglu, B., & Uzbay, T. (2008). Escitalopram increases cortical nitric oxide synthase (NOS) in rat brain during ethanol withdrawal. *Nitric Oxide: Biology and Chemistry*, *19*(3), 284–288. https://doi.org/10.1016/j.niox.2008.06.222.

Saleh, L. A., Hamza, M., El Gayar, N. H., Abd El-Samad, A. A., Nasr, E. A., & Masoud, S. I. (2014). Ibuprofen suppresses depressive like behavior induced by BCG inoculation in mice: Role of nitric oxide and prostaglandin. *Pharmacology Biochemistry and Behavior*, *125*, 29–39. https://doi.org/10.1016/j.pbb.2014.07.013.

Sales, A. J., Hiroaki-Sato, V. A., & Joca, S. R. (2017). Participation of hippocampal nitric oxide synthase and soluble guanylate cyclase in the modulation of behavioral responses elicited by the rat forced swimming test. *Behavioural Pharmacology*, *28*(1), 19–29. https://doi.org/10.1097/fbp.0000000000000263.

Savegnago, L., Jesse, C. R., Pinto, L. G., Rocha, J. B., Barancelli, D. A., Nogueira, C. W., et al. (2008). Diphenyl diselenide exerts antidepressant-like and anxiolytic-like effects in mice: Involvement of L-arginine-nitric oxide-soluble guanylate cyclase pathway in its antidepressant-like action. *Pharmacology, Biochemistry, and Behavior*, *88*(4), 418–426. https://doi.org/10.1016/j.pbb.2007.09.015.

Schildkraut, J. J. (1965). The catecholamine hypothesis of affective disorders: A review of supporting evidence. *The American Journal of Psychiatry, 122*(5), 509–522.

Selley, M. L. (2004). Increased (E)-4-hydroxy-2-nonenal and asymmetric dimethylarginine concentrations and decreased nitric oxide concentrations in the plasma of patients with major depression. *Journal of Affective Disorders, 80*(2-3), 249–256.

Sherwin, E., Gigliucci, V., & Harkin, A. (2017). Regional specific modulation of neuronal activation associated with nitric oxide synthase inhibitors in an animal model of antidepressant activity. *Behavioural Brain Research, 316*, 18–28. https://doi.org/10.1016/j.bbr.2016.08.049.

Shibakawa, Y. S., Sasaki, Y., Goshima, Y., Echigo, N., Kamiya, Y., Kurahashi, K., et al. (2005). Effects of ketamine and propofol on inflammatory responses of primary glial cell cultures stimulated with lipopolysaccharide. *British Journal of Anaesthesia, 95*(6), 803–810. https://doi.org/10.1093/bja/aei256.

Shibuki, K., & Okada, D. (1991). Endogenous nitric oxide release required for long-term synaptic depression in the cerebellum. *Nature, 349*(6307), 326–328. https://doi.org/10.1038/349326a0.

Shintani, F., Kanba, S., Nakaki, T., Nakamura, R., Sato, K., Yagi, G., et al. (1994). Inhibition by lithium of cyclic GMP formation without inhibition of nitric oxide generation in the mouse neuroblastoma cell (N1E-115). *Neuropsychopharmacology, 11*(2), 119–124.

Skolnick, P. (1999). Antidepressants for the new millennium. *European Journal of Pharmacology, 375*(1-3), 31–40.

Sloane, R. B., Hughes, W., & Haust, H. L. (1966). Catecholamine excretion in manic-depressive and schizophrenic psychosis and its relationship to symptomatology. *Canadian Psychiatric Association Journal, 11*(1), 6–19.

Soczynska, J. K., Kennedy, S. H., Goldstein, B. I., Lachowski, A., Woldeyohannes, H. O., & McIntyre, R. S. (2009). The effect of tumor necrosis factor antagonists on mood and mental health-associated quality of life: Novel hypothesis-driven treatments for bipolar depression? *Neurotoxicology, 30*(4), 497–521. https://doi.org/10.1016/j.neuro.2009.03.004.

Sperner-Unterweger, B., Kohl, C., & Fuchs, D. (2014). Immune changes and neurotransmitters: Possible interactions in depression? *Progress in Neuro-Psychopharmacology & Biological Psychiatry, 48*, 268–276. https://doi.org/10.1016/j.pnpbp.2012.10.006.

Srivastava, N., Barthwal, M. K., Dalal, P. K., et al. (2002). A study of nitric oxide, beta-adrenergic receptors and antioxidant status in the polymorphonuclear leukocytes from the patients of depression. *Journal of Affective Disorders, 72*, 45–52.

Stamler, J. S., Simon, D. I., Jaraki, O., Osborne, J. A., Francis, S., Mullins, M., et al. (1992). S-nitrosylation of tissue-type plasminogen activator confers vasodilatory and antiplatelet properties on the enzyme. *Proceedings of the National Academy of Sciences of the United States of America, 89*(17), 8087–8091.

Steinert, J. R., Chernova, T., & Forsythe, I. D. (2010). Nitric oxide signaling in brain function, dysfunction, and dementia. *The Neuroscientist, 16*(4), 435–452. https://doi.org/10.1177/1073858410366481.

Strawbridge, R., Young, A. H., & Cleare, A. J. (2017). Biomarkers for depression: Recent insights, current challenges and future prospects. *Neuropsychiatric Disease and Treatment, 13*, 1245–1262. https://doi.org/10.2147/ndt.s114542.

Stuehr, D. J. (1999). Mammalian nitric oxide synthases. *Biochimica et Biophysica Acta, 1411*(2-3), 217–230.

Suzuki, E., Nakaki, T., Kanba, S., Shintani, F., & Miyaoka, H. (2003). Long-term imipramine treatment increases nitrate levels in the rat hypothalamus. *Cellular and Molecular Neurobiology, 23*(6), 953–962.

Suzuki, E., Nakaki, T., Shintani, F., Kanba, S., & Miyaoka, H. (2002). Antipsychotic, antidepressant, anxiolytic, and anticonvulsant drugs induce type II nitric oxide synthase mRNA in rat brain. *Neuroscience Letters, 333*(3), 217–219.

Suzuki, E., Yagi, G., Nakaki, T., Kanba, S., & Asai, M. (2001). Elevated plasma nitrate levels in depressive states. *Journal of Affective Disorders, 63*, 221–224.

Suzuki, E., Yoshida, Y., Shibuya, A., & Miyaoka, H. (2003). Nitric oxide involvement in depression during interferon-alpha therapy. *The International Journal of Neuropsychopharmacology, 6*, 415–419.

Szewczyk, B., Poleszak, E., Sowa-Kucma, M., Wrobel, A., Slotwinski, S., Listos, J., et al. (2010). The involvement of NMDA and AMPA receptors in the mechanism of antidepressant-like action of zinc in the forced swim test. *Amino Acids, 39*(1), 205–217. https://doi.org/10.1007/s00726-009-0412-y.

Tanda, K., Nishi, A., Matsuo, N., Nakanishi, K., Yamasaki, N., Sugimoto, T., et al. (2009). Abnormal social behavior, hyperactivity, impaired remote spatial memory, and increased D1-mediated dopaminergic signaling in neuronal nitric oxide synthase knockout mice. *Molecular Brain, 2*(1), 19. https://doi.org/10.1186/1756-6606-2-19.

Tarazi, F. I., Zhang, K., & Baldessarini, R. J. (2002). Long-term effects of newer antipsychotic drugs on neuronal nitric oxide synthase in rat brain. *Nitric Oxide: Biology and Chemistry*, 7(4), 297–300. doi:S108986030200126X [pii].

Tomaz, V. S., Cordeiro, R. C., Costa, A. M., de Lucena, D. F., Nobre Junior, H. V., de Sousa, F. C., et al. (2014). Antidepressant-like effect of nitric oxide synthase inhibitors and sildenafil against lipopolysaccharide-induced depressive-like behavior in mice. *Neuroscience, 268*, 236–246. https://doi.org/10.1016/j.neuroscience.2014.03.025.

Trueba, A. F., Smith, N. B., Auchus, R. J., & Ritz, T. (2013). Academic exam stress and depressive mood are associated with reductions in exhaled nitric oxide in healthy individuals. *Biological Psychology, 93*(1), 206–212. https://doi.org/10.1016/j.biopsycho.2013.01.017.

Ulak, G., Mutlu, O., Akar, F. Y., Komsuoğlu, F. I., Tanyeri, P., & Erden, B. F. (2008). Neuronal NOS inhibitor 1-(2-trifluoromethylphenyl)-imidazole augment the effects of antidepressants acting via serotonergic system in the forced swimming test in rats. *Pharmacology, Biochemistry and Behavior, 90*, 563–568.

Umathe, S. N., Bhutada, P. S., Jain, N. S., Mundhada, Y. R., Borkar, S. S., & Dhumal, B. (2009). Role of nitric oxide in obsessive–compulsive behavior and its involvement in the anti-compulsive effect of paroxetine in mice. *Nitric Oxide: Biology and Chemistry, 21*, 140–147. https://doi.org/10.1016/j.niox.2009.07.001.

van Amsterdam, J. G. C., & Opperhuisen, A. (1999). Nitric oxide and biopterin in depression and stress. *Psychiatry Research, 85*, 33–38.

van Zyl, L. T., Lesperance, F., Frasure-Smith, N., Malinin, A. I., Atar, D., Laliberte, M. A., et al. (2009). Platelet and endothelial activity in comorbid major depression and coronary artery disease patients treated with citalopram: The Canadian Cardiac Randomized Evaluation of Antidepressant and Psychotherapy Efficacy Trial (CREATE) biomarker substudy. *Journal of Thrombosis and Thrombolysis, 27*(1), 48–56. https://doi.org/10.1007/s11239-007-0189-3.

Volke, V., Wegener, G., Bourin, M., & Vasar, E. (2003). Antidepressant and anxiolytic-like effects of selective neuronal NOS inhibitor 1-(2-trifluoromethylphenyl)-imidazole in mice. *Behavioural Brain Research, 140*, 141–147.

Wang, D., An, S. C., & Zhang, X. (2008). Prevention of chronic stress-induced depression-like behavior by inducible nitric oxide inhibitor. *Neuroscience Letters, 433*(1), 59–64. https://doi.org/10.1016/j.neulet.2007.12.041.

Wang, M., Duan, F., Wu, J., Min, Q., Huang, Q., Luo, M., et al. (2018). Effect of cyclooxygenase-2 inhibition on the development of posttraumatic stress disorder in rats. *Molecular Medicine Reports, 17*(4), 4925–4932. https://doi.org/10.3892/mmr.2018.8525.

Wang, C. H., Hsiao, C. J., Lin, Y. N., Wu, J. W., Kuo, Y. C., Lee, C. K., et al. (2014). Carbamazepine attenuates inducible nitric oxide synthase expression through Akt inhibition in activated microglial cells. *Pharmaceutical Biology*, *52*(11), 1451–1459. https://doi.org/10.3109/13880209.2014.898074.

Wegener, G., Bandpey, Z., Heiberg, I. L., Volke, V., Trabace, L., Rosenberg, R., et al. (2004). Combined chronic treatment with citalopram and lithium does not modify the regional neurochemistry of nitric oxide in rat brain. *Journal of Physiology and Pharmacology*, *55*(3), 575–586.

Wegener, G., Volke, V., Harvey, B. H., & Rosenberg, R. (2003). Local, but not systemic, administration of serotonergic antidepressants decreases hippocampal nitric oxide synthase activity. *Brain Research*, *959*(1), 128–134.

Wei, Y. C., Zhou, F. L., He, D. L., Bai, J. R., Hui, L. Y., Wang, X. Y., et al. (2009). The level of oxidative stress and the expression of genes involved in DNA-damage signaling pathways in depressive patients with colorectal carcinoma. *Journal of Psychosomatic Research*, *66*(3), 259–266.

Xing, G., Chavko, M., Zhang, L.-X., Yang, S., & Post, R. M. (2002). Decreased calcium-dependent constitutive nitric oxide synthase (cNOS) activity in prefrontal cortex in schizophrenia and depression. *Schizophrenia Research*, *58*, 21–30.

Yaron, I., Shirazi, I., Judovich, R., Levartovsky, D., Caspi, D., & Yaron, M. (1999). Fluoxetine and amitriptyline inhibit nitric oxide, prostaglandin E2, and hyaluronic acid production in human synovial cells and synovial tissue cultures. *Arthritis and Rheumatism*, *42*(12), 2561–2568. https://doi.org/10.1002/1529-0131(199912)42:12<2561::AID-ANR8>3.0.CO;2-U.

Yildiz, F., Erden, B. F., Ulak, G., Utkan, T., & Gacar, N. (2000). Antidepressant-like effect of 7-nitroindazole in the forced swimming test in rats. *Psychopharmacology (Berlin)*, *149*(1), 41–44.

Yoshimura, R., Yanagihara, N., Terao, T., Minami, K., Abe, K., & Izumi, F. (1995). Inhibition by carbamazepine of various ion channels-mediated catecholamine secretion in cultured bovine adrenal medullary cells. *Naunyn-Schmiedebergs Archiv für Pharmakologie*, *352*(3), 297–303.

Yoshino, Y., Ochi, S., Yamazaki, K., Nakata, S., Abe, M., Mori, Y., et al. (2015). Antidepressant action via the nitric oxide system: A pilot study in an acute depressive model induced by arginin. *Neuroscience Letters*, *599*, 69–74. https://doi.org/10.1016/j.neulet.2015.05.043.

Yuen, E., Swanson, S., & Witkin, J. M. (2017). Prediction of human efficacious antidepressant doses using the mouse forced swim test. *Pharmacology, Biochemistry, and Behavior*, *161*, 22–29. https://doi.org/10.1016/j.pbb.2017.09.002.

Yuskaitis, C. J., & Jope, R. S. (2009). Glycogen synthase kinase-3 regulates microglial migration, inflammation, and inflammation-induced neurotoxicity. *Cellular Signalling*, *21*, 264–273.

Zhang, J., Huang, X.-Y., Ye, C.-X., Wu, H.-Y., Hu, Y., Zhou, Q.-G., et al. (2010). Neuronal nitric oxide alteration for the role of 5-HT_{1A} receptor in modulating anxiety-related behaviors. *The Journal of Neuroscience*, *30*(7), 2433–2441.

Zhou, Q. G., Hu, Y., Hua, Y., Hu, M., Luo, C. X., Han, X., et al. (2007). Neuronal nitric oxide synthase contributes to chronic stress-induced depression by suppressing hippocampal neurogenesis. *Journal of Neurochemistry*, *103*(5), 1843–1854. https://doi.org/10.1111/j.1471-4159.2007.04914.x.

Zhou, X. Y., Zhang, F., Ying, C. J., Chen, J., Chen, L., Dong, J., et al. (2017). Inhibition of iNOS alleviates cognitive deficits and depression in diabetic mice through down-regulating the NO/sGC/cGMP/PKG signal pathway. *Behavioural Brain Research*, *322*(Pt A), 70–82. https://doi.org/10.1016/j.bbr.2016.12.046.

Zomkowski, A. D., Engel, D., Cunha, M. P., Gabilan, N. H., & Rodrigues, A. L. (2012). The role of the NMDA receptors and L-arginine-nitric oxide-cyclic guanosine monophosphate pathway in the antidepressant-like effect of duloxetine in the forced swimming test. *Pharmacology, Biochemistry, and Behavior*, *103*(2), 408–417. https://doi.org/10.1016/j.pbb.2012.09.011.

Zomkowski, A. D., Engel, D., Gabilan, N. H., & Rodrigues, A. L. (2010). Involvement of NMDA receptors and L-arginine-nitric oxide-cyclic guanosine monophosphate pathway in the antidepressant-like effects of escitalopram in the forced swimming test. *European Neuropsychopharmacology*, *20*(11), 793–801. https://doi.org/10.1016/j.euroneuro.2010.07.011.

Zomkowski, A. D., Hammes, L., Lin, J., Calixto, J. B., Santos, A. R., & Rodrigues, A. L. (2002). Agmatine produces antidepressant-like effects in two models of depression in mice. *Neuroreport*, *13*(4), 387–391.

Zorrilla, E. P., Luborsky, L., McKay, J. R., Rosenthal, R., Houldin, A., Tax, A., et al. (2001). The relationship of depression and stressors to immunological assays: A meta-analytic review. *Brain, Behavior, and Immunity*, *15*, 199–226.

CHAPTER SIX

Selective allosteric modulation of muscarinic acetylcholine receptors for the treatment of schizophrenia and substance use disorders

Laura B. Teal[a,b], Robert W. Gould[a,b], Andrew S. Felts[a,b], Carrie K. Jones[a,b,*]
[a]Department of Pharmacology, Vanderbilt University, Nashville, TN, United States
[b]Vanderbilt Center for Neuroscience Drug Discovery, Vanderbilt University, Nashville, TN, United States
*Corresponding author: e-mail address: carrie.jones@vanderbilt.edu

Contents

1. Introduction 155
2. Cholinergic innervation and regions implicated in schizophrenia and SUD 160
3. Muscarinic acetylcholine receptors and schizophrenia 162
   3.1 M_1/M_4-preferring orthosteric agonist xanomeline showed antipsychotic effects 167
   3.2 Allosteric modulation of M_1 mAChR and schizophrenia 170
   3.3 Allosteric modulation of M_4 mAChR and schizophrenia 171
4. Muscarinic acetylcholine receptors and substance use disorders 173
   4.1 Allosteric modulation of M_4 mAChR and substance use 178
   4.2 Allosteric modulation of M_5 mAChR and substance use 179
5. Potential challenges with mAChR allosteric modulation 179
6. Conclusion 181
Acknowledgments 182
Conflict of interest statement 182
References 182
Further reading 196

Abstract

Muscarinic acetylcholine receptor (mAChRs) subtypes represent exciting new targets for the treatment of schizophrenia and substance use disorder (SUD). Recent advances in the development of subtype-selective allosteric modulators have revealed promising effects in preclinical models targeting the different symptoms observed in schizophrenia and SUD. M_1 PAMs display potential for addressing the negative and cognitive symptoms of schizophrenia, while M_4 PAMs exhibit promise in treating preclinical models predictive of antipsychotic-like activity. In SUD, there is increasing support for

Advances in Pharmacology, Volume 86
ISSN 1054-3589
https://doi.org/10.1016/bs.apha.2019.05.001

modulation of mesocorticolimbic dopaminergic circuitry involved in SUD with selective M_4 mAChR PAMs or M_5 mAChR NAMs. Allosteric modulators of these mAChR subtypes have demonstrated efficacy in rodent models of cocaine and ethanol seeking, with indications that these ligand may also be useful for other substances of abuse, as well as in various stages in the cycle of addiction. Importantly, allosteric modulators of the different mAChR subtypes may provide viable treatment options, while conferring greater subtype specificity and corresponding enhanced therapeutic index than orthosteric muscarinic ligands and maintaining endogenous temporo-spatial ACh signaling. Overall, subtype specific mAChR allosteric modulators represent important novel therapeutic mechanisms for schizophrenia and SUD.

Abbreviations

ACh	acetylcholine
AChEI	acetylcholinesterase inhibitor
AD	Alzheimer's Disease
BQCA	benzyl quinolone carboxylic acid
CNS	central nervous system
CPP	conditioned place preference
DA	dopamine
DBB	diagonal band of Broca
DSM-5	diagnostic and statistical manual, 5th edition
EtOH	ethanol
GLU	glutamate
GPCR	G protein-coupled receptor
KO	knockout (genetic)
LTD	long-term depression
LTP	long-term potentiation
LDTg	laterodorsal tegmental nucleus
mAChR	muscarinic acetylcholine receptor
MS	medial septum
NAM	negative allosteric modulator
NA	nucleus accumbens
nBM	nucleus basalis magnocellularis
NMDAR	*N*-methyl-D-aspartate receptor
NOR	novel object recognition
PAM	positive allosteric modulator
PFC	prefrontal cortex
PNS	peripheral nervous system
PPI	prepulse inhibition
PPTg	pedunculopontine tegmental nucleus
REM	rapid eye movement
SA	self-administration
SNP	single nucleotide polymorphism
SPNs	spiny projection neurons
SUD	substance use disorder
TMD	transmembrane domain
VTA	ventral tegmental area

1. Introduction

Acetylcholine (ACh) represents an important neurotransmitter in both the central and peripheral nervous systems (CNS and PNS, respectively). Previous studies have shown that ACh signaling is dysregulated in many neuropsychiatric disorders, including substance use disorder (SUD), schizophrenia, and Alzheimer's Disease (AD; Langmead, Watson, & Reavill, 2008; Jones, Byun, & Bubser, 2012). ACh receptors fall broadly into two families of receptors: nicotinic ionotropic receptors and muscarinic metabotropic G protein-coupled receptors (GPCRs) (Jones et al., 2012; Rahman, Engleman, & Bell, 2015, respectively). For the purposes of this review, we will examine the roles of different muscarinic acetylcholine receptor (mAChR) subtypes in the underlying pathophysiology of schizophrenia and SUD and the potential development of selective modulators of these mAChR subtypes as novel therapeutics for these disorders. Structurally, mAChRs resemble other class A (rhodopsin-like) GPCRs (Fig. 1) with seven helical transmembrane domains (TMDs; Caulfield & Birdsall, 1998; Kruse et al., 2012; Kubo, Fukuda, et al., 1986; Kubo, Maeda, et al., 1986). The

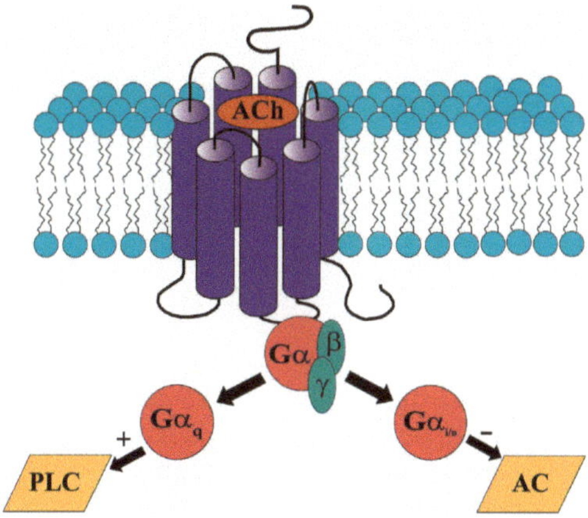

Fig. 1 Muscarinic Acetylcholine Receptor Structure and Coupling. These mAChRs are seven transmembrane domain class A GPCRs. The G_α subunit associates with the third intracellular domain of the protein which shows the lowest subtype homology, and the ACh binding pore within the receptor is the region of highest homology. M_1, M_3, and M_5 selectively couple to $G_{q/11}$ G-proteins leading to activation of PLC and subsequent increases in DAG and IP_3, leading to increased intracellular calcium. M_2 and M_4 preferentially activate $G_{i/o}$ G-proteins, inhibiting adenylyl cyclase and therefore reducing intracellular cAMP concentrations.

orthosteric ACh binding pocket resides within the TMDs and is highly conserved across the muscarinic subtypes, whereas intracellular and extracellular loops are less highly conserved and thus serve as potential targets for design of subtype selective compounds (Kruse et al., 2012; Wess, Gdula, & Brann, 1991; Wess, Maggio, Palmer, & Vogel, 1992).

Five distinct subtypes of mAChRs (M_1-M_5) have been identified, which differ in their functional coupling to heterotrimeric G proteins as well as synaptic and anatomical localization (Fig. 2). M_1, $M_{3,}$ and M_5 mAChRs primarily couple through G_q effector proteins, increasing inositol 1,4,5-phosphate signaling and downstream Ca^{2+} mobilization, while M_2 and M_4 mAChRs act through $G_{i/o}$ and inhibit adenylyl cyclase activation (Offermanns et al., 1994; Parker, Kameyama, Higashijima, & Ross, 1991; Peralta, Ashkenazi, Winslow, Ramachandran, & Capon, 1988). These

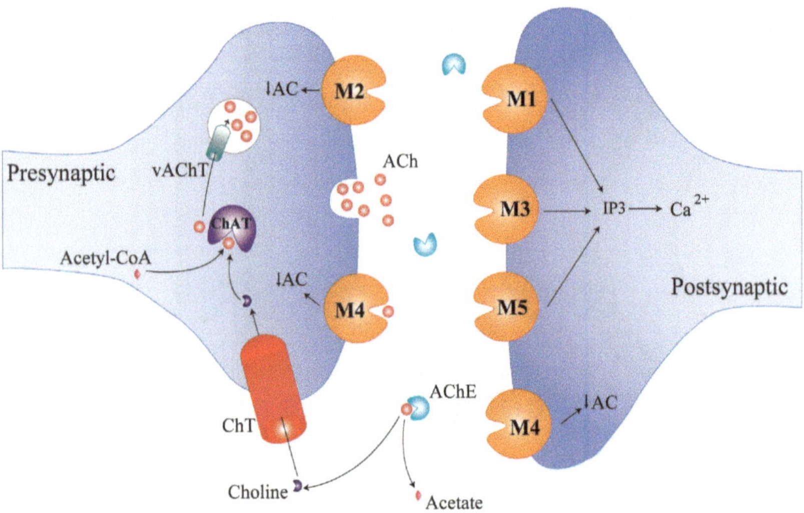

Fig. 2 Representation of a Hypothetical Cholinergic Synapse. mAChR subtypes M2 and M4 localize presynaptically (left neuron) and serve as autoreceptors on cholinergic terminals (and also heteroreceptors on non-cholinergic pre-synaptic terminals, such as DA, which is not shown). These autoreceptors inhibit neurotransmission via decreasing adenylyl cyclase. ACh is synthesized in cholinergic neurons from choline and acetyl-CoA. Choline uptake is mediated by choline transporters on the membrane. After synthesis via choline acetyltransferase, ACh is packaged into vesicles via a vesicular acetylcholine transporter. After release, ACh is hydrolyzed by acetylcholinesterase, and choline is subsequently taken back up into the presynaptic neuron. The postsynaptic intracellular messengers are also shown. *Abbreviations*: AC, adenylyl cyclase; AChE, acetylcholinesterase; ChAT, choline acyltransferase; ChT, choline transporter; vAChT, vesicular acetylcholine transporter.

differences in G protein coupling between the mAChR subtypes are mediated by differences in the third intracellular domain of the protein sequence, where the G_α subunit associates with the receptor (Liu, Conklin, Blin, Yun, & Wess, 1995).

M_1 is the predominant mAChR subtype expressed in the central nervous system (CNS), with localization post-synaptically within the striatum, hippocampus, amygdala, and all layers of the cortex (Buckley, Bonner, & Brann, 1988; Levey, Edmunds, Koliatsos, Wiley, & Heilman, 1995; Levey, Kitt, Simonds, Price, & Brann, 1991; Vilaró, Wiederhold, Palacios, & Mengod, 1991). The M_1 mAChR is also expressed in several peripheral tissues, including vas deferens, aortic smooth muscle, sympathetic ganglia, submaxillary gland, and at very low levels in the ileum (Levey, 1993; Tracey & Peach, 1992). In addition, M_1 mAChRs physically and functionally couple to the *N*-methyl-D-aspartate receptor (NMDAR), a subtype of glutamate (GLU)-gated ion channel, leading to the potentiation of glutamatergic signaling throughout the hippocampus and forebrain regions (Calabresi, Centonze, Gubellini, Pisani, & Bernardi, 1998; Marino, Rouse, Levey, Potter, & Conn, 1998; Sur et al., 2003). A reduction of function of these NMDARs is thought to underlie some of the pathological changes and associated symptoms in schizophrenia, making the coupling of M_1 mAChR physiology to NMDAR function of particular interest.

In contrast, M_2 mAChRs are primarily found on cholinergic neurons and act as presynaptic autoreceptors to control ACh release (Zhang, Basile, et al., 2002, Zhang, Yamada, Gomeza, Basile, & Wess, 2002; Rouse, Edmunds, Yi, Gilmor, & Levey, 2000; Rouse, Gilmor, & Levey, 1998). This mAChR subtype is expressed throughout the CNS, specifically within the basal forebrain, parts of the striatum, cranial motor nuclei, non-pyramidal neurons of the hippocampus, and the pedunculopontine and laterodorsal tegmental nuclei (PPTg and LDTg, respectively) of the brainstem. M_2 mAChRs are also expressed in high abundance in endothelial cells of the heart, the ileum, the uterus, and sympathetic ganglia (Dorje, Levey, & Brann, 1991; Levey et al., 1991, 1995; Li, Yasuda, Wall, Wellstein, & Wolfe, 1991; Vilaró, Wiederhold, Palacios, & Mengod, 1992).

M_3 is generally expressed at lower levels than the other mAChR subtypes within several regions of the CNS, including the cortex, hippocampus, and striatum. In contrast, M_3 mAChRs have higher levels of expression within the submaxillary gland, aortic smooth muscle, lung, ileum, pancreas, and bladder (Buckley et al., 1988; Dorje et al., 1991; Tracey & Peach, 1992; Wall, Yasuda, Li, & Wolfe, 1991). While there is comparatively less known about the function of M_3 receptors within the CNS, this mAChR subtype is localized in brain regions that regulate insulin homeostasis, including the hypothalamus and dorsal vagal complex of the brainstem (Weston-Green, Huang, Lian, & Deng, 2012).

Notably, M_4 mAChRs are expressed both presynaptically and postsynaptically within the CNS (Zang & Creese, 1997; Zhang, Basile, et al., 2002; Zhang, Yamada, et al., 2002). Presynaptically, they function as autoreceptors on cholinergic projections, as well as modulating the function of cholinergic interneurons within the striatum (Hersch, Gutekunst, Flees, Heilman, & Levey, 1994). The M_4 mAChR subtype is also found presynaptically on glutamatergic projections, where it plays a modulatory role in cortico-striatal glutamatergic signaling (Pancani et al., 2014). In addition, M_4 mAChRs are colocalized with D_1 dopamine receptors on medium spiny GABAergic neurons within the striatum and act to regulate GABAergic signaling within the direct pathway of the basal ganglia circuitry (Ince, Ciliax, & Levey, 1997; Tzavara et al., 2004). Peripherally, M_4 mAChRs have been reported to be localized predominantly in the lung, with very low expression in the ileum and salivary glands (Levey, 1993).

M_5 mAChRs, interestingly, have a far less widespread distribution than the other mAChR subtypes, making them a potentially important drug target for modulation of specific CNS circuits without associated potential side effects. In particular, M_5 mRNA is found in low density in the ventral tegmental area (VTA) as well as the substantia nigra, with little to no expression in other regions of the CNS (Vilaró, Palacios, & Mengod, 1990; Weiner, Levey, & Brann, 1990). Previous studies have reported that the M_5 receptor protein is localized somatodendritically within the VTA (Garzón & Pickel, 2013), coupled with functional evidence that M_5 may act within the striatum to modulate DA release in the accumbens (Bendor et al., 2010; Foster et al., 2014; Zhang, Basile, et al., 2002; Zhang, Yamada, et al., 2002). In addition to expression within the brain, there is evidence that M_5 mAChRs are expressed within the cerebral vasculature, particularly the circle of Willis and pial arteries (Tayebati, Di Tullio, Tomassoni, & Amenta, 2003; Yamada et al., 2001).

Overall as shown in Table 1, the five mAChR subtypes exhibit diverse localization and expression patterns throughout the CNS (see Table 1). As such, several of these mAChR subtypes, particularly M1, M4, and M5, have been increasingly recognized as viable drug targets for a variety of CNS disorders (see Bock, Schrage, & Mohr, 2018; Kruse et al., 2014), with increasing emphasis on the identification of subtype specific compounds as the different roles of each mAChR subtype are further elucidated.

Table 1 Muscarinic subtype receptor regional expression.

Receptor	High expression	Moderate expression	Low expression
M_1	Cortex, hippocampus	Striatum, basolateral amygdala, olfactory nuclei, bulb, and tubercle, piriform cortex	Caudate putamen
M_2	Pontine nuclei, olfactory bulb, medial septal nuclei, diagonal band,		Thalamus (habenulae)
M_3	Hippocampus, olfactory tubercle, piriform cortex	Cortex, cerebellum, thalamus	Striatum, lateral septal nuclei, caudate putamen, superior colliculus, pontine nuclei, central grey
M_4	Caudate putamen, nucleus accumbens and striatum, olfactory bulb and tubercle	Cortex, hippocampus, medial septal nuclei, diagonal band, nucleus basalis magnocellularis, substantia innominata	Thalamus, cerebellum
M_5	Substantia nigra, ventral tegmental area		Hippocampus, lateral habenula, ventromedial hypothalamic nucleus, mamillary nucleus

Sources: Brann, M. R., Buckley, N. J., & Bonner, T. I. (1988). The striatum and cerebral cortex express different muscarinic receptor mRNAs. *FEBS Letters, 230*(1–2), 90–94.
Buckley, N. J., Bonner, T. I., & Brann, M. R. (1988). Localization of a family of muscarinic receptor mRNAs in rat brain. *The Journal of Neuroscience, 8*(12), 4646–4652.
Vilaró, M. T., Palacios, J. M., & Mengod, G. (1990). Localization of m5 muscarinic receptor mRNA in rat brain examined by in situ hybridization histochemistry. *Neuroscience Letters, 114*(2), 154–159.
Weiner, D. M., Levey, A. I., & Brann, M. R. (1990). Expression of muscarinic acetylcholine and dopamine receptor mRNAs in rat basal ganglia. *Proceedings of the National Academy of Sciences of the United States of America, 87*, 7050–7054.

Early evidence for the possible roles of these different mAChR subtypes in various neuropsychiatric conditions has accumulated from characterization of subtype-specific mAChR knockout (KO) mouse strains (for a thorough review of mAChR knockout lines, see Thomsen, Sørensen, & Dencker, 2018; Wess, Eglen, & Gautam, 2007) and from pharmacologic challenge studies with non-selective muscarinic ligands, including the non-selective muscarinic antagonist scopolamine and the subtype-preferring muscarinic orthosteric agonists xanomeline (M_1/M_4) and pirenzepine (M_1) (Jones et al., 2012). However, progress has been hindered by the lack of highly mAChR subtype selective compounds. Due to the high degree of homology at the orthosteric ACh binding site across the five mAChR subtypes, it has been historically difficult to develop subtype specific ligands that do not exhibit dose-limiting side effects through non-selective activation of peripherally expressed mAChR subtypes (Thakurathi, Vincenzi, & Henderson, 2013).

More recently, an alternative approach has been taken to discover mAChR ligands that activate a particular mAChR subtype by actions at sites that are topographically distinct and less highly conserved than the orthosteric binding site of ACh, termed allosteric sites (see Burger, Sexton, Christopoulos, & Thal, 2018; Christopoulos, 2002; Conn, Lindsley, Meiler, & Niswender, 2014). Allosteric activators of mAChRs possess high subtype selectivity and display different modes of action. Allosteric agonists or negative allosteric modulators (NAMs) can activate or antagonize the mAChR subtype directly; while positive allosteric modulators (PAMs) do not directly activate the receptor, but bind to an allosteric site distinct from the ACh-binding site and potentiate the effects of endogenous ACh. Since mAChR PAMs have no intrinsic activity and can only exert their effects in the presence of ACh at a given synapse, these ligands provide a potential advantage by maintaining some level of activity dependence on the endogenous receptor activation.

2. Cholinergic innervation and regions implicated in schizophrenia and SUD

Cholinergic projections within the CNS can be broadly divided into the basal forebrain and the caudal mesencephalic regions. Within these two regions, six major groups of cholinergic projections have been classified based on location and projection (Mesulam, Mufson, Wainer, & Levey, 1983), with each region playing distinct roles in various neurological functions (see Fig. 3A). Ch1-Ch4 comprise the basal forebrain cholinergic system and are thought to be involved in the processes of attention, learning, and memory (Everitt & Robbins, 1997). Ch1 (the medial septum; MS) and Ch2 (the vertical limb of the diagonal band of Broca; DBB) project to the hippocampal formation and medial cortex (Eckenstein, Baughman, & Quinn, 1988). In contrast, Ch3 (the horizontal limb of the DBB) projects to the olfactory bulb, while Ch4 (the nuclear basalis magnocellularis;

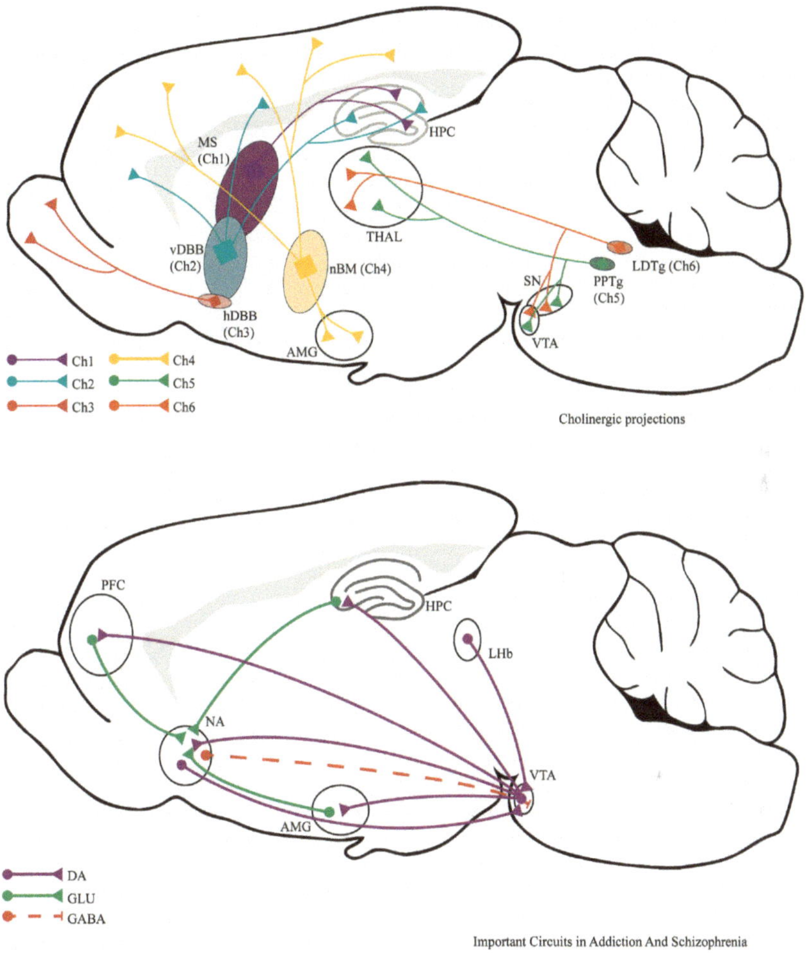

Fig. 3 (A) Cholinergic regions in the mouse brain and their projections. Cholinergic regions are widely organized into the basal forebrain and the caudal mesencephalon. The basal forebrain is comprised of the medial septum (MS; Ch1) and its hippocampal (HPC) projections, the vertical limb of the diagonal band of Broca (vDBB; Ch2) and its cortical and hippocampal projections, the horizontal limb of the diagonal band of Broca (hDBB; Ch3) and its olfactory projections, and the nucleus basalis magnocellularis (nBM; Ch4) and its projections to the cortex and amygdala (AMG). The caudal mesencephalon is comprised of only two cholinergic nuclei: the pedunculopontine tegmental nucleus (PPTg; Ch5) and the laterodorsal tegmental nucleus (LDTg; Ch6), both of which project to the thalamus (THAL), substantia nigra (SN), and ventral tegmental area (VTA). (B) Prominent circuits implicated in schizophrenia and SUD. Major dopaminergic, glutamatergic, and GABAergic projections. *Other abbreviations*: LHb, lateral habenula; NA, nucleus accumbens; PFC, prefrontal cortex. *Panel (A): Image adapted from Bubser, M., Byun, N. E., Wood, M. R., & Jones, C. K. (2011). Muscarinic receptor pharmacology and circuitry for the modulation of cognition.* Handbook of Experimental Pharmacology, 208, *121–166 with permission.*

nBM) neurons project to the amygdala as well as widely throughout the cerebral cortex, and these cortical projections are known to selectively degenerate in Alzheimer's Disease (AD; McGeer, McGeer, Kamo, & Wong, 1986; Mesulam et al., 1983; Price & Stern, 1983). In addition, Ch5-Ch6 comprise the caudal mesencephalon cholinergic system and are involved in sleep, arousal, and regulation of dopaminergic neuronal signaling (Datta & Siwek, 1997; Steidl, Wasserman, Blaha, & Yeomans, 2017; Van Dort et al., 2015). Ch5 (the pedunculopontine tegmental nucleus; PPTg) and Ch6 (the laterodorsal tegmental nucleus; LDTg) project to the thalamus, pontine reticular formation, ventral tegmental area (VTA), and substantia nigra (Clarke, Hommer, Pert, & Skirboll, 1987; Gould, Woolf, & Butcher, 1989; Hallanger, Levey, Lee, Rye, & Wainer, 1987; Satoh & Fibiger, 1986; Semba, Reiner, & Fibiger, 1990). Taken together, these different cholinergic neurons project to a wide array of brain areas, many of which directly modulate circuitry relevant to schizophrenia and/or SUD, as will be discussed below.

3. Muscarinic acetylcholine receptors and schizophrenia

Schizophrenia is a chronic neuropsychiatric disorder that is characterized by three major symptom clusters: (1) positive symptoms, such as delusions and hallucinations, (2) negative symptoms, including anhedonia, social withdrawal, and blunted affect, and (3) cognitive impairments, including deficits in executive function, working memory, and/or attention (American Psychiatric Association, 2013). These core symptom clusters are often accompanied by comorbid depression and sleep disturbances (Buckley, Miller, Lehrer, & Castle, 2009). In the case of sleep disruption, decreases in Rapid Eye Movement (REM) sleep latency are often seen before and during acute psychosis (Pritchett et al., 2012; Sprecher, Ferrarelli, & Benca, 2015). In addition, decreases in slow wave sleep quality and duration have been associated with both the negative and cognitive symptoms of schizophrenia (Göder et al., 2004; Keshavan et al., 1995; Koch et al., 2014; Yang & Winkelman, 2006). Current pharmacological treatments include typical, atypical, and dopamine partial agonist antipsychotics (Li, Snyder, & Vanover, 2016; Miyamoto, Duncan, Marx, & Lieberman, 2005). With regard to the efficacy and side effect profile of first generation typical antipsychotics like haloperidol, these drugs selectively antagonize the D_2 DA receptor subtype to attenuate primarily the positive symptoms of schizophrenia within a dose range that also induces a high proportion of extrapyramidal side effects, including dystonia, akathisia, and/or parkinsonism (Kurz, Hummer, Oberbauer, & Fleischhacker, 1995). In the case of second-generation atypical antipsychotics, these medications antagonize a broader range of receptors resulting in reduction of the positive symptoms with fewer associated extrapyramidal side effects than the first-generation antipsychotics. For example, the atypical antipsychotic clozapine displays low affinity for dopamine receptor subtypes, primarily D_4 and D_2, with higher affinity for a number of serotonin receptors, including 5-HT_2, 5-HT_3, 5-HT_6, and 5-HT_7. However, atypical antipsychotics still induce other dose-limiting adverse effects, including weight gain, type II diabetes mellitus, hyperlipidemia, and in the case of clozapine, agranulocytosis (Naheed & Green, 2001). The representative third generation antipsychotic Aripiprazole is a partial dopamine agonist with high D_2 and D_3 DA receptor affinity and moderate affinity for serotonin 5-HT_{1A} receptors (where it acts as a partial agonist) and 5-HT_{2A} receptors (where it acts as an antagonist). Because of its activity as a partial agonist, it is attenuated the positive symptoms with decreased frequency of extrapyramidal and metabolic side effects, although akathisia is common (Burris et al., 2002; Li et al., 2016; Stark et al., 2007). Unfortunately, all currently approved antipsychotics have little to no *efficacy in ameliorating* the negative and/or cognitive symptoms observed in schizophrenia. Thus, there is a critical need to develop novel treatment mechanisms targeting these other symptoms clusters of schizophrenia, while providing a broader therapeutic index.

Neuropsychiatric disorders such as schizophrenia present with such a complex set of neurobiological changes that it becomes difficult to implicate a single brain area or circuit in the etiology of the disease. Nonetheless, certain regions and circuits have emerged as key players in the pathophysiology of schizophrenia (Fig. 3B). Both the mesolimbic and mesocortical dopaminergic projections are generally accepted to be dysregulated in schizophrenia, although the exact nature of these dopaminergic signaling imbalances has been an ever-evolving hypothesis (Howes & Kapur, 2009). In addition to altered dopaminergic signaling, the prefrontal cortex (PFC) shows decreased connectivity to a variety of other regions, including limbic and striatal regions (see Sakurai & Gamo, 2018; Zhou, Fan, Qiu, & Jiang, 2015 for review). The PFC also shows alterations in GABAergic interneuron populations, which directly correlate with the cognitive impairments in patients with schizophrenia (Dienel & Lewis, 2018). Cholinergic inputs targeting mAChRs serve to modulate striatal dopamine circuits as well as directly impacting both pyramidal and GABAergic interneuron populations neuronal within the PFC (Raedler, Bymaster, Tandon, Copolov, & Dean, 2007). In addition, NMDAR hypofunction has long been associated with schizophrenic symptoms (Olney, Newcomer, & Farber, 1999), suggesting that the interaction between glutamatergic and cholinergic circuits may also be critical in schizophrenia. Taken together, this yields a variety of potential mechanisms by which muscarinic modulation may serve to impact circuit level dysregulation in schizophrenia. The specific roles of different mAChR subtypes in modulating these circuits will be discussed in more depth below.

Early evidence for the role of mAChRs in schizophrenia stems from multiple studies including genetic associations in patient populations, assessment of mAChR densities in postmortem brains, neuroimaging, neuropharmacological challenge and subtype-specific mAChR KO mouse studies. Polymorphisms in the human M_1 mAChR gene CHRM1 have been associated with cognitive symptoms in patients diagnosed with schizophrenia; specifically individuals with a homozygous single nucleotide polymorphism (SNP) at the CHRM1 locus 267 showed poorer performance on cognitive tests than those with heterozygous alleles (Liao et al., 2003; Scarr et al., 2012). This same polymorphism was also associated with decreased grey matter in the precentral gyrus of patients with schizophrenia, with no accompanying changes in cortical thickness (Carruthers et al., 2018; Cropley et al., 2015). In addition, two SNPs in the human M_4 mAChR gene CHRM4 have been associated with increased risk for schizophrenia (Scarr, Craig, et al., 2013; Scarr, Um, Cowie, & Dean, 2013), implying a potential genetic role for M_4, as well as M_1, in patients with schizophrenia.

Binding studies using postmortem brain tissues from individuals with schizophrenia have also been used to assess alterations in the expression of different mAChRs, specifically M_1 and/or M_4. These studies were conducted by measuring changes in the binding of the M_1-preferring orthosteric antagonist [^{3}H]pirenzepine (relative binding affinity M1 > M4 > M2,3,5), under low doses thought to confer M_1 specificity (Bolden, Cusack, & Richelson, 1992; Giachetti, Giraldo, Ladinsky, & Montagna, 1986; Moriya et al., 1999; Zang & Creese, 1997). In patients with schizophrenia compared to age-matched controls, these postmortem binding studies showed decreased levels of M_1 in the prefrontal cortex (PFC), caudate putamen, hippocampus, and superior temporal gyrus (Crook et al.,1999; Crook, Tomaskovic-Crook, Copolov, & Dean, 2000, 2001; Dean et al., 1996; Dean, McLeod, Keriakous, McKenzie, & Scarr, 2002; Deng & Huang, 2005; Zavitsanou, Katsifis, Mattner, & Xu-Feng, 2004). These decreased levels of [^{3}H]pirenzepine binding also correlated with increased efficacy of $G\alpha_{q/11}$ coupling to the M_1 mAChR, as measured by $G\alpha_{q/11}$-[^{35}S]-GTPγS (Salah-Uddin et al., 2009). In contrast, alterations in M_1 mAChR levels were not mimicked in bipolar disorder or major depression patient populations (Zavitsanou et al., 2004), suggesting that M_1 mAChRs may have a key role in schizophrenia, rather than a more general function across various neuropsychiatric disorders. Analysis of the [^{3}H]pirenzepine binding studies using a kernel density estimation followed by distribution fitting separated patients with schizophrenia into different groups. One of the cohorts, representing 26% of all subjects with the disorder, showed a 74% decrease in mean cortical [^{3}H]pirenzepine binding compared to controls, or a so called "muscarinic receptor-deficit schizophrenia" (MRDS) (Scarr et al., 2009). Subsequently, it was found that the micro RNA-107, which targets CHRM1, was increased specifically in this muscarinic-deficient population of schizophrenia, while levels of M_1 mRNA were decreased across all populations of patients with schizophrenia, implying there may be a complex, differential regulation of M_1 in these subpopulations (Scarr, Craig, et al., 2013; Scarr, Um, et al., 2013). Of note, when hippocampal [^{3}H]pirenzepine-binding was combined with *in situ* hybridization of M_1 and M_4 oligonucleotides from the same brain region of schizophrenia patients, decreased pirenzepine binding was only associated with decreases in M_4, but not M_1 receptor expression (Scarr, Sundram, Keriakous, & Dean, 2007). These studies indicate that the development of subtype-specific mAChR radioligands is critically needed to further understand the relative distribution of the different mAChR subtypes across the stages of schizophrenia illness.

Pharmacologic challenge studies in animals and clinical populations have also provided evidence for altered mAChR signaling in schizophrenia. For example, when non-selective muscarinic antagonists were administered to individuals with schizophrenia in an attempt to treat the extrapyramidal motor side-effects associated with typical antipsychotics, these drugs resulted in a worsening of the positive symptoms in these schizophrenia patients (Johnstone et al., 1983; Singh, Kay, & Opler, 1987; Tandon et al., 1991). These non-selective mAChR antagonists also induced schizophrenia-like symptoms, such as transient hallucinations and cognitive impairments, in healthy individuals (Hamborg-Petersen, Nielsen, & Thordal, 1984; McEvoy, 1987; Osterholm & Camoriano, 1982; Rusted & Warburton, 1988). Moreover, treatment with the indirect-acting mAChR agonist physostigmine, an acetylcholinesterase inhibitor (AChEI), has been shown

Table 2 Muscarinic knock-out mice show support for mAChRs in schizophrenia.

Receptor	Observed KO phenotype	Source
M_1	Impaired working memory	Anagnostaras et al. (2003)
	Impaired long-term potentiation	
M_1/M_4 double KO	Impaired PPI (not seen in individual M_1 or M_4 KO in this study)	Thomsen, Wess, Fulton, Fink-Jensen, and Caine (2010)
M_4	Impaired PPI	Felder et al. (2001)
	Abnormal social behavior	Koshimizu, Leiter, and Miyakawa (2012)
	Abolished antipsychotic function	Dencker et al. (2011) and Woolley, Carter, Gartlon, Watson, and Dawson (2009)
	Hyperexcitability of accumbal D_1 dopaminergic neurons	Tzavara et al. (2004)
	Abolished striatal DA release	Zhang, Yamada, et al. (2002)
M_5	Changes in PPI? (conflicting results)	Thomsen et al. (2007) and Wang et al. (2004)
	Reduced striatal DA release	Zhang, Yamada, et al. (2002)

to improve some cognitive and positive symptoms observed schizophrenia patients (Janowsky, El-Yousef, & Davis, 1973; Edelstein, Schultz, Hirschowitz, Kanter, & Garver, 1981; Kirrane, Mitropoulou, Nunn, Silverman, & Siever, 2001). In addition, the direct-acting, non-selective muscarinic agonist oxotremorine produced efficacy comparable to haloperidol and clozapine in several preclinical models of antipsychotic-like activity (Maehara, Hikichi, Satow, Okuda, & Ohta, 2008). However, because of their lack of specificity, these direct and indirect mAChR activators induced dose-related adverse effects that limited their clinical utility for the treatment of schizophrenia.

Extensive studies using subtype selective mAChR KO mice have substantially contributed to the body of evidence implicating different mAChRs in the various symptom domains of schizophrenia (see Table 2). For example, M_1 KO mice show prefrontal cortical cognitive dysfunctions similar to those observed in schizophrenia (Anagnostaras et al., 2003; Gould et al., 2015), while M_4 KO mice show disruptions in mesolimbic DA signaling consistent with the neurochemical changes that underlie many of the positive symptoms in schizophrenia (Tzavara et al., 2004). Interestingly, when M_4 mAChRs are specifically knocked out in D_1 dopamine receptor expressing medium spiny neurons (MSNs) within the striatum, mice show a hyperlocomotive phenotype and an abolishment of antipsychotic-like effects of the M_1- and M_4-preferring mAChR agonist xanomeline (discussed in detail below; Dencker et al., 2011; Jeon et al., 2010); supporting a role for the M_4 mAChR as a potential antipsychotic target. More recently, M_4 KO mice were also reported to exhibit cognitive impairments in both contextual and cue-mediated fear conditioning (Bubser et al., 2014) and prepulse inhibition (PPI) of the acoustic startle reflex (Felder et al., 2001; Koshimizu et al., 2012). Taken together, these studies suggest a role for both the M_1 and M_4 mAChRs in schizophrenia. It has been hypothesized that M_1 may play a larger role in the underlying pathophysiology of the negative and/or cognitive symptoms of schizophrenia based on its high expression within cortical regions and functional coupling to NMDARs, while M_4 may have a greater impact on the positive symptoms based on its high striatal expression. Studies using M_1 and M_4 selective PAMs have provided support for this hypothesis as will be discussed below. In the case of the M_5 mAChRs, previous studies have established a genetic association between CHRM5, the gene encoding M_5, and an increased incidence of schizophrenia (De Luca et al., 2004). In addition, abnormalities in mesolimbic DA signaling and PPI have been reported in M_5 KO mice (Thomsen et al., 2007; Wang et al., 2004). Collectively, these findings from preclinical and human genetic, anatomic, pharmacologic, and/or behavioral studies offer further confirmation for the development of subtype selective mAChR ligands for the treatment of different symptom clusters in schizophrenia.

3.1 M_1/M_4-preferring orthosteric agonist xanomeline showed antipsychotic effects

Further support for the development of subtype selective mAChR compounds for treating symptoms of schizophrenia comes from earlier studies targeting mAChRs as treatments for Alzheimer's Disease (AD). The currently approved treatments for AD target the cholinergic system and include acetylcholinesterase inhibitors (AChEIs), which inhibit the breakdown of acetylcholine. In the search for better treatments of the cognitive symptoms of AD, M_1/M_4-preferring muscarinic orthosteric agonist xanomeline (see Fig. 4) was developed (Bymaster et al., 1997; Grant & El-Fakahany, 2005). In a large multicenter trial evaluating the effects of the xanomeline

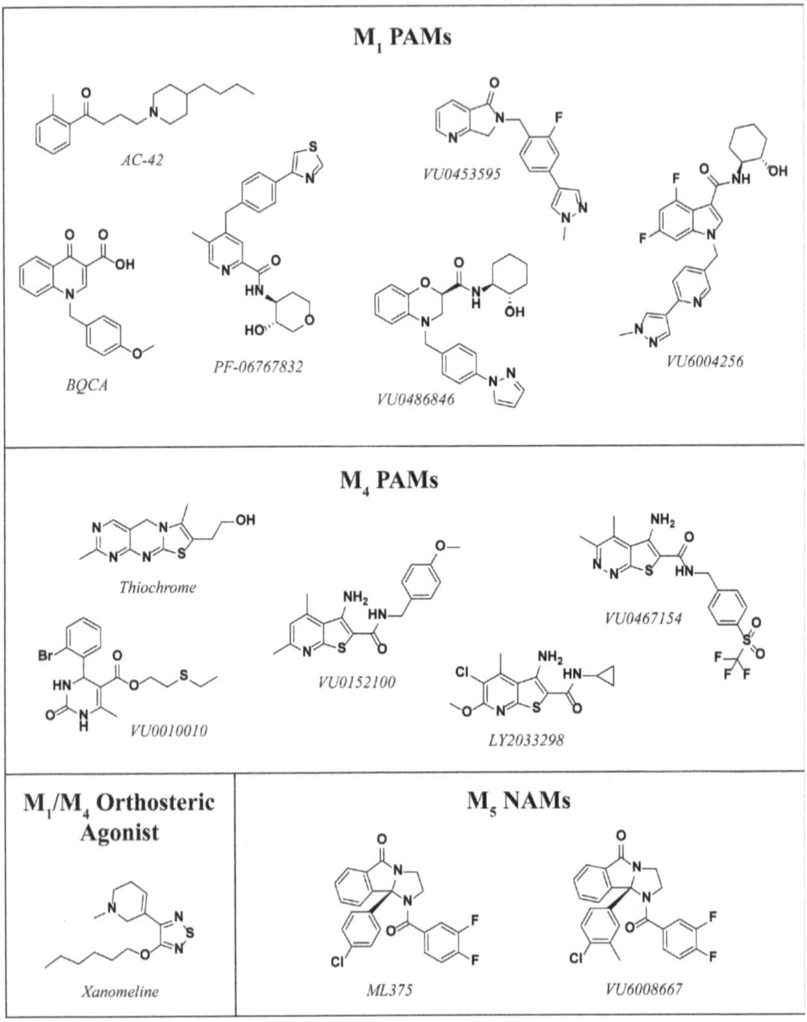

Fig. 4 Muscarinic modulators with subtype selectivity.

in AD patients, significant effects were observed on a range of different behavioral disturbances with a trend toward improvements in cognitive performance (Bodick, Offen, Levey, et al., 1997, Bodick, Offen, Shannon, et al., 1997; Veroff, Bodick, Offen, Sramek, & Cutler, 1998). Of particular note, xanomeline produced robust dose-dependent decreases in agitation, vocal outbursts, suspiciousness, delusions and hallucinations, while also enhancing blunted affect and other AD-related behavioral disturbances that share similarities to those observed in schizophrenia. These promising clinical findings raised the possibility that xanomeline might represent a novel treatment approach for schizophrenia. This supposition was supported by preclinical studies showing that xanomeline produced a similar antipsychotic-like activity profile to drugs like haloperidol or clozapine in behavioral measures, including conditioned avoidance and reversals of amphetamine-induced hyperlocomotion and apomorphine-induced PPI (Barak & Weiner, 2011; Brown et al., 2014; Perry et al., 2001; Stanhope et al., 2001), and in neurochemical studies demonstrating increased dopamine release in the prefrontal cortex (Perry et al., 2001). Moreover, xanomeline failed to attenuate amphetamine-induced hyperlocomotion in the M_4 KO mice and only partially attenuated it in the M_1 KO mice (Woolley et al., 2009), further reinforcing the involvement of M_4 and M_1 in the efficacy of this ligand.

In a subsequent 4-week, double-blind, placebo-controlled proof-of-concept trial the potential antipsychotic efficacy of xanomeline was evaluated in subjects with schizophrenia ($n=20$) (Shekhar et al., 2008). In these studies, xanomeline produced robust improvements in schizophrenic patients as compared with the placebo group, as measured by the Positive and Negative Syndrome Scale (PANSS), Clinical Global Impression Scale, and the Brief Psychiatric Rating Scale (BPRS) (Shekhar et al., 2008). Xanomeline also significantly enhanced verbal learning and short-term memory in schizophrenia patients, indicating efficacy in aspects of cognition performance (Shekhar et al., 2008). However, xanomeline still produced dose-limiting adverse gastrointestinal effects consistent with non-selective activation of peripheral mAChR subtypes, thus limiting its further clinical development. Recently, Karuna Pharmaceuticals completed a Phase I, double-blind, randomized, multiple-dose pilot study in normal healthy volunteers to evaluate the feasibility of administration of xanomeline in combination with the peripheral mAChR antagonist trospium chloride (KarXT; Karuna-Xanomeline-Trospium) in an effort to mitigate previously observed peripheral adverse side effects with xanomeline alone (ClinicalTrials.gov, NCT02831231, 2017). Based on these preliminary results, Karuna Pharmaceuticals is currently evaluating the efficacy, safety, and tolerability profile of KarXT in a Phase 2, randomized, double-blind, placebo-controlled, inpatient study in adult patients with schizophrenia who are in an acute exacerbation phase (ClinicalTrials.gov, NCT03697252, 2018). Future results from this study will help to determine if there is a viable therapeutic path for further development of mAChR orthosteric agonists like xanomeline. Alternatively, our group and others have focused on the development of highly subtype selective allosteric modulations of different mAChRs, particularly M_1 and M_4 as a novel therapeutic approach for schizophrenia.

3.2 Allosteric modulation of M_1 mAChR and schizophrenia

Over the last decade, there have been extensive efforts to discover and characterize selective M_1 allosteric modulators as tool compounds to further understand M_1 biology in general and as potential novel therapeutics. The first generation of M_1 allosteric modulators included AC-42 (see Fig. 4), which was the first ligand confirmed to bind at an allosteric site on the M_1 mAChR (Langmead et al., 2006; Spalding et al., 1989). These first-generation allosteric modulators represented important tool compounds in cell-based assays, but lacked sufficient physiochemical properties to progress to evaluation in animals. Second-generation allosteric modulators (both allosteric agonists and PAMs) have been developed that are systemically active and more suitable for *in vivo* dosing. Both the M_1 PAMs BQCA (benzyl quinolone carboxylic acid) and PF-06767832 (see Fig. 4) produced enhanced performance in acquisition of learning and memory tasks when administered alone as well as reversal of scopolamine-induced memory impairments and/or blockade of amphetamine-induced disruptions in PPI in wild-type mice (Chambon, Jatzke, Wegener, Gravius, & Danysz, 2012; Davoren et al., 2016; Gould et al., 2015; Shirey et al., 2009). BQCA also increased Fos expression (a marker of neuronal activity) in the PFC similar to xanomeline (Ma et al., 2009). Finally, BQCA has been shown to potentiate the effects of current atypical (but not typical) antipsychotic treatments in both PPI and a Y-maze model of spatial memory (Choy et al., 2016). The M_1 allosteric agonist TBPB [1-(1′-2-methylbenzyl)-1,4′-bipiperidin-4-yl)-1*H*-benzo[*d*]imidazol-2(3*H*)-one] was also shown to produce antipsychotic activity in rats and to potentiate NMDAR currents in hippocampal pyramidal cells in slice physiology (Jones et al., 2008). With the third generation of M_1 PAMs, the highly optimized VU6004256 (see Fig. 4) was shown to attenuate prefrontal cortical cognitive abnormalities found in a genetic mouse model of NMDAR hypofunction: specifically the global knockdown in the NR1 subunit of the NMDAR (Grannan et al., 2016). Consistent with these findings, another optimized M_1 PAM VU0453595 (see Fig. 4) was reported to restore impaired long-term depression (LTD) in the prefrontal cortex induced by chronic treatment with the NMDAR antagonist phencyclidine (PCP), as well as prefrontal cortical cognitive deficits and social impairments in mice (Ghoshal et al., 2016). More recently, the high potency M_1 PAM VU0486846 (see Fig. 4) was also reported to produce robust efficacy in a novel-object recognition (NOR) working memory test in wild-type mice as well as reverse cognitive deficits in the NOR assay induced by the atypical antipsychotic risperidone

(Rook et al., 2018). Taken together, evidence from studies using these M_1 allosteric agonists and PAMs indicates that selective positive modulation of M_1 mAChRs enhances PFC-dependent memory functions and decreases some psychotomimetic-like symptoms across preclinical models of schizophrenia. Thus, M_1 PAMs provide a promising target for developing new treatments for schizophrenia, particularly in terms of treating cognitive and/or negative symptoms. This treatment approach is especially intriguing given the current lack of treatments for this aspect as well as the known association between cognitive function in schizophrenia and decreased quality of life and long-term functional outcome measures (Bobes, Garcia-Portilla, Bascaran, Saiz, & Bousoño, 2007; Green, 1996; Green, Kern, & Heaton, 2004).

3.3 Allosteric modulation of M_4 mAChR and schizophrenia

Based on known distribution and ability to modulate DAergic function, M_4 receptors have been hypothesized to mediate the antipsychotic effects of xanomeline via modulation of D_1 expressing GABAergic MSNs in the striatum. Thiochrome, as shown in Fig. 4, is an oxidation product and metabolite of thiamine and was the first M_4 PAM to be described in the literature, representing an early tool compound for cell based work (Lazareno, Dolě, Popham, & Birdsall, 2004). The first highly selective M_4 PAM suitable for *in vivo* dosing was LY2033298 (see Fig. 4; Chan et al., 2008) which, based on site-directed mutagenesis studies, robustly potentiated the response of ACh through binding at residue F186 in the third extracellular loop (E3) of the receptor (Nawaratne, Leach, Felder, Sexton, & Christopoulos, 2010). When administered alone, LY2033298 had no effects *in vivo*, but potentiated the effects of a sub-threshold dose of the non-selective muscarinic orthosteric agonist oxotremorine to reduce apomorphine-induced PPI and inhibit conditioned avoidance response, two preclinical models predictive of antipsychotic-like activity (Chan et al., 2008; Leach et al., 2010). Interestingly, the lower potency of LY2033298 at the rat M_4 mAChR was thought to explain in part the lack of efficacy observed with the compound alone when used *in vivo*. Another important early M_4 PAM tool compound, VU0010010 (see Fig. 4), was reported to act through an allosteric site to enhance the affinity of the M_4 mAChR for ACh and increase the coupling efficiency of the M_4 mAChR to its G-proteins (Shirey et al., 2008). This M_4 tool compound, developed primarily for cell-based and electrophysiological assays, was used to demonstrate potentiation of a depression of synaptic transmission induced by carbachol (a non-selective cholinergic agonist) at excitatory but not inhibitory CA1 hippocampal synapses (Shirey et al., 2008), providing a strong indication that within the hippocampus M_4 regulates specifically glutamatergic synapses.

VU0152100 and VU0467154 (see Fig. 4) followed VU0010010, with more ideal physiochemical properties with suitability for *in vivo* studies. VU0152100 attenuated amphetamine-induced behaviors, including hyperlocomotion and disruptions in both conditioned freezing and PPI (Brady et al., 2008; Byun et al., 2014). This compound also improved memory on an object recognition task in wild-type rats (Galloway, Lebois, Shagarabi, Hernandez, & Manns, 2014). With the recent advances in M_4 PAM development, VU0467154 represents the most highly optimized M_4 PAM tool compound to date with enhanced *in vitro* potency and pharmacokinetic properties suitable for extensive acute and chronic *in vivo* pharmacologic characterization. As such, VU0467154 has shown robust efficacy across several preclinical models of antipsychotic-like activity, including reversal of amphetamine- and the NMDAR antagonist MK-801-induced hyperlocomotion (Bubser et al., 2014). More importantly, selective activation of the M_4 mAChR by VU0467154 results in dose-related attenuation of MK-801-induced deficits of associative learning and memory function (Bubser et al., 2014; Wood et al., 2017) as well as improved acquisition of memory when dosed alone in rodents after acute and repeated dosing (Gould et al., 2018). These recent findings indicate that M_4 PAMs may perhaps be useful for the treatment of the cognitive symptoms observed in schizophrenia, as well as for amelioration of the positive symptoms via modulation of striatal DA.

More recently, VU0467154 was shown to induce state-dependent alterations in sleep/wake architecture and arousal, including delayed Rapid Eye Movement (REM) sleep onset, increased cumulative duration of total and Non-Rapid Eye Movement (NREM) sleep, and increased arousal during waking periods in rats (Gould et al., 2016). By contrast in the same study, the atypical antipsychotic clozapine reduced arousal during wake, increased cumulative NREM, and decreased REM sleep. VU0467154 like clozapine also attenuated MK-801-induced increases in high frequency gamma power consistent with an APD-like mechanism of action (Gould et al., 2016). These data indicate that selective positive allosteric modulation of M4 may represent a novel mechanism for treating multiple symptoms of schizophrenia, including the disruptions in sleep architecture without a sedative profile.

Finally, the purported mechanism of action for the antipsychotic-like activity of M_4 PAMs is believed to be through M_4 mAChR inhibition of striatal dopamine release. Using VU0467154, it has been demonstrated that the inhibition of striatal DA by M_4 PAMs also requires CB_2 cannabinoid signaling to be intact (Foster et al., 2016), and that this cannabinoid signaling is mediated through co-activation of $mGlu_1$, a metabotropic glutamate receptor (Yohn et al., 2018). These studies serve to highlight the interconnectivity of cholinergic and glutamatergic striatal dopaminergic signaling critical for development of novel antipsychotics.

4. Muscarinic acetylcholine receptors and substance use disorders

According to the Diagnostic and Statistical Manual, 5th Edition (DSM-5), the hallmark of Substance Use Disorders (SUD) is a cluster of cognitive, behavioral, and physiological symptoms including craving, social isolation, and tolerance, wherein a person continues to use the substance despite related consequences (American Psychiatric Association, 2013). In addition, the DSM-5 recognizes for the first time substance-induced disorders that include schizophrenia and associated disorders, bipolar disorder, depressive and anxiety disorders, and sleep-wake disorders, among others (American Psychiatric Association, 2013). SUD is commonly described as an addiction cycle, which is characterized by initial drug use (recreational or prescription opioids), abuse (including increased frequency and/or dose of drug use), followed by periods of abstinence (voluntary or involuntary), and frequent and often repeated periods of relapse to drug abuse (Kourrich, Calu, & Bonci, 2015). This cycle can be robustly modeled in animals with the most common method being self-administration, a behavioral paradigm in which animals are allowed access to a lever which, upon being pressed, will deliver a rewarding stimulus, usually by intravenous administration (see Lynch, Nicholson, Dance, Morgan, & Foley, 2010). This allows the animal to be dosed contingently upon performing an action, and to titrate the dose over the course of the session. Furthermore, it is possible to examine the potential for relapse with a saline-extinction version of the self-administration model—wherein a lever previously associated with a reinforcing drug is paired with saline, and the time taken to extinguish drug-seeking behaviors is measured, as well as the effects of a drug-paired cue on this extinguished responding.

Dysfunction in neurological processes related to reward, executive function and inhibitory control, memory and learning, and motivation are all involved in SUD (Volkow, Wang, Fowler, Tomasi, & Telang, 2011). It is true that drugs of abuse converge on common mesolimbic DA reward pathways through a variety of direct cellular mechanisms that result in increased dopamine transmission within the nucleus accumbens (NA; Di Chiara & Imperato, 1988; see Nestler, 2005 for review). The mesolimbic DA pathway plays a central role in reward behavior, both through direct dopaminergic input as well as indirect glutamatergic pathways (Fig. 3B; Cooper, Robison, & Mazei-Robison, 2017; Hamid et al., 2016; Luscher, 2016; Quintero, 2013; Salamone & Correa, 2012; Yang et al., 2018). Thus, if it is possible to modulate this convergent mechanism, it may be possible to produce a pan-addiction treatment useful for many substances of abuse.

While this mesolimbic dopaminergic pathway is the best characterized pathway in SUD, it is only one of many implicated in the full pathology of the disorder. Greater reward circuitry involves a balance between activation of rewarding and aversive pathways, and it has been shown that activating cholinergic neurons in the LDTg stimulates mesolimbic DAergic neurons and this action is rewarding, while glutamatergic neurons from the lateral habenula activate mesocortical DAergic projections (VTA DA neurons which project to the PFC) and that this activation is aversive (Lammel et al., 2012; Lammel, Ion, Roeper, & Malenka, 2011). Mesocorticolimbic glutamate circuits have been implicated as critical in both learned response to drug cues (a circuit which also includes the hippocampus and the amygdala) and in impaired executive function/inhibitory control, and show neuroplastic changes particularly in maintenance of addiction (see Kalivas, 2009; van Huijstee & Mansvelder, 2015 for reviews).

Based on previously mentioned anatomical and physiological studies, multiple mAChR subtypes have been shown to directly or indirectly modulate the mesolimbic DA pathway. In particular, several mAChR subtypes are located within the NA, which receives inputs from many of addiction-related neural circuits (see Fig. 3B), suggesting that there may be a variety of mechanisms by which mAChRs could modulate one or more of these addiction circuits; though most of which are not yet completely understood. In addition, mAChRs have also displayed potential for modulating other regions that are critical in SUD, including PFC, which is the major region implicated in executive dysfunction aspects of SUD.

Accumulating human genetics studies provide evidence to link various mAChRs with SUD. One SNP in the CHRM1 was positively associated with risk of nicotine dependence (Lou et al., 2006). In addition, another study found an association between polymorphisms in CHRM2, the gene for M_2, and for the severity of, but not risk for, alcohol dependence (Jung et al., 2010). In another study, a polymorphism in CHRM4 was associated with increased incidence of cocaine dependence (Levran et al., 2016); while a SNP in CHRM5 was associated with increase in cigarette consumption, but not risk for addiction (Anney et al., 2007). While interestingly, the broader significant of these polymorphisms in each of mAChRs and potential links to the under pathophysiology of SUD remains unclear at this time.

Early anatomical evidence connecting mAChRs to substance use showed an increase in mAChR levels in the hippocampus and cortex following acute ethanol administration in mice (Rabin et al., 1980). However, after 10 days of ethanol administration, mAChR binding in the cortex of rats was shown to decrease, while binding in the striatum increased (Muller, Britton, & Seeman, 1980). After chronic alcohol abuse in humans, however, postmortem evaluation showed a decrease in mAChR binding sites using the non-selective muscarinic antagonist [^{3}H]quinuclidinyl benzilate ([^{3}H]QNB) in the thalamus as compared to age-matched controls, specifically in older subjects (Hellstrom-Lindahl, Winblad, & Nordberg, 1993). It is clear that ethanol exposure impacts mAChR availability, though the exact time course in different brain regions type is not completely understood. In addition to the effects of ethanol on mAChRs, other studies have examined the effects of substances of abuse on gene expression in rodents. Extended access to oxycodone resulted in a 1.65-fold increase in M_5 mRNA in the dorsal striatum (Zhang et al., 2014), a result that also merits further investigation. Seven days of investigator-administered cocaine also showed increases in M_1, M_3, and M_5 mRNA in the NA (Eipper-Mains et al., 2013), while self-administered oxycodone showed an increase only in M_3 in the dorsal striatum (Mayer-Blackwell et al., 2014). The impact of drugs of abuse on mAChRs is not yet fully understood and provides an exciting route for further exploration.

Studies using subtype-selective mAChR KO mouse lines have substantially contributed to understanding the role(s) of muscarinic cholinergic modulation in SUD (see Table 3). Because of the relatively specific localization of M_5 in the ventral tegmental area (VTA) of the mesolimbic DA pathway, M_5 mAChRs are thought to be activated by cholinergic input from both the LDTg and PPTg of the pons to modulate VTA dopaminergic neurons, which mediate the rewarding effects of many drugs of abuse (Steidl et al., 2017; Yeomans, Kofman, & McFarlane, 1985). In the absence of M_5

Table 3 Muscarinic knock-out mice show support for mAChRs in SUD.

Receptor	Observed KO phenotype	Source
M_1	Enhanced DA transmission in the accumbens	Gerber et al. (2001)
	Increased response to amphetamine	
	Decreased morphine CPP	Carrigan and Dykstra (2007))
	Decreased cocaine CPP	
	Attenuated discriminatory stimulus of cocaine	Joseph and Thomsen (2017)) and Thomsen et al. (2012)
M_4	Increased cocaine SA	Schmidt et al. (2011)
	Impaired cocaine-induced DA release in the NA	
	Hyperexcitability of accumbal D_1 dopaminergic neurons	Tzavara et al. (2004)
	Partially attenuated discriminatory stimulus of cocaine	Thomsen et al. (2012)
M_5	Impaired morphine CPP	Basile et al. (2002)
	Impaired cocaine CPP	Fink-Jensen et al. (2003)
	Reduced cocaine SA	Fink-Jensen et al. (2003)
	Reduced naloxone-induced withdrawal symptoms	Basile et al. (2002) and Fink-Jensen et al. (2003)
	Reduced morphine-induced locomotion	Steidl and Yeomans (2009))
	Abolished prolonged accumbal DA release	Forster, Yeomans, Takeuchi, and Blaha (2001)
	Abolished morphine-induced accumbal DA release	Steidl, Miller, Blaha, and Yeomans (2011)
	No change in analgesia	Basile et al. (2002)
	No change in food self-administration	Thomsen et al. (2005)

mAChRs, pons stimulation still produced acute dopamine release in the NA, but prolonged accumbal dopamine release was abolished (Forster et al., 2001), demonstrating the importance of M_5 in dopamine reward pathways. Early studies on M_5 KO mice revealed an impairment in morphine-induced condition place preference (CPP), as well as a reduction in both somatic and affective naloxone-induced withdrawal symptoms without altering the analgesic response (Basile et al., 2002). M_5 KO mice also displayed reductions in morphine-induced (Steidl & Yeomans, 2009) and amphetamine-induced locomotion (Wang et al., 2004). Consistent with these findings, virally transfecting M_5 mAChRs into the VTA (but not other regions) of M_5 KO mice increased morphine-induced locomotion (Wasserman, Wang, Rashid, Josselyn, & Yeomans, 2013). Additionally, intra-VTA administered morphine in M_5 KO mice showed no ability to yield an increase in accumbal DA efflux, implying that M_5 is not just modulatory, but necessary (Steidl et al., 2011). However, effects of M_5 mAChR activation on dopamine release are at least partially dependent on the location of the M_5 mAChRs (Foster et al., 2014), demonstrating the need to further understand the full localization and function of M_5 mAChRs within the mesolimbic DA pathway.

In addition to effects on opioids, knockout mouse models have elucidated the role of mAChRs in psychostimulant effects. M_5 KO mice evaluated in a cocaine self-administration (SA) paradigm administered cocaine at a lower rate and exhibited a decreased cocaine-mediated CPP as well as withdrawal symptoms (Fink-Jensen et al., 2003), but showed no deficits in food maintained SA (Thomsen et al., 2005). M_1 KO mice also showed decreased cocaine and morphine SA. In contrast, when M_4 mAChRs were knocked out, mice self-administered *more* cocaine than their wild-type counterparts (Schmidt et al., 2011). Cocaine-induced dopamine efflux within the NA was also increased in M_4 KO mice, in accordance with these results. These results are consistent with the previously mentioned high expression of the M_4 within the striatum and its physiological control of DA neurotransmission in the mesolimbic DA pathway.

Historically, nonspecific muscarinic agents have also served to elucidate the role of mAChRs in SUD. For example, injection of scopolamine into the basolateral amygdala of mice disrupted cocaine stimulus-reward conditioning, but not condition-cued reinstatement (See, McLaughlin, & Fuchs, 2003), implying that mAChRs in the amygdala are necessary for reward learning. AChEI administration was also shown to decrease the lethal effects of cocaine, possibly due to a direct interaction between cocaine and mAChRs, though the exact mechanism of this remains unclear (Flynn, Vaishnav, & Mash, 1992; Witkin, Goldberg, Katz, & Kuhar, 1989). Moreover, xanomeline produced a rightward shift in the cocaine dose-response curve, therefore attenuating cocaine's discriminatory stimulus in wild type, but not M_1, M_4, or M_1/M_4 double KO mice (Thomsen et al., 2010, 2012), suggesting that enhancement at either M_1 or M_4 could provide a potential treatment approach for psychostimulant addiction. Importantly, these effects were also seen under a repeated dosing regimen, increasing the translatability of the initial acute challenge observations given that pharmacological treatment for psychostimulant addiction would be administered chronically (Thomsen, Fulton, & Caine, 2014). Although to date, less research has investigated the therapeutic potential of selective M_1 PAMs for SUD, M_1 mAChR modulation of circuits involved in regulating cognition, arousal, or sleep may hold promise for treating lesser investigated symptoms associated with abstinence following chronic substance use.

4.1 Allosteric modulation of M_4 mAChR and substance use

Several of the M_4 PAMs described above have shown promise in preclinical models of SUD, with research to date focused on psychostimulants, such as cocaine. Acute administration of VU0152100 decreased cocaine self-administration in mice, cocaine-induced hyperlocomotion, and cocaine-induced increases in dopamine release within the striatum, results which were absent in M_4 KO animals (Dencker et al., 2012). In addition, selective deletion of M_4 mAChRs in D_1-DA receptor expressing MSNs resulted in a partial reduction of these effects, implying that the effects of cocaine are partially mediated by M_4 regulation of DA transmission. When tested in a saline-extinction model of cocaine self-administration, VU0152100 in combination with VU0357017 (an M_1 selective PAM) reduced the number of sessions necessary to meet extinction criteria by more than half, while xanomeline-treated mice showed no cocaine-induced reinstatement (Lebois et al., 2010; Stoll, Hart, Lindsley, & Thomsen, 2018). The highly optimized M_4 PAM VU0467154 produced a similar reduction in both cocaine-induced hyperlocomotion and dopamine efflux within the NA, as well as facilitating extinction of and preventing reinstatement of cocaine mediated CPP (Dall et al., 2017). Collectively, these results indicate that M_4 PAMs have potential to reduce cocaine intake, as well as decrease cocaine craving/drug seeking and prevention of relapse. To date, research has focused on preclinical models of cocaine use disorder; however, given that M_4 mAChR modulation attenuates DAergic function, an underlying contribution to the rewarding effects of all substances of abuse, M_4 mAChR PAMs have the potential for treating some symptoms associated with all SUDs.

4.2 Allosteric modulation of M_5 mAChR and substance use

Based on the previously mentioned anatomical localization of M_5 in the VTA of the mesolimbic DA pathway and the decreased cocaine and morphine drug seeking behaviors in the M_5 KO mice studies, these studies have resulted in the development of selective M_5 negative allosteric modulators (NAMs) as potential treatments for SUD. ML375 represents the first highly selective and centrally penetrant M_5 NAM suitable for *in vivo* studies (see Fig. 4; Berizzi et al., 2016; Gentry et al., 2013). Recent results have shown that ML375 dose-dependently decreased self-administration of cocaine under multiple schedules of reinforcement (Gunter et al., 2017). In addition, ML375 also decreased self-administration and attenuated cue-induced reinstatement of ethanol (Berizzi et al., 2018). Interestingly, when administered via intra-striatal microinjection, ML375 reduced ethanol SA when injected into the intra-dorsolateral striatum, but not into the intra-dorsomedial striatum, implicating the intra-dorsolateral striatum in particular in cholinergic modulation of reward. However, ML375 has an *in vivo* half-life of approximately 80 h in the rat, making it difficult for use in repeated dosing studies. Recently VU6008667 (see Fig. 4), a short-acting M_5 NAM, has been reported with an *in vivo* half-life of approximately 2.5 h in rats, which will allow for future chronic dosing studies (McGowan et al., 2017). Though much is yet not understood in terms of M_5 and cholinergic modulation of reward circuits in substance use disorders, it is clear that M_5 NAMs are a promising mechanism for multiple stages in the cycle of SUD.

5. Potential challenges with mAChR allosteric modulation

The advantages with allosteric modulators are such that, along with increased subtype specificity, PAMs do not induce activation of the receptor without the presence of an orthosteric activator such as the endogenous ligand. This means that, unlike an agonist, PAMs enhance signaling of a receptor on the same temporo-spatial scale as endogenous signaling, likely leading to less overall disruption in the system. For example, an M_5 NAM provides promise for blocking cue-associated increases in dopamine release which may attenuate relapse, *without* reducing basal dopaminergic tone, which could result in anhedonia or precipitation of a withdrawal state. However, if overall cholinergic tone is decreased, a PAM may not be sufficient to compensate for this loss, because it only has impact if endogenous signaling is occurring.

This reliance on endogenous signaling means that the impact of allosteric modulation must be considered within the context of the disease or disorder progression, with an understanding of relevant changes in endogenous signaling that occur. For example, as noted above, many patients with schizophrenia show decreased levels in muscarinic receptors, particularly within the cortex and hippocampus. To date, it remains unknown whether these alterations in receptor expression are accompanied by changes in cortical or hippocampal cholinergic tone with the stage of illness in schizophrenia. However, if cholinergic tone varies with the stage of disease, then a PAM may only be beneficial when tone is sufficiently high enough to be potentiated. Otherwise, an allosteric agonist would be more suitable for treatment of a hypocholinergic state. In SUD, like schizophrenia, it remains unknown whether cholinergic tone on the various mAChRs in key regions of the mesocorticolimbic DA circuitry fluctuates with the stage of the addiction cycle. Thus, if cholinergic tone is not sufficiently high, allosteric agonists may produce better improvements in the various stages of SUD as well. It is known that initial stages of addiction are marked by excessive DA release in the NA and a similar state is produce in relapse conditions (see Di Chiara & Bassareo, 2007; Spanagel & Weiss, 1999 for review). Under these conditions, an M_5 NAM would turn down this excessive release, and would thus be ideal. However, with chronic use on certain substance of abuse such as cocaine, periods of abstinence or withdrawal are marked by a hypodopaminergic state (see Di Chiara & Bassareo, 2007; Spanagel & Weiss, 1999 for review), under which conditions an M_5 NAM might be actually be contraindicated. In summary, because of their dependence on endogenous tone, allosteric modulators are particularly susceptible to changes over disease progression, and therefore understanding these changes in endogenous ACh tone will be critical in future studies.

In addition, because allosteric modulators bind to less conserved regions on the receptor, there is a greater challenge in ensuring both PAMs and NAMs will have the same specificity and efficacy across different model systems. For example, M_4 PAM VU0467154 was found to be 35 times less potent at human M_4 as compared to rodent, preventing it from advancing to a clinical candidate (Wood et al., 2017). Thus, allosteric modulators must be thoroughly examined for selectivity and efficacy in the system in question in order to interpret any results. Allosteric modulators are also particularly susceptible to probe dependence, or differential selectivity in the presence of different orthosteric ligands (Kenakin, 2008), which must be taken into account both when translating to an endogenous system and when considering co-administration with an orthosteric agonist.

Finally, the majority of our current understanding of allosteric modulators is based on acute single-dose studies rather than after chronic administration, so much remains to be understood about the potential for development of tolerance. However, benzodiazepines act as known allosteric modulators of ionotropic $GABA_A$ receptors and have been shown to induce tolerance in some preclinical and clinical chronic dosing paradigms (File, 1985). It is speculated that because mAChR PAMs only boost endogenous ACh signaling that these PAMs will be less likely to induce tolerance via receptor desensitization or downregulation than allosteric or orthosteric after chronic administration. Evidence supporting this hypothesis has recently been provided from a study demonstrating that neither the robust efficacy in preclinical models nor the plasma and brain levels of the M_4 PAM VU0467154 were not altered after 10 days of repeated (Gould et al., 2018). Thus overall, allosteric modulation remains a promising strategy to increase receptor subtype specificity for pharmacological drug targets.

6. Conclusion

The current level of understanding of mAChRs is rapidly expanding as these receptor subtypes are recognized as viable targets for multiple CNS disorders. The development of subtype specific allosteric modulators has advanced our understanding of the function of different mAChR subtypes in various neuropsychiatric processes, as well as provided promising novel pharmacotherapies for various neuropsychiatric disorders, especially for schizophrenia and SUD.

Importantly, similar therapeutic strategies might be effective in the seemingly disparate disorders of schizophrenia and SUD; a fact which is highlighted by shared genetic liabilities and similar neural circuity involvement. In particular, a shared polygenetic liability is evident between schizophrenia and SUD, including tobacco, alcohol, cannabis, and cocaine use disorders (Carey et al., 2016; Hartz et al., 2017; Mallard, Paige Harden, & Fromme, 2018). Comorbidity between schizophrenia and SUD is estimated between 19 and 51%, depending on the substances examined, the country, and the method of sampling, with the highest comorbidity currently observed in alcohol use disorder (Brunette et al., 2018; Carrà et al., 2012; Hunt, Large, Cleary, Lai, & Saunders, 2018; Nesvåg et al., 2015; Toftdahl, Nordentoft, & Hjorthøj, 2016). Whether this comorbidity is due to self-medication with substances of abuse in patients with schizophrenia, shared reward deficiencies, substance use increasing risk for schizophrenia, or some combination of these factors remains unclear (see Dwiel,

Henricks, & Doucette, 2018 for review). Recent evidence suggests that current antipsychotic drugs, in particular clozapine and risperidone, may have some efficacy in reducing substance use and craving (Krause et al., 2019). Because mesocorticolimbic circuitry is relevant to both disorders, selective mAChR allosteric modulator therapies may be useful in schizophrenia, SUD, or in cases of comorbidity.

In summary, with the increasing development of subtype selective allosteric modulators for the different mAChRs, we are now poised to further investigate the role of specific mAChRs in more complex preclinical models of various aspects of schizophrenia and SUD and the potential efficacy of mAChR modulators in schizophrenia and SUD clinical populations. Because of the lack of peripheral activation via other muscarinic subtypes, allosteric modulators of mAChRs will potential display a broader therapeutic index than current muscarinic drugs, allowing for much more efficacious treatment without deleterious side-effects. Findings in rodent models with current tool compounds show immense promise in the treatment of positive, negative, and cognitive symptoms of schizophrenia, as well as providing evidence for potential pan-addiction treatments that show efficacy across multiple stages in the cycle of addiction.

Acknowledgments

The authors are supported via funding from Ono Pharmaceuticals, Lundbeck Pharmaceuticals, and Ancora Pharmaceuticals, as well as from the National Institutes of Health (T32 GM07628 and NIDA Grant R01DA37207).

Conflict of interest statement

The authors report no conflicts of interest in regards to this review.

References

American Psychiatric Association. (2013). *Diagnostic and statistical manual of mental disorders* (5th ed.). Washington DC: American Psychiatric Association.

Anagnostaras, S. G., Murphy, G. G., Hamilton, S. E., Mitchell, S. L., Rahnama, N. P., Nathanson, N. M., et al. (2003). Selective cognitive dysfunction in acetylcholine M1 muscarinic receptor mutant mice. *Nature Neuroscience*, *6*(1), 51–58.

Anney, R. J., Lotfi-Miri, M., Olsson, C. A., Reid, S. C., Hemphill, S. A., & Patton, G. C. (2007). Variation in the gene coding for the M5 muscarinic receptor (CHRM5) influences cigarette dose but is not associated with dependence to drugs of addiction: Evidence from a prospective population based cohort study of young adults. *BMC Genetics*, *8*(1), 46.

Barak, S., & Weiner, I. (2011). The M1/M4 preferring agonist xanomeline reverses amphetamine-, MK801- and scopolamine-induced abnormalities of latent inhibition: Putative efficacy against positive, negative and cognitive symptoms in schizophrenia. *International Journal of Neuropsychopharmacology*, *14*(9), 1233–1246.

Basile, A. S., Fedorova, I., Zapata, A., Liu, X., Shippenberg, T., Duttaroy, A., et al. (2002). Deletion of the M5 muscarinic acetylcholine receptor attenuates morphine reinforcement and withdrawal but not morphine analgesia. *Proceedings of the National Academy of Sciences of the United States of America*, *99*(17), 11452–11457.

Bendor, J., Lizardi-Ortiz, J. E., Westphalen, R. I., Brandstetter, M., Hemmings, H. C., Sulzer, D., et al. (2010). AGAP1/AP-3-dependent endocytic recycling of M5 muscarinic receptors promotes dopamine release. *The EMBO Journal*, *29*, 2813–2826.

Berizzi, A. E., Gentry, P. R., Rueda, P., Den Hoedt, S., Sexton, P. M., Langmead, C. J., et al. (2016). Molecular mechanisms of action of M5 muscarinic acetylcholine receptor allosteric modulators. *Molecular Pharmacology*, *90*(4), 427–436.

Berizzi, A. E., Perry, C. J., Shackleford, D. M., Lindsley, C. W., Jones, C. K., Chen, N. A., et al. (2018). Muscarinic M5 receptors modulate ethanol seeking in rats. *Neuropsychopharmacology*, *43*, 1510–1517.

Bobes, J., Garcia-Portilla, M. P., Bascaran, M. T., Saiz, P. A., & Bousoño, M. (2007). Quality of life in schizophrenic patients. *Dialogues in Clinical Neuroscience*, *9*(2), 215–226.

Bock, A., Schrage, R., & Mohr, K. (2018). Allosteric modulators targeting CNS muscarinic receptors. *Neuropharmacology*, *136*, 427–437.

Bodick, N. C., Offen, W. W., Levey, A. I., Cutler, N. R., Gauthier, S. G., Satlin, A., et al. (1997). Effects of xanomeline, a selective muscarinic receptor agonist, on cognitive function and behavioral symptoms in Alzheimer disease. *Archives of Neurology*, *54*(4), 465–473.

Bodick, N. C., Offen, W. W., Shannon, H. E., Satterwhite, J., Lucas, R., van Lier, R., et al. (1997). The selective muscarinic agonist xanomeline improves both the cognitive deficits and behavioral symptoms of Alzheimer disease. *Alzheimer Disease and Associated Disorders*, *11*(Suppl. 4), S16–S22.

Bolden, C., Cusack, B., & Richelson, E. (1992). Antagonism by antimuscarinic and neuroleptic compounds at the five cloned human muscarinic cholinergic receptors expressed in Chinese hamster ovary cells. *The Journal of Pharmacology and Experimental Therapeutics*, *260*(2), 576–580.

Brady, A. E., Jones, C. K., Bridges, T. M., Kennedy, J. P., Thompson, A. D., Heiman, J. U., et al. (2008). Centrally active allosteric potentiators of the M4 muscarinic acetylcholine receptor reverse amphetamine-induced hyperlocomotor activity in rats. *The Journal of Pharmacology and Experimental Therapeutics*, *327*(3), 941–953.

Brown, J. W., Rueter, L. E., & Zhang, M. (2014). Predictive validity of a MK-801-induced cognitive impairment model in mice: Implications on the potential limitations and challenges of modeling cognitive impairment associated with schizophrenia preclinically. *Progress in Neuro-Psychopharmacology and Biological Psychiatry*, *49*, 53–62.

Brunette, M. F., Mueser, K. T., Babbin, S., Meyer-Kalos, P., Rosenheck, R., Correll, C. U., et al. (2018). Demographic and clinical correlates of substance use disorders in first episode psychosis. *Schizophrenia Research*, *194*, 4–12.

Bubser, M., Bridges, T. M., Dencker, D., Gould, R. W., Grannan, M., Noetzel, M. J., et al. (2014). Selective activation of M4 muscarinic acetylcholine receptors reverses MK-801-induced behavioral impairments and enhances associative learning in rodents. *ACS Chemical Neuroscience*, *5*(10), 920–942.

Buckley, N. J., Bonner, T. I., & Brann, M. R. (1988). Localization of a family of muscarinic receptor mRNAs in rat brain. *The Journal of Neuroscience*, *8*(12), 4646–4652.

Buckley, P. F., Miller, B. J., Lehrer, D. S., & Castle, D. J. (2009). Psychiatric comorbidities and schizophrenia. *Schizophrenia Bulletin*, *35*(2), 383–402.

Burger, W. A. C., Sexton, P. M., Christopoulos, A., & Thal, D. M. (2018). Toward an understanding of the structural basis of allostery in muscarinic acetylcholine receptors. *The Journal of General Physiology*, *150*(10), 1360–1372.

Burris, K. D., Molski, T. F., Xu, C., Ryan, E., Tottori, K., Kikuchi, T., et al. (2002). Aripiprazole, a novel antipsychotic, is a high-affinity partial agonist at human dopamine D2 receptors. *The Journal of Pharmacology and Experimental Therapeutics*, *302*, 381–389.

Bymaster, F. P., Whitesitt, C. A., Shannon, H. E., DeLapp, N., Ward, J. S., Calligaro, D. O., et al. (1997). Xanomeline: A selective muscarinic agonist for the treatment of Alzheimer's disease. *Drug Development Research, 40*(2), 158–170.

Byun, N. E., Grannan, M., Bubser, M., Barry, R. L., Thompson, A., Rosanelli, J., et al. (2014). Antipsychotic drug-like effects of the selective M4 muscarinic acetylcholine receptor positive allosteric modulator VU0152100. *Neuropsychopharmacology, 39*(7), 1578–1593.

Calabresi, P., Centonze, D., Gubellini, P., Pisani, A., & Bernardi, G. (1998). Endogenous ACh enhances striatal NMDA-responses via M1-like muscarinic receptors and PKC activation. *European Journal of Neuroscience, 10*, 2887–2895.

Carey, C. E., Agrawal, A., Bucholz, K. K., Hartz, S. M., Lynskey, M. T., Nelson, E. C., et al. (2016). Associations between polygenic risk for -psychiatric disorders and substance involvement. *Frontiers in Genetics, 7*, 149.

Carrà, G., Johnson, S., Bebbington, P., Angermeyer, M. C., Heider, D., Brugha, T., et al. (2012). The lifetime and past-year prevalence of dual diagnosis in people with schizophrenia across Europe: Findings from the European Schizophrenia Cohort (EuroSC). *European Archives of Psychiatry and Clinical Neuroscience, 262*(7), 607–616.

Carrigan, K. A., & Dykstra, L. A. (2007). Behavioral effects of morphine and cocaine in M1 muscarinic acetylcholine receptor-deficient mice. *Psychopharmacology, 191*(4), 985–993.

Carruthers, S. P., Gurvich, C. T., Cropley, V. L., Pantelis, C., Bousman, C. A., Lenroot, R. K., et al. (2018). The effects of a muscarinic receptor 1 gene variant on cortical thickness and surface area in schizophrenia. *Psychiatry Research: Neuroimaging, 280*, 62–64.

Caulfield, M. P., & Birdsall, N. J. M. (1998). International Union of Pharmacology. XVII. Classification of muscarinic acetylcholine receptors. *Pharmacological Reviews, 50*(2), 279–290.

Chambon, C., Jatzke, C., Wegener, N., Gravius, A., & Danysz, W. (2012). Using cholinergic M1 receptor positive allosteric modulators to improve memory via enhancement of brain cholinergic communication. *European Journal of Pharmacology, 697*(1–3), 73–80.

Chan, W. Y., Mckinzie, D. L., Bose, S., Mitchell, S. N., Witkin, J. M., Thompson, R. C., et al. (2008). Allosteric modulation of the muscarinic M4 receptor as an approach to treating schizophrenia. *Proceedings of the National Academy of Sciences of the United States of America, 105*(31), 10978–10983.

Choy, K. H. C., Shackleford, D. M., Malone, D. T., Mistry, S. N., Patil, R. T., Scammells, P. J., et al. (2016). Positive allosteric modulation of the muscarinic M1 receptor improves efficacy of antipsychotics in mouse glutamatergic deficit models of behavior. *The Journal of Pharmacology and Experimental Therapeutics, 359*(2), 354–365.

Christopoulos, A. (2002). Allosteric binding sites on cell-surface receptors: Novel targets for drug discovery. *Nature Reviews Drug Discovery, 1*, 198–210.

Clarke, P. B. S., Hommer, D. W., Pert, A., & Skirboll, L. R. (1987). Innervation of substantia nigra neurons by cholinergic afferents from pedunculopontine nucleus in the rat: Neuroanatomical and electrophysiological evidence. *Neuroscience, 23*(3), 1011–1019.

ClinicalTrials.gov. (2017). *Pilot study comparing effects of xanomeline alone to xanomeline plus trospium*. National Library of Medicine, [Identification No. NCT02831231].

ClinicalTrials.gov. (2018). *A study to assess safety and efficacy of KarXT in adult patients with schizophrenia*. National Library of Medicine, [Identification No. NCT03697252].

Conn, P. J., Lindsley, C. W., Meiler, J., & Niswender, C. M. (2014). Opportunities and challenges in the discovery of allosteric modulators of GPCRs for treating CNS disorders. *Nature Reviews. Drug Discovery, 13*(9), 692–708.

Cooper, S., Robison, A. J., & Mazei-Robison, M. S. (2017). Reward circuitry in addiction. *Neurotherapeutics, 14*(3), 687–697.

Crook, J. M., Dean, B., Pavey, G., & Copolov, D. L. (1999). The binding of [3H]AF-DX 384 is reduced in the caudate-putamen of subjects with schizophrenia. *Life Sciences*, *64*(19), 1761–1771.

Crook, J. M., Tomaskovic-Crook, E., Copolov, D. L., & Dean, B. (2000). Decreased muscarinic receptor binding in subjects with schizophrenia: A study of the human hippocampal formation. *Biological Psychiatry*, *48*(5), 381–388.

Crook, J. M., Tomaskovic-Crook, E., Copolov, D. L., & Dean, B. (2001). Low muscarinic receptor binding in prefrontal cortex from subjects with schizophrenia: A study of Brodmann's areas 8, 9, 10, and 46 and the effects of neuroleptic drug treatment. *American Journal of Psychiatry*, *158*, 918–925.

Cropley, V. L., Scarr, E., Fornito, A., Klauser, P., Bousman, C. A., Scott, R., et al. (2015). The effect of a muscarinic receptor 1 gene variant on grey matter volume in schizophrenia. *Psychiatry Research: Neuroimaging*, *234*(2), 182–187.

Dall, C., Weikop, P., Dencker, D., Molander, A. C., Wörtwein, G., Conn, P. J., et al. (2017). Muscarinic receptor M4 positive allosteric modulators attenuate central effects of cocaine. *Drug and Alcohol Dependence*, *176*, 154–161.

Datta, S., & Siwek, D. F. (1997). Excitation of the brain stem pedunculopontine tegmentum cholinergic cells induces wakefulness and REM sleep. *Journal of Neurophysiology*, 77(6), 2975–2988.

Davoren, J. E., Lee, C.-W., Garnsey, M., Brodney, M. A., Cordes, J., Dlugolenski, K., et al. (2016). Discovery of the potent and selective M1 PAM-agonist N-[(3R,4S)-3-hydroxytetrahydro-2H -pyran-4-yl]-5-methyl-4-[4-(1,3-thiazol-4-yl)benzyl]pyridine-2-carboxamide (PF-06767832): Evaluation of efficacy and cholinergic side effects. *Journal of Medicinal Chemistry*, *59*(13), 6313–6328.

De Luca, V., Wang, H., Squassina, A., Wong, G. W. H., Yeomans, J., & Kennedy, J. L. (2004). Linkage of M5 muscarinic and (alpha)7-nicotinic receptor genes on 15q13 to schizophrenia. *Neuropsychobiology*, *50*, 124–127.

Dean, B., Crook, J. M., Opeskin, K., Hill, C., Keks, N., & Copolov, D. L. (1996). The density of muscarinic M1 receptors is decreased in the caudate-putamen of subjects with schizophrenia. *Molecular Psychiatry*, *1*(1), 54–58.

Dean, B., McLeod, M., Keriakous, D., McKenzie, J., & Scarr, E. (2002). Decreased muscarinic1 receptors in the dorsolateral prefrontal cortex of subjects with schizophrenia. *Molecular Psychiatry*, 7, 1083–1091.

Dencker, D., Weikop, P., Sørensen, G., Woldbye, D. P. D., Wörtwein, G., Wess, J., et al. (2012). An allosteric enhancer of M4 muscarinic acetylcholine receptor function inhibits behavioral and neurochemical effects of cocaine. *Psychopharmacology*, *224*, 277–287.

Dencker, D., Wörtwein, G., Weikop, P., Jeon, J., Thomsen, M., Sager, T. N., et al. (2011). Involvement of a subpopulation of neuronal M4 muscarinic acetylcholine receptors in the antipsychotic-like effects of the M1/M4 preferring muscarinic receptor agonist xanomeline. *The Journal of Neuroscience*, *31*(16), 5905–5908.

Deng, C., & Huang, X.-F. (2005). Decreased density of muscarinic receptors in the superior temporal gyrusin schizophrenia. *Journal of Neuroscience Research*, *81*(6), 883–890.

Di Chiara, G., & Bassareo, V. (2007). Reward system and addiction: What dopamine does and doesn't do. *Current Opinion in Pharmacology*, 7(1), 69–76.

Di Chiara, G., & Imperato, A. (1988). Drugs abused by humans preferentially increase synaptic dopamine concentrations in the mesolimbic system of freely moving rats. *Proceedings of the National Academy of Sciences of the United States of America*, *85*(14), 5274–5278.

Dienel, S. J., & Lewis, D. A. (2018). Alterations in cortical interneurons and cognitive function in schizophrenia. *Neurobiology of Disease*, (in press).

Dorje, F., Levey, A. I., & Brann, M. R. (1991). Immunological detection of muscarinic receptor subtype proteins (m1-m5) in rabbit peripheral tissues. *Molecular Pharmacology*, *40*, 459–462.

Dwiel, L. L., Henricks, A. M., & Doucette, W. T. (2018). The link between schizophrenia and substance use disorder: A unifying hypothesis. *Schizophrenia Research*, *194*, 78–85.

Eckenstein, F. P., Baughman, R. W., & Quinn, J. (1988). An anatomical study of cholinergic innervation in rat cerebral cortex. *Neuroscience*, *25*(2), 457–474.

Edelstein, P., Schultz, J. R., Hirschowitz, J., Kanter, D. R., & Garver, D. L. (1981). Physostigmine and lithium response in the schizophrenias. *American Journal of Psychiatry*, *138*(8), 1078–1081.

Eipper-Mains, J. E., Kiraly, D. D., Duff, M. O., Horowitz, M. J., McManus, C. J., Eipper, B. A., et al. (2013). Effects of cocaine and withdrawal on the mouse nucleus accumbens transcriptome. *Genes, Brain and Behavior*, *12*(1), 21–33.

Everitt, B. J., & Robbins, T. W. (1997). Central cholinergic system and cognition. *Annual Review of Psychology*, *48*, 649–684.

Felder, C. C., Porter, A. C., Skillman, T. L., Zhang, L., Bymaster, F. P., Nathanson, N. M., et al. (2001). Elucidating the role of muscarinic receptors in psychosis. *Life Sciences*, *68*, 2605–2613.

File, S. E. (1985). Tolerance to the behavioral actions of benzodiazepines. *Neuroscience & Biobehavioral Reviews*, *9*(1), 113–121.

Fink-Jensen, A., Fedorova, I., Wörtwein, G., Woldbye, D. P. D., Rasmussen, T., Thomsen, M., et al. (2003). Role for M5 muscarinic acetylcholine receptors in cocaine addiction. *Journal of Neuroscience Research*, *74*(1), 91–96.

Flynn, D. D., Vaishnav, A. A., & Mash, D. C. (1992). Interactions of cocaine with primary and secondary recognition sites on muscarinic receptors. *Molecular Pharmacology*, *41*, 736–742.

Forster, G. L., Yeomans, J. S., Takeuchi, J., & Blaha, C. D. (2001). M5 muscarinic receptors are required for prolonged accumbal dopamine release after electrical stimulation of the pons in mice. *The Journal of Neuroscience*, *21*, 1–6.

Foster, D. J., Gentry, P. R., Lizardi-Ortiz, J. E., Bridges, T. M., Wood, M. R., Niswender, C. M., et al. (2014). M5 receptor activation produces opposing physiological outcomes in dopamine neurons depending on the receptor's location. *Journal of Neuroscience*, *34*(9), 3253–3262.

Foster, D. J., Wilson, J. M., Remke, D. H., Mahmood, M. S., Uddin, M. J., Wess, J., et al. (2016). Antipsychotic-like effects of M4 positive allosteric modulators are mediated by CB2 receptor-dependent inhibition of dopamine release. *Neuron*, *91*(6), 1244–1252.

Galloway, C. R., Lebois, E. P., Shagarabi, S. L., Hernandez, N. A., & Manns, J. R. (2014). Effects of selective activation of M1 and M4 muscarinic receptors on object recognition memory performance in rats. *Pharmacology*, *93*, 57–64.

Garzón, M., & Pickel, V. M. (2013). Somatodendritic targeting of M5 muscarinic receptor in the rat ventral tegmental area: Implications for mesolimbic dopamine transmission. *Journal of Comparative Neurology*, *521*(13), 2927–2946.

Gentry, P. R., Kokubo, M., Bridges, T. M., Kett, N. R., Harp, J. M., Cho, H. P., et al. (2013). Discovery of the first M5-selective and CNS penetrant negative allosteric modulator (NAM) of a muscarinic acetylcholine receptor: (S)-9b-(4-chlorophenyl)-1-(3,4-difluorobenzoyl)-2,3-dihydro-1 H -imidazo[2,1- a]isoindol-5(9b H)-one (ML375). *Journal of Medicinal Chemistry*, *56*(22), 9351–9355.

Gerber, D. J., Sotnikova, T. D., Gainetdinov, R. R., Huang, S. Y., Caron, M. G., & Tonegawa, S. (2001). Hyperactivity, elevated dopaminergic transmission, and response to amphetamine in M1 muscarinic acetylcholine receptor-deficient mice. *Proceedings of the National Academy of Sciences of the United States of America*, *98*(26), 15312–15317.

Ghoshal, A., Rook, J. M., Dickerson, J. W., Roop, G. N., Morrison, R. D., Jalan-Sakrikar, N., et al. (2016). Potentiation of M1 muscarinic receptor reverses plasticity deficits and negative and cognitive symptoms in a schizophrenia mouse model. *Neuropsychopharmacology*, *41*(2), 598–610.

Giachetti, A., Giraldo, E., Ladinsky, H., & Montagna, E. (1986). Binding and functional profiles of the selective M1 muscarinic receptor antagonists trihexyphenidyl and dicyclomine. *British Journal of Pharmacology, 89*(1), 83–90.

Göder, R., Boigs, M., Braun, S., Friege, L., Fritzer, G., Aldenhoff, J. B., et al. (2004). Impairment of visuospatial memory is associated with decreased slow wave sleep in schizophrenia. *Journal of Psychiatric Research, 38*(6), 591–599.

Gould, R. W., Dencker, D., Grannan, M. D., Bubser, M., Zhan, X., Wess, J., et al. (2015). Role for the M1 muscarinic acetylcholine receptor in top-down cognitive processing using a touchscreen visual discrimination task in mice. *ACS Chemical Neuroscience, 6*(10), 1683–1695.

Gould, R. W., Grannan, M. D., Gunter, B. W., Ball, J., Bubser, M., Bridges, T. M., et al. (2018). Cognitive enhancement and antipsychotic-like activity following repeated dosing with the selective M4 PAM VU0467154. *Neuropharmacology, 128*, 492–502.

Gould, R. W., Nedelcovych, M. T., Gong, X., Tsai, E., Bubser, M., Bridges, T. M., et al. (2016). State-dependent alterations in sleep/wake architecture elicited by the M4 PAM VU0467154—Relation to antipsychotic-like drug effects. *Neuropharmacology, 102*, 244–253.

Gould, E., Woolf, N. J., & Butcher, L. L. (1989). Cholinergic projections to the substantia nigra from the pedunculopontine and laterodorsal tegmental nuclei. *Neuroscience, 28*(3), 611–623.

Grannan, M. D., Mielnik, C. A., Moran, S. P., Gould, R. W., Ball, J., Lu, Z., et al. (2016). Prefrontal cortex-mediated impairments in a genetic model of NMDA receptor hypofunction are reversed by the novel M1 PAM VU6004256. *ACS Chemical Neuroscience*, 7(12), 1706–1716.

Grant, M. K. O., & El-Fakahany, E. E. (2005). Persistent binding and functional antagonism by xanomeline at the muscarinic M5 receptor. *Journal of Pharmacology and Experimental Therapeutics, 315*, 313–319.

Green, M. F. (1996). What are the functional consequences of neurocognitive deficits in schizophrenia? *American Journal of Psychiatry, 153*, 321–330.

Green, M. F., Kern, R. S., & Heaton, R. K. (2004). Longitudinal studies of cognition and functional outcome in schizophrenia: Implications for MATRICS. *Schizophrenia Research*, 72(1), 41–51.

Gunter, B. W., Gould, R. W., Bubser, M., Mcgowan, K. M., Lindsley, C. W., & Jones, C. K. (2017). Selective inhibition of M5 muscarinic acetylcholine receptors attenuates cocaine self-administration in rats. *Addiction Biology, 23*(5), 1106–1116.

Hallanger, A. E., Levey, A. I., Lee, H. J., Rye, D. B., & Wainer, B. H. (1987). The origins of cholinergic and other subcortical afferents to the thalamus in the rat. *The Journal of Comparative Neurology, 262*(1), 105–124.

Hamborg-Petersen, B., Nielsen, M. M., & Thordal, C. (1984). Toxic effect of scopolamine eye drops in children. *Acta Ophthalmologica, 62*(3), 485–488.

Hamid, A. A., Pettibone, J. R., Mabrouk, O. S., Hetrick, V. L., Schmidt, R., Vander Weele, C. M., et al. (2016). Mesolimbic dopamine signals the value of work. *Nature Neuroscience, 19*(1), 117–126.

Hartz, S. M., Horton, A. C., Oehlert, M., Carey, C. E., Agrawal, A., Bogdan, R., et al. (2017). Association between substance use disorder and polygenic liability to schizophrenia. *Biological Psychiatry, 82*(10), 709–715.

Hellstrom-Lindahl, E., Winblad, B., & Nordberg, A. (1993). Muscarinic and nicotinic receptor changes in the cortex and thalamus of brains of chronic alcoholics. *Brain Research, 620*(1), 42–48.

Hersch, S. M., Gutekunst, C.-A., Flees, H. D., Heilman, C. J., & Levey, A. I. (1994). Distribution of m1-m4 muscarinic receptor proteins in the rat striatum: Light and electron microscopic immunocytochemistry using subtype-specific antibodies. *The Journal of Neuroscience, 14*(5), 3351–3363.

Howes, O. D., & Kapur, S. (2009). The dopamine hypothesis of schizophrenia: Version III—The final common pathway. *Schizophrenia Bulletin*, *35*(3), 549–562.

Hunt, G. E., Large, M. M., Cleary, M., Lai, H. M. X., & Saunders, J. B. (2018). Prevalence of comorbid substance use in schizophrenia spectrum disorders in community and clinical settings, 1990–2017: Systematic review and meta-analysis. *Drug and Alcohol Dependence*, *191*, 234–258.

Ince, E., Ciliax, B. J., & Levey, A. I. (1997). Differential expression of D1 and D2 dopamine and m4 muscarinic acetylcholine receptor proteins in identified striatonigral neurons. *Synapse*, *27*, 357–366.

Janowsky, D. S., El-Yousef, M. K., & Davis, J. M. (1973). Antagonistic effects of physostigmine and methylphenidate in man. *American Journal of Psychiatry*, *130*, 1370–1376.

Jeon, J., Dencker, D., Wörtwein, G., Woldbye, D. P. D., Cui, Y., Davis, A. A., et al. (2010). A subpopulation of neuronal M4 muscarinic acetylcholine receptors plays a critical role in modulating dopamine-dependent behaviors. *The Journal of Neuroscience*, *30*(6), 2396–2405.

Johnstone, E. C., Crow, T. J., Ferrier, I. N., Frith, C. D., Owens, D. G. C., Bourne, R. C., et al. (1983). Adverse effects of anticholinergic medication on positive schizophrenic symptoms. *Psychological Medicine*, *13*(3), 513–527.

Jones, C. K., Brady, A. E., Davis, A. A., Xiang, Z., Bubser, M., Tantawy, M. N., et al. (2008). Novel selective allosteric activator of the M1 muscarinic acetylcholine receptor regulates amyloid processing and produces antipsychotic-like activity in rats. *Journal of Neuroscience*, *28*(41), 10422–10433.

Jones, C. K., Byun, N. E., & Bubser, M. (2012). Muscarinic and nicotinic acetylcholine receptor agonists and allosteric modulators for the treatment of schizophrenia. *Neuropsychopharmacology*, *37*(10), 16–42.

Joseph, L., & Thomsen, M. (2017). Effects of muscarinic receptor antagonists on cocaine discrimination in wild-type mice and in muscarinic receptor M1, M2, and M4 receptor knockout mice. *Behavioural Brain Research*, *329*, 75–83.

Jung, M. H., Park, B. L., Lee, B.-C., Ro, Y., Park, R., Shin, H. D., et al. (2010). Association of CHRM2 polymorphisms with severity of alcohol dependence. *Genes, Brain and Behavior*, *10*(2), 253–256.

Kalivas, P. W. (2009). The glutamate homeostasis hypothesis of addiction. *Nature Reviews Neuroscience*, *10*, 561–572.

Kenakin, T. (2008). Functional selectivity in GPCR modulator screening. *Combinatorial Chemistry & High Throughput Screening*, *11*(5), 337–343.

Keshavan, M. S., Miewald, J., Haas, G., Sweeney, J., Ganguli, R., & Reynolds, C. F. (1995). Slow-wave sleep and symptomatology in schizophrenia and related psychotic disorders. *Journal of Psychiatric Research*, *29*(4), 303–314.

Kirrane, R. M., Mitropoulou, V., Nunn, M., Silverman, J., & Siever, L. J. (2001). Physostigmine and cognition in schizotypal personality disorder. *Schizophrenia Research*, *48*(1), 1–5.

Koch, J., Aldenhoff, J. B., Göder, R., Boigs, M., Braun, S., & Fritzer, G. (2014). Delta power in sleep in relation to neuropsychological performance in healthy subjects and schizophrenia patients. *The Journal of Neuropsychiatry and Clinical Neurosciences*, *18*(4), 529–535.

Koshimizu, H., Leiter, L. M., & Miyakawa, T. (2012). M4 muscarinic receptor knockout mice display abnormal social behavior and decreased prepulse inhibition. *Molecular Brain*, *5*, 10.

Kourrich, S., Calu, D. J., & Bonci, A. (2015). Intrinsic plasticity: An emerging player in addiction. *Nature Reviews Neuroscience*, *16*, 173–184.

Krause, M., Huhn, M., Schneider-Thoma, J., Bighelli, I., Gutsmiedl, K., & Leucht, S. (2019). Efficacy, acceptability and tolerability of antipsychotics in patients with schizophrenia and comorbid substance use. A systematic review and meta-analysis. *European Neuropsychopharmacology*, *29*, 32–45.

Kruse, A. C., Hu, J., Pan, A. C., Arlow, D. H., Rosenbaum, D. M., Rosemond, E., et al. (2012). Structure and dynamics of the M3 muscarinic acetylcholine receptor. *Nature, 482*, 552–556.

Kruse, A. C., Kobilka, B. K., Gautam, D., Sexton, P. M., Christopoulos, A., & Wess, J. (2014). Muscarinic acetylcholine receptors: Novel opportunities for drug development. *Nature Reviews Drug Discovery, 13*(7), 549–560.

Kubo, T., Fukuda, K., Mikami, A., Maeda, A., Takahashi, H., Mishina, M., et al. (1986). Cloning, sequencing, and expression of complementary DNA encoding the muscarinic acetylcholine receptor. *Nature, 323*, 411–416.

Kubo, T., Maeda, A., Sugimoto, K., Akiba, I., Mikami, A., Takahashi, H., et al. (1986). Primary structure of porcine cardiac muscarinic acetylcholine receptor deduced from the cDNA sequence. *FEBS Letters, 209*(2), 367–372.

Kurz, M., Hummer, M., Oberbauer, H., & Fleischhacker, W. W. (1995). Extrapyramidal side effects of clozapine and haloperidol. *Psychopharmacology, 118*(1), 52–56.

Lammel, S., Ion, D. I., Roeper, J., & Malenka, R. C. (2011). Projection-specific modulation of dopamine neuron synapses by aversive and rewarding stimuli. *Neuron, 70*(5), 855–862.

Lammel, S., Lim, B. K., Ran, C., Huang, K. W., Betley, M. J., Tye, K. M., et al. (2012). Input-specific control of reward and aversion in the ventral tegmental area. *Nature, 491*(7423), 212–217.

Langmead, C. J., Fry, V. A. H., Forbes, I. T., Branch, C. L., Christopoulos, A., Wood, M. D., et al. (2006). Probing the molecular mechanism of interaction between 4-n-butyl-1-[4-(2-methylphenyl)-4-oxo-1-butyl]-piperidine (AC-42) and the muscarinic M1 receptor: Direct pharmacological evidence that AC-42 is an allosteric agonist. *Molecular Pharmacology, 69*, 236–246.

Langmead, C. J., Watson, J., & Reavill, C. (2008). Muscarinic acetylcholine receptors as CNS drug targets. *Pharmacology and Therapeutics, 117*(2), 232–243.

Lazareno, S., Dolě, V., Popham, A., & Birdsall, N. J. M. (2004). Thiochrome enhances acetylcholine affinity at muscarinic M4 receptors: Receptor subtype selectivity via cooperativity rather than affinity. *Molecular Pharmacology, 65*(1), 257–266.

Leach, K., Loiacono, R. E., Felder, C. C., McKinzie, D. L., Mogg, A., Shaw, D. B., et al. (2010). Molecular mechanisms of action and in vivo validation of an M4 muscarinic acetylcholine receptor allosteric modulator with potential antipsychotic properties. *Neuropsychopharmacology, 35*(4), 855–869.

Lebois, E. P., Bridges, T. M., Lewis, L. M., Dawson, E. S., Kane, A. S., Xiang, Z., et al. (2010). Discovery and characterization of novel subtype-selective allosteric agonists for the investigation of M1 receptor function in the central nervous system. *ACS Chemical Neuroscience, 1*(2), 104–121.

Levey, A. I. (1993). Immunological localization of m1-m5 muscarinic acetylcholine receptors in peripheral tissues and brain. *Life Sciences, 52*, 441–448.

Levey, A. I., Edmunds, S. M., Koliatsos, V., Wiley, R. G., & Heilman, C. J. (1995). Expression of ml-m4 muscarinic acetylcholine receptor proteins in rat hippocampus and regulation by cholinergic innervation. *The Journal of Neuroscience, 15*(5), 4077–4092.

Levey, A. I., Kitt, C. A., Simonds, W. F., Price, D. L., & Brann, M. R. (1991). Identification and localization of muscarinic acetylcholine receptor proteins in brain with subtype-specific antibodies. *The Journal of Neuroscience, 1*(10), 3218–3228.

Levran, O., Randesi, M., Peles, E., Correa da Rosa, J., Ott, J., Rotrosen, J., et al. (2016). African-specific variability in the acetylcholine muscarinic receptor M4: Association with cocaine and heroin addiction. *Pharmacogenomics, 17*(9), 995–1003.

Li, P., Snyder, G. L., & Vanover, K. E. (2016). Dopamine targeting drugs for the treatment of schizophrenia: Past, present and future. *Current Topics in Medicinal Chemistry, 16*, 3385–3403.

Li, M., Yasuda, R. P., Wall, S. J., Wellstein, A., & Wolfe, B. B. (1991). Distribution of m2 muscarinic receptors in rat brain using antisera selective for m2 receptors. *Molecular Pharmacology, 40*, 28–35.

Liao, D., Hong, C., Chen, H., Chen, Y., Lee, S., & Chang, C. (2003). Association of muscarinic m1 receptor genetic polymorphisms with psychiatric symptoms and cognitive function in schizophrenic patients. *Neuropsychobiology*, *48*(2), 72–76.

Liu, J., Conklin, B. R., Blin, N., Yun, J., & Wess, J. (1995). Identification of a receptor/G-protein contact site critical for signaling specificity and G-protein activation. *Proceedings of the National Academy of Sciences of the United States of America*, *92*(25), 11642–11646.

Lou, X.-Y., Ma, J. Z., Payne, T. J., Beuten, J., Crew, K. M., & Li, M. D. (2006). Gene-based analysis suggests association of the nicotinic acetylcholine receptor β1 subunit (CHRNB1) and M1 muscarinic acetylcholine receptor (CHRM1) with vulnerability for nicotine dependence. *Human Genetics*, *120*(3), 381–389.

Luscher, C. (2016). The emergence of a circuit model for addiction. *Annual Review of Neuroscience*, *39*, 257–276.

Lynch, W. J., Nicholson, K. L., Dance, M. E., Morgan, R. W., & Foley, P. L. (2010). Animal models of substance abuse and addiction: Implications for science, animal welfare, and society. *Comparative Medicine*, *60*(3), 177–188.

Ma, L., Seager, M. A., Seager, M., Wittmann, M., Jacobson, M., Bickel, D., et al. (2009). Selective activation of the M1 muscarinic acetylcholine receptor achieved by allosteric potentiation. *Proceedings of the National Academy of Sciences of the United States of America*, *106*(37), 15950–15955.

Maehara, S., Hikichi, H., Satow, A., Okuda, S., & Ohta, H. (2008). Antipsychotic property of a muscarinic receptor agonist in animal models for schizophrenia. *Pharmacology Biochemistry and Behavior*, *91*(1), 140–149.

Mallard, T. T., Paige Harden, K., & Fromme, K. (2018). Genetic risk for schizophrenia is associated with substance use in emerging adulthood: An event-level polygenic prediction model. *Psychological Medicine*, 1–9.

Marino, M. J., Rouse, S. T., Levey, A. I., Potter, L. T., & Conn, P. J. (1998). Activation of the genetically defined m1 muscarinic receptor potentiates N-methyl-D-aspartate (NMDA) receptor currents in hippocampal pyramidal cells. *Proceedings of the National Academy of Sciences of the United States of America*, *95*, 11465–11470.

Mayer-Blackwell, B., Schlussman, S. D., Butelman, E. R., Ho, A., Ott, J., Kreek, M. J., et al. (2014). Self administration of oxycodone by adolescent and adult mice affects striatal neurotransmitter receptor gene expression. *Neuroscience*, *258*, 280–291.

McEvoy, J. P. (1987). A double-blind crossover comparison of antiparkinson drug therapy: Amantadine versus anticholinergics in 90 normal volunteers, with an emphasis on differential effects on memory function. *The Journal of Clinical Psychiatry*, *48*(Suppl. 1), 20–23.

McGeer, P. L., McGeer, E. G., Kamo, H., & Wong, K. (1986). Positron emission tomography and the possible origins of cytopathology in Alzheimer's disease. *Progress in Neuro-Psychopharmacology and Biological Psychiatry*, *10*, 501–518.

McGowan, K. M., Nance, K. D., Cho, H. P., Bridges, T. M., Jeffrey Conn, P., Jones, C. K., et al. (2017). Continued optimization of the M5NAM ML375: Discovery of VU6008667, an M5NAM with high CNS penetration and a desired short half-life in rat for addiction studies. *Bioorganic and Medicinal Chemistry Letters*, *27*(6), 1356–1359.

Mesulam, M.-M., Mufson, E. J., Wainer, B. H., & Levey, A. I. (1983). Central cholinergic pathways in the rat: An overview based on an alternative nomenclature (Ch1–Ch6). *Neuroscience*, *10*(4), 1185–1201.

Miyamoto, S., Duncan, G. E., Marx, C. E., & Lieberman, J. A. (2005). Treatments for schizophrenia: A critical review of pharmacology and mechanisms of action of antipsychotic drugs. *Molecular Psychiatry*, *10*(1), 79–104.

Moriya, H., Takagi, Y., Nakanishi, T., Hayashi, M., Tani, T., & Hirotsu, I. (1999). Affinity profiles of various muscarinic antagonists for cloned human muscarinic acetylcholine receptor (mAChR) subtypes and mAChRs in rat heart and submandibular gland. *Life Sciences*, *64*(25), 2351–2358.

Muller, P., Britton, R. S., & Seeman, P. (1980). The effects of long-term ethanol on brain receptors for dopamine, acetylcholine, serotonin and noradrenaline. *European Journal of Pharmacology*, *65*(1), 31–37.

Naheed, M., & Green, B. (2001). Focus on clozapine. *Current Medical Research and Opinion*, *17*(3), 223–229.

Nawaratne, V., Leach, K., Felder, C. C., Sexton, P. M., & Christopoulos, A. (2010). Structural determinants of allosteric agonism and modulation at the M4 muscarinic acetylcholine receptor. *The Journal of Biological Chemistry*, *285*(25), 19012–19021.

Nestler, E. J. (2005). Is there a common molecular pathway for addiction? *Nature Neuroscience*, *8*(11), 1445–1449.

Nesvåg, R., Knudsen, G. P., Bakken, I. J., Høye, A., Ystrom, E., Surén, P., et al. (2015). Substance use disorders in schizophrenia, bipolar disorder, and depressive illness: A registry-based study. *Social Psychiatry and Psychiatric Epidemiology*, *50*(8), 1267–1276.

Offermanns, S., Wieland, T., Homann, D., Sandmann, J., Bombien, E., Spicher, K., et al. (1994). Transfected muscarinic acetyicholine receptors selectively couple to Gi-type G proteins and Gq/11. *Molecular Pharmacology*, *45*, 890–898.

Olney, J. W., Newcomer, J. W., & Farber, N. B. (1999). NMDA receptor hypofunction model of schizophrenia. *Journal of Psychiatric Research*, *33*(6), 523–533.

Osterholm, R. K., & Camoriano, J. K. (1982). Transdermal scopolamine psychosis. *The Journal of the American Medical Association*, *247*(22), 3081.

Pancani, T., Bolarinwa, C., Smith, Y., Lindsley, C. W., Conn, P. J., & Xiang, Z. (2014). M4 mAChR-mediated modulation of glutamatergic transmission at corticostriatal synapses. *ACS Chemical Neuroscience*, *5*(4), 318–324.

Parker, E. M., Kameyama, K., Higashijima, T., & Ross, E. M. (1991). Reconstitutively active G protein-coupled receptors purified from baculovirus-infected insect cells. *Journal of Biological Chemistry*, *266*(1), 519–527.

Peralta, E. G., Ashkenazi, A., Winslow, J. W., Ramachandran, J., & Capon, D. J. (1988). Differential regulation of PI hydrolysis and adenylyl cyclase by muscarinic receptor subtypes. *Nature*, *334*(4), 434–437.

Perry, K. W., Nisenbaum, L. K., George, C. A., Shannon, H. E., Felder, C. C., & Bymaster, F. P. (2001). The muscarinic agonist xanomeline increases monoamine release and immediate early gene expression in the rat prefrontal cortex. *Biological Psychiatry*, *49*(8), 716–725.

Price, J. L., & Stern, R. (1983). Individual cells in the nucleus basalis-diagonal band complex have restricted axonal projections to the cerebral cortex in the rat. *Brain Research*, *269*(2), 352–356.

Pritchett, D., Wulff, K., Oliver, P. L., Bannerman, D. M., Davies, K. E., Harrison, P. J., et al. (2012). Evaluating the links between schizophrenia and sleep and circadian rhythm disruption. *Journal of Neural Transmission*, *119*(10), 1061–1075.

Quintero, G. C. (2013). Role of nucleus accumbens glutamatergic plasticity in drug addiction. *Neuropsychiatric Disease and Treatment*, *9*, 1499–1512.

Rabin, R. A., Wolfe, B. B., Dibner, M. D., Zahniser, N. R., Melchior, C., & Molinoff, P. B. (1980). Effects of ethanol administration and withdrawal on neurotransmitter receptor systems in C57 mice. *Journal of Pharmacology and Experimental Therapeutics*, *213*(3), 491–496.

Raedler, T. J., Bymaster, F. P., Tandon, R., Copolov, D. L., & Dean, B. (2007). Towards a muscarinic hypothesis of schizophrenia. *Molecular Psychiatry*, *12*, 232–246.

Rahman, S., Engleman, E. A., & Bell, R. L. (2015). Nicotinic receptor modulation to treat alcohol and drug dependence. *Frontiers in Neuroscience*, *8*, 426.

Rook, J. M., Bertron, J. L., Cho, H. P., Garcia-Barrantes, P. M., Moran, S. P., Maksymetz, J. T., et al. (2018). A novel M1 PAM VU0486846 exerts efficacy in cognition models without displaying agonist activity or cholinergic toxicity. *ACS Chemical Neuroscience*, *9*(9), 2274–2285.

Rouse, S. T., Edmunds, S. M., Yi, H., Gilmor, M. L., & Levey, A. I. (2000). Localization of M2 muscarinic acetylcholine receptor protein in cholinergic and non-cholinergic terminals in rat hippocampus. *Neuroscience Letters*, *284*, 182–186.

Rouse, S. T., Gilmor, M. L., & Levey, A. I. (1998). Differential presynaptic and postsynaptic expression of m1–m4 muscarinic acetylcholine receptors at the perforant pathway/granule cell synapse. *Neuroscience*, *86*(1), 221–232.

Rusted, J. M., & Warburton, D. M. (1988). The effects of scopolamine on working memory in healthy young volunteers. *Psychopharmacology*, *96*, 145–152.

Sakurai, T., & Gamo, N. J. (2018). Cognitive functions associated with developing prefrontal cortex during adolescence and developmental neuropsychiatric disorders. *Neurobiology of Disease*, (in press).

Salah-Uddin, H., Scarr, E., Pavey, G., Harris, K., Hagan, J. J., Dean, B., et al. (2009). Altered M1 muscarinic acetylcholine receptor (CHRM1)-Gαq/11 coupling in a schizophrenia endophenotype. *Neuropsychopharmacology*, *34*, 2156–2166.

Salamone, J. D., & Correa, M. (2012). The mysterious motivational functions of mesolimbic dopamine. *Neuron*, *76*(3), 470–485.

Satoh, K., & Fibiger, H. C. (1986). Cholinergic neurons of the laterodorsal tegmental nucleus: Efferent and afferent connections. *The Journal of Comparative Neurology*, *253*(3), 277–302.

Scarr, E., Cowie, T. F., Kanellakis, S., Sundram, S., Pantelis, C., & Dean, B. (2009). Decreased cortical muscarinic receptors define a subgroup of subjects with schizophrenia. *Molecular Psychiatry*, *14*(11), 1017–1023.

Scarr, E., Craig, J. M., Cairns, M. J., Seo, M. S., Galati, J. C., Beveridge, N. J., et al. (2013). Decreased cortical muscarinic M1 receptors in schizophrenia are associated with changes in gene promoter methylation, mRNA and gene targeting microRNA. *Translational Psychiatry*, *3*, e230.

Scarr, E., Sundram, S., Deljo, A., Cowie, T. F., Gibbons, A. S., Juzva, S., et al. (2012). Muscarinic M1 receptor sequence: Preliminary studies on its effects on cognition and expression. *Schizophrenia Research*, *138*(1), 94–98.

Scarr, E., Sundram, S., Keriakous, D., & Dean, B. (2007). Altered hippocampal muscarinic M4, but not M1, receptor expression from subjects with schizophrenia. *Biological Psychiatry*, *61*(10), 1161–1170.

Scarr, E., Um, J. Y., Cowie, T. F., & Dean, B. (2013). Cholinergic muscarinic M4 receptor gene polymorphisms: A potential risk factor and pharmacogenomic marker for schizophrenia. *Schizophrenia Research*, *146*(1–3), 279–284.

Schmidt, L. S., Thomsen, M., Weikop, P., Dencker, D., Wess, J., Woldbye, D. P. D., et al. (2011). Increased cocaine self-administration in M4 muscarinic acetylcholine receptor knockout mice. *Psychopharmacology*, *216*(3), 367–378.

See, R., McLaughlin, J., & Fuchs, R. (2003). Muscarinic receptor antagonism in the basolateral amygdala blocks acquisition of cocaine-stimulus association in a model of relapse to cocaine-seeking behavior in rats. *Neuroscience*, *117*(2), 477–483.

Semba, K., Reiner, P. B., & Fibiger, H. C. (1990). Single cholinergic mesopontine tegmental neurons project to both the pontine reticular formation and the thalamus in the rat. *Neuroscience*, *38*(3), 643–654.

Shekhar, A., Potter, W. Z., Lightfoot, J., Lienemann, J., Dubé, S., Mallinckrodt, C., et al. (2008). Selective muscarinic receptor agonist xanomeline as a novel treatment approach for schizophrenia. *American Journal of Psychiatry*, *165*(8), 1033–1039.

Shirey, J. K., Brady, A. E., Jones, P. J., Davis, A. A., Bridges, T. M., Kennedy, J. P., et al. (2009). A selective allosteric potentiator of the M1 muscarinic acetylcholine receptor increases activity of medial prefrontal cortical neurons and restores impairments in reversal learning. *Journal of Neuroscience*, *29*(45), 14271–14286.

Shirey, J. K., Xiang, Z., Orton, D., Brady, A. E., Johnson, K. A., Williams, R., et al. (2008). An allosteric potentiator of M4 mAChR modulates hippocampal synaptic transmission. *Nature Chemical Biology*, *4*(1), 42–50.

Singh, M. M., Kay, S. R., & Opler, L. A. (1987). Anticholinergic-neuroleptic antagonism in terms of positive and negative symptoms of schizophrenia: Implications for psychobiological subtyping. *Psychological Medicine*, *17*(1), 39–48.

Spalding, T. A., Trotter, C., Skjaerbaek, N., Messier, T. L., Currier, E. A., Burstein, E. S., et al. (1989). Discovery of an ectopic activation site on the M1 muscarinic receptor. *Molecular Pharmacology*, *61*(6), 1297–1302.

Spanagel, R., & Weiss, F. (1999). The dopamine hypothesis of reward: Past and current status. *Trends in Neurosciences*, *22*(11), 521–527.

Sprecher, K. E., Ferrarelli, F., & Benca, R. M. (2015). Sleep and plasticity in schizophrenia. In P. Meerlo, R. Benca, & T. Abel (Eds.), *Current topics in behavioral neuroscience. Sleep, neuronal plasticity, and brain function* (pp. 433–458). Berlin, Heidelberg: Springer.

Stanhope, K. J., Mirza, N. R., Bickerdike, M. J., Bright, J. L., Harrington, N. R., Hesselink, M. B., et al. (2001). The muscarinic receptor agonist xanomeline has an antipsychotic-like profile in the rat. *The Journal of Pharmacology and Experimental Therapeutics*, *299*, 782–792.

Stark, A. D., Jordan, S., Allers, K. A., Bertekap, R. L., Chen, R., Mistry Kannan, T., et al. (2007). Interaction of the novel antipsychotic aripiprazole with 5-HT1A and 5-HT2A receptors: Functional receptor-binding and in vivo electrophysiological studies. *Psychopharmacology*, *190*(3), 373–382.

Steidl, S., Miller, A. D., Blaha, C. D., & Yeomans, J. S. (2011). M5 muscarinic receptors mediate striatal dopamine activation by ventral tegmental morphine and pedunculopontine stimulation in mice. *PLoS One*, *6*(11), e27538.

Steidl, S., Wasserman, D. I., Blaha, C. D., & Yeomans, J. S. (2017). Opioid-induced rewards, locomotion, and dopamine activation: A proposed model for control by mesopontine and rostromedial tegmental neurons. *Neuroscience and Biobehavioral Reviews*, *83*(September), 72–82.

Steidl, S., & Yeomans, J. S. (2009). M5 muscarinic receptor knockout mice show reduced morphine-induced locomotion but increased locomotion after cholinergic antagonism in the ventral tegmental area. *Journal of Pharmacology and Experimental Therapeutics*, *328*(1), 263–275.

Stoll, K., Hart, R., Lindsley, C. W., & Thomsen, M. (2018). Effects of muscarinic M1 and M4 acetylcholine receptor stimulation on extinction and reinstatement of cocaine seeking in male mice, independent of extinction learning. *Psychopharmacology*, *235*(3), 815–827.

Sur, C., Mallorga, P. J., Wittmann, M., Jacobson, M. A., Pascarella, D., Williams, J. B., et al. (2003). N-desmethylclozapine, an allosteric agonist at muscarinic 1 receptor, potentiates N-methyl-D-aspartate receptor activity. *Proceedings of the National Academy of Sciences of the United States of America*, *100*(23), 13674–13679.

Tandon, R., Shipley, J. E., Greden, J. F., Mann, N. A., Eisner, W. H., & Goodson, J. (1991). Muscarinic cholinergic hyperactivity in schizophrenia: Relationship to positive and negative symptoms. *Schizophrenia Research*, *4*(1), 23–30.

Tayebati, S., Di Tullio, M., Tomassoni, D., & Amenta, F. (2003). Localization of the m5 muscarinic cholinergic receptor in rat circle of Willis and pial arteries. *Neuroscience*, *122*(1), 205–211.

Thakurathi, N., Vincenzi, B., & Henderson, D. C. (2013). Assessing the prospect of donepezil in improving cognitive impairment in patients with schizophrenia. *Expert Opinion on Investigational Drugs*, *22*(2), 259–265.

Thomsen, M., Conn, P. J., Lindsley, C., Wess, J., Boon, J. Y., Fulton, B. S., et al. (2010). Attenuation of cocaine's reinforcing and discriminative stimulus effects via muscarinic M1 acetylcholine receptor stimulation. *The Journal of Pharmacology and Experimental Therapeutics*, *332*(3), 959.

Thomsen, M., Fulton, B. S., & Caine, S. B. (2014). Acute and chronic effects of the M1/M4-preferring muscarinic agonist xanomeline on cocaine vs. food choice in rats. *Psychopharmacology*, *231*(3), 469–479.

Thomsen, M., Lindsley, C. W., Conn, P. J., Wessell, J. E., Fulton, B. S., Wess, J., et al. (2012). Contribution of both M1 and M4 receptors to muscarinic agonist-mediated attenuation of the cocaine discriminative stimulus in mice. *Psychopharmacology*, *220*(4), 673–685.

Thomsen, M., Sørensen, G., & Dencker, D. (2018). Physiological roles of CNS muscarinic receptors gained from knockout mice. *Neuropharmacology*, *136*, 411–420.

Thomsen, M., Wess, J., Fulton, B. S., Fink-Jensen, A., & Caine, S. B. (2010). Modulation of prepulse inhibition through both M1 and M4 muscarinic receptors in mice. *Psychopharmacology*, *208*(3), 401–416.

Thomsen, M., Woldbye, D. P. D., Wörtwein, G., Fink-Jensen, A., Wess, J., & Caine, S. B. (2005). Reduced cocaine self-administration in muscarinic M5 acetylcholine receptor-deficient mice. *The Journal of Neuroscience*, *25*(36), 8141–8149.

Thomsen, M., Wörtwein, G., Fink-Jensen, A., Woldbye, D. P. D., Wess, J., & Caine, S. B. (2007). Decreased prepulse inhibition and increased sensitivity to muscarinic, but not dopaminergic drugs in M5 muscarinic acetylcholine receptor knockout mice. *Psychopharmacology*, *192*(1), 97–110.

Toftdahl, N. G., Nordentoft, M., & Hjorthøj, C. (2016). Prevalence of substance use disorders in psychiatric patients: A nationwide Danish population-based study. *Social Psychiatry and Psychiatric Epidemiology*, *51*(1), 129–140.

Tracey, W. R., & Peach, M. J. (1992). Differential muscarinic receptor mRNA expression by freshly isolated and cultured bovine aortic endothelial cells. *Circulation Research*, *70*, 234–240.

Tzavara, E. T., Bymaster, F. P., Davis, R. J., Wade, M. R., Perry, K. W., Wess, J., et al. (2004). M4 muscarinic receptors regulate the dynamics of cholinergic and dopaminergic neurotransmission: Relevance to the pathophysiology and treatment of related central nervous system pathologies. *The FASEB Journal*, *18*(12), 1–18.

Van Dort, C. J., Zachs, D. P., Kenny, J. D., Zheng, S., Goldblum, R. R., Gelwan, N. A., et al. (2015). Optogenetic activation of cholinergic neurons in the PPT or LDT induces REM sleep. *Proceedings of the National Academy of Sciences of the United States of America*, *112*(2), 584–589.

van Huijstee, A. N., & Mansvelder, H. D. (2015). Glutamatergic synaptic plasticity in the mesocorticolimbic system in addiction. *Frontiers in Cellular Neuroscience*, *8*, 466.

Veroff, A. E., Bodick, N. C., Offen, W. W., Sramek, J. J., & Cutler, N. R. (1998). Efficacy of xanomeline in Alzheimer disease: Cognitive improvement measured using the Computerized Neuropsychological Test Battery (CNTB). *Alzheimer Disease and Associated Disorders*, *12*(4), 304–312.

Vilaró, M. T., Palacios, J. M., & Mengod, G. (1990). Localization of m5 muscarinic receptor mRNA in rat brain examined by in situ hybridization histochemistry. *Neuroscience Letters*, *114*(2), 154–159.

Vilaró, M. T., Wiederhold, K., Palacios, J. M., & Mengod, G. (1991). Muscarinic cholinergic receptors in the rat caudate-putamen and olfactory tubercle belong predominantly to the m4 class: In situ hybridization and receptor autoradiography evidence. *Neuroscience*, *40*(1), 159–167.

Vilaró, M. T., Wiederhold, K., Palacios, J. M., & Mengod, G. (1992). Muscarinic M2 receptor mRNA expression and receptor binding in cholinergic and non-cholinergic cells in

the rat brain: A correlative study using in situ hybridization histochemistry and receptor autoradiography. *Neuroscience*, *47*(2), 367–393.
Volkow, N. D., Wang, G.-J., Fowler, J. S., Tomasi, D., & Telang, F. (2011). Addiction: Beyond dopamine reward circuitry. *Proceedings of the National Academy of Sciences of the United States of America*, *108*(37), 15037–15042.
Wall, S. J., Yasuda, R. P., Li, M., & Wolfe, B. B. (1991). Development of an antiserum against m3 muscarinic receptors: Distribution of m3 receptors in rat tissues and clonal cell lines. *Molecular Pharmacology*, *40*, 783–789.
Wang, H., Ng, K., Hayes, D., Gao, X., Forster, G., Blaha, C. D., et al. (2004). Decreased amphetamine-induced locomotion and improved latent inhibition in mice mutant for the M5 muscarinic receptor gene found in the human 15q schizophrenia region. *Neuropsychopharmacology*, *29*, 2126–2139.
Wasserman, D. I., Wang, H. G., Rashid, A. J., Josselyn, S. A., & Yeomans, J. S. (2013). Cholinergic control of morphine-induced locomotion in rostromedial tegmental nucleus versus ventral tegmental area sites. *European Journal of Neuroscience*, *38*(5), 2774–2785.
Weiner, D. M., Levey, A. I., & Brann, M. R. (1990). Expression of muscarinic acetylcholine and dopamine receptor mRNAs in rat basal ganglia. *Proceedings of the National Academy of Sciences of the United States of America*, *87*, 7050–7054.
Wess, J., Eglen, R. M., & Gautam, D. (2007). Muscarinic acetylcholine receptors: Mutant mice provide new insights for drug development. *Nature Reviews Drug Discovery*, *6*(9), 721–733.
Wess, J., Gdula, D., & Brann, M. R. (1991). Site-directed mutagenesis of the m3 muscarinic receptor: Identification of a series of threonine and tyrosine residues involved in agonist but not antagonist binding. *The EMBO Journal*, *10*(12), 3729–3734.
Wess, J., Maggio, R., Palmer, J. R., & Vogel, Z. (1992). Role of conserved threonine and tyrosine residues in acetylcholine binding and muscarinic receptor activation. *The Journal of Biological Chemistry*, *267*(27), 19313–19319.
Weston-Green, K., Huang, X. F., Lian, J., & Deng, C. (2012). Effects of olanzapine on muscarinic M3 receptor binding density in the brain relates to weight gain, plasma insulin and metabolic hormone levels. *European Neuropsychopharmacology*, *22*(5), 364–373.
Witkin, J. M., Goldberg, S. R., Katz, J. L., & Kuhar, M. J. (1989). Modulation of the lethal effects of cocaine by cholinomimetics. *Life Sciences*, *45*(24), 2295–2301.
Wood, M. W. R., Noetzel, M. J., Poslusney, M. S., Melancon, B. J., Tarr, J. C., Lamsal, A., et al. (2017). Challenges in the development of an M4 PAM in vivo tool compound: The discovery of VU0467154 and unexpected DMPK profiles of close analogs. *Bioorganic & Medicinal Chemistry Letters*, *27*(2), 171–175.
Woolley, M. L., Carter, H. J., Gartlon, J. E., Watson, J. M., & Dawson, L. A. (2009). Attenuation of amphetamine-induced activity by the non-selective muscarinic receptor agonist, xanomeline, is absent in muscarinic M4 receptor knockout mice and attenuated in muscarinic M1 receptor knockout mice. *European Journal of Pharmacology*, *603*(1–3), 147–149.
Yamada, M., Lamping, K. G., Duttaroy, A., Zhang, W., Cui, Y., Bymaster, F. P., et al. (2001). Cholinergic dilation of cerebral blood vessels is abolished in M5 muscarinic acetylcholine receptor knockout mice. *Proceedings of the National Academy of Sciences of the United States of America*, *98*(24), 14096–14101.
Yang, H., de Jong, J. W., Tak, Y., Peck, J., Bateup, H. S., & Lammel, S. (2018). Nucleus accumbens subnuclei regulate motivated behavior via direct inhibition and disinhibition of VTA dopamine subpopulations. *Neuron*, *97*, 434–449.
Yang, C., & Winkelman, J. W. (2006). Clinical significance of sleep EEG abnormalities in chronic schizophrenia. *Schizophrenia Research*, *82*(2–3), 251–260.
Yeomans, J. S., Kofman, O., & McFarlane, V. (1985). Cholinergic involvement in lateral hypothalamic rewarding brain stimulation. *Brain Research*, *329*(1–2), 19–26.

Yohn, S. E., Foster, D. J., Covey, D. P., Moehle, M. S., Galbraith, J., Garcia-Barrantes, P. M., et al. (2018). Activation of the mGlu1 metabotropic glutamate receptor has antipsychotic-like effects and is required for efficacy of M4 muscarinic receptor allosteric modulators. *Molecular Psychiatry*.

Zang, Z., & Creese, I. (1997). Differential regulation of expression of rat hippocampal muscarinic receptor subtypes following fimbria-fornix lesion. *Biochemical Pharmacology*, *53*(9), 1379–1382.

Zavitsanou, K., Katsifis, A., Mattner, F., & Xu-Feng, H. (2004). Investigation of M1/M4 muscarinic receptors in the anterior cingulate cortex in schizophrenia, bipolar disorder and major depression disorder. *Neuropsychopharmacology*, *29*(3), 619–625.

Zhang, W., Basile, A. S., Gomeza, J., Volpicelli, L. A., Levey, A. I., & Wess, J. (2002). Characterization of central inhibitory muscarinic autoreceptors by the use of muscarinic acetylcholine receptor knock-out mice. *The Journal of Neuroscience*, *22*(5), 1709–1717.

Zhang, Y., Mayer-Blackwell, B., Schlussman, S. D., Randesi, M., Butelman, E. R., Ho, A., et al. (2014). Extended access oxycodone self-administration and neurotransmitter receptor gene expression in the dorsal striatum of adult C57BL/6 J mice. *Psychopharmacology*, *231*(7), 1277–1287.

Zhang, W., Yamada, M., Gomeza, J., Basile, A. S., & Wess, J. (2002). Multiple muscarinic acetylcholine receptor subtypes modulate striatal dopamine release, as studied with M1-M5 muscarinic receptor knock-out mice. *The Journal of Neuroscience*, *22*(15), 6347–6352.

Zhou, Y., Fan, L., Qiu, C., & Jiang, T. (2015). Prefrontal cortex and the dysconnectivity hypothesis of schizophrenia. *Neuroscience Bulletin*, *31*(2), 207–219.

Further reading

Diana, M. (2011). The dopamine hypothesis of drug addiction and its potential therapeutic value. *Frontiers in Psychiatry*, *2*, 64.

Jones, C. K., Eberle, E. L., Shaw, D. B., Mckinzie, D. L., & Shannon, H. E. (2005). Pharmacologic interactions between the muscarinic cholinergic and dopaminergic systems in the modulation of prepulse inhibition in rats. *The Journal of Pharmacology and Experimental Therapeutics*, *312*, 1055–1063.

CHAPTER SEVEN

Medications development for food-based and drug use disorders

Fernando B. de Moura[a,b], **Stephen J. Kohut**[a,b], **Jack Bergman**[a,b,*]
[a]Behavioral Biology Program, McLean Hospital, Boston, MA, United States
[b]Department of Psychiatry, Harvard Medical School, Boston, MA, United States
*Corresponding author: e-mail address: jack_bergman@hms.harvard.edu

Contents

1. Introduction 198
2. Drug and food addiction 201
3. Gut-brain axis peptides in addiction 203
   3.1 Ghrelin 203
   3.2 Leptin 204
   3.3 Cholecystokinin 205
   3.4 Cocaine- and amphetamine-regulated transcript peptide 206
   3.5 Pancreatic peptides (insulin and glucagon) 207
   3.6 Conclusion 208
4. Neurotransmitter systems as modulators of food and drug reward processes 209
   4.1 Opioids 209
   4.2 Acetylcholine 210
   4.3 Cannabinoids 212
   4.4 Dopamine 213
   4.5 Serotonin 216
   4.6 Summary 218
5. Non-pharmacological approaches to the management of substance use disorders 219
6. Conclusion 220
Acknowledgment 220
Conflict of interest statement 221
References 221
Further reading 235

Abstract

Despite decades of research, few medications have gained Food and Drug Administration (FDA) approval for the management of substance abuse disorder. The paucity of successful medications can be attributed, in part, to the lack of clearly identified

Advances in Pharmacology, Volume 86
ISSN 1054-3589
https://doi.org/10.1016/bs.apha.2019.04.005

neurobiological targets for addressing the core pathology of addictive behavior. Commonalities in the behavioral and brain processes involved in the rewarding effects of drugs and foods has prompted the evaluation of candidate medications that target neural pathways involved in both drug and eating disorders. Here, pharmacological strategies for the development of novel medications for drug addiction are presented in the context of potential overlapping neurobiological targets identified for eating disorders (e.g., obesity, overeating, binge-eating) and substance abuse. Mechanisms discussed in this chapter include modulators of the gut-brain axis (e.g., leptin, ghrelin, cholecystokinin, cocaine- and amphetamine-regulated transcript, and pancreatic peptides) and neurotransmitter systems (e.g., opioids, cannabinoids, dopamine, serotonin, and acetylcholine).

Abbreviations

CART cocaine- and amphetamine-regulated transcript
CCK cholecystokinin
GLP-1 glucagon-like peptide-1
MOR μ-opioid receptor

1. Introduction

Pharmacological strategies in identifying candidate medications for the management of substance use disorders and, in particular, the reduction of drug use or relapse prevention, generally employ one of two therapeutic approaches. First, agonist replacement therapy (either direct or indirect) underlies the search for medications that share some of the behavioral and/or neurochemical effects of the abused drug but that exhibit lesser abuse potential. This approach is exemplified by the development and current use of the mu-opioid receptor agonists methadone and buprenorphine (Volkow, 2017) for opioid dependence and nicotine or the nicotinic receptor partial agonist varenicline for smoking cessation (Rollema et al., 2007). The second approach is the development of drugs that, by reducing or blocking the pharmacological actions of the abused drug, provide antagonist therapy. For example, a long-acting formulation of naltrexone (Vivitrol), which is a competitive antagonist at the mu-opioid receptor, was recently introduced for the prevention of relapse to opioid dependence (Volkow, 2017). An interesting alternative but, as yet, unrealized approach to the development of medications for relapse prevention is immunological: vaccines that target the offending molecule and, by binding it, prevent its entry into the brain and consequent receptor activation. This approach has been actively investigated for the development of anti-nicotine and anti-opioid medications (Montoya, 2012) but, thus far, safe and effective vaccines for any type of substance use disorder have not been identified.

As the above examples suggest, receptor-based strategies have focused principally on the neurotransmitter system that is directly implicated in the behavioral effects of the specific drug of abuse—e.g., the nicotinic acetylcholine system for nicotine and mu-opioid mechanisms for heroin. This is not to disregard other strategies that have been useful in the management of substance use disorders. For example, the adrenoceptor agonists clonidine or lofexidine, by attenuating the adverse physiological effects of abstinence, can be valuable in achieving successful opioid withdrawal (Kosten & Baxter, 2019). Nevertheless, to date, the medications that are most effective for managing substance use disorders—and that have managed to gain FDA-approval for that purpose—target the receptor mechanisms that are directly engaged by drugs of abuse (Kohut & Bergman, 2017).

While targeting receptor systems that are directly activated by the abused drug has proven to be a profitable medications development approach for some drug classes—e.g., nicotine and opioids—the application of this approach to abused drugs from other pharmacological classes (and, in particular, psychomotor stimulants) remains a formidable challenge. Strategically, defining potential targets has been a difficult first step. Monoaminergic stimulants such as cocaine or methamphetamine are indirect agonists, i.e., do not directly activate a particular receptor mechanism but, rather, produce behavioral effects by increasing synaptic levels of dopamine that, in turn, increase dopamine receptor activity (Rothman & Baumann, 2003). Historically, considerable effort has been expended in evaluating dopamine receptor agonists and antagonists as candidate medications. Unfortunately, and with few exceptions, the development of dopamine receptor antagonists has virtually ceased, due to unwanted extrapyramidal side effects (Coffin, Latranyi, & Chipkin, 1989; Gerlach, Lublin, & Peacock, 1996; Knable, Heinz, Raedler, & Weinberger, 1997; but see Kumar et al., 2016). As well, the preponderance of research indicates that directly-acting agonists (both D1 and D2) unfortunately produce unacceptable adverse effects (Kohut & Bergman, 2017). As a consequence, the development of candidate medications for stimulant use disorders necessarily has focused on indirect agonist therapy. Despite some glimmers of positive results with this approach, the development of medications nevertheless has proceeded only haltingly, stalling over concerns regarding the stimulant-like effects and potential diversion of currently available candidates (Negus & Henningfield, 2015).

The realization that abused drugs come from various pharmacological classes that act through dissimilar neurochemical mechanisms has led to the view that a common underlying neurobiological mechanism, or neural pathway, may be engaged by all drugs of abuse. In turn, this has raised interest in the potential value of candidate medications that, rather than being mechanistically selective for the abused drug, might modulate activity in such a common pathway. Early on, the mesolimbic dopamine system, comprised of ventral and dorsal striatal brain regions including the nucleus accumbens, caudate, and putamen, emerged as a strong candidate for such neural circuitry (Di Chiara & Imperato, 1988; Spanagel & Weiss, 1999; Wise & Rompre, 1989; Yokel & Wise, 1975). Indeed, studies in rodents and monkeys have repeatedly demonstrated that a wide range of abused drugs preferentially increase synaptic dopamine levels in striatum (Bradberry, Barrett-Larimore, Jatlow, & Rubino, 2000; Di Chiara & Imperato, 1988; Drevets et al., 1999; reviewed by Di Chiara et al., 2004), whereas human positron emission tomography (PET) imaging studies have shown that striatal dopamine levels can be correlated with drug-induced subjective reports of "high" and "drug-liking" (Volkow et al., 1996). Although more recent evidence has accumulated to suggest that this view—i.e., that the mesolimbic dopamine system serves as the common pathway for drug abuse—may be overly simplistic (Brown, Kupchik, & Kalivas, 2013; Kalivas, 2009; Pierce & Kumaresan, 2006), it remains highly popular. Thus, for at least the last quarter century, the dopamine system has been spotlighted as a primary target for medication development efforts. As noted in the preceding paragraph, however, the results of studies with drugs that directly target dopamine receptors either through direct agonist or antagonist actions, have not been promising and, consequently, such dopamine receptor-based efforts have not yet been profitable (see above; reviewed by Bergman, 2008; Bergman & Rheingold, 2015; Kohut & Bergman, 2017). Though there continues to be interest in identifying and exploiting elements of dopamine pharmacology, e.g., D3 receptor subtype antagonism, toward the development of novel candidate medications for cocaine or opioid abuse (Bergman & Rheingold, 2015; Newman et al., 2012), the future success of such endeavors remains uncertain.

2. Drug and food addiction

Theoretical foundations for the classification of eating disorders (overeating, binge-eating, overconsumption of foods high in refined sugar and fat, etc.) and drug use as addictive disorders have been presented elsewhere (DiLeone, Taylor, & Picciotto, 2012; Grigson, 2002; Ifland et al., 2009; Volkow, 2017; Volkow & Wise, 2005; Wise, 1997), and a comprehensive analysis of this topic is far beyond the scope of this review. Nevertheless, it is worth noting overlap in the neural concomitants of drug- and food-based rewarding effects and in these two categories of behavioral disorders (reviewed by Dagher, 2009; DiLeone et al., 2012; Gordon, Ariel-Donges, Bauman, & Merlo, 2018; Hebebrand et al., 2014). Clearly, substance and food addictions share a number of clinical features and diagnostic criteria (DSM-V; Dimitrijevic, Popovic, Sabljak, Skodric-Trifunovic, & Dimitrijevic, 2015). Both are thought to be chronic relapsing disorders and are characterized by compulsive intake that persists despite clear adverse consequences (health, economic, etc.; Volkow & Wise, 2005). Comorbidity is also common in patients with drug and eating disorders, the most recognizable being concurrent eating and alcohol use disorders (Wolfe & Maisto, 2000). Finally, both substance- and food-based addictions are often inadequately addressed by the medical community in part due to continued stigma of addiction per se as a moral failing (Barry, McGinty, Pescosolido, & Goldman, 2014; DePierre, Puhl, & Luedicke, 2013; Puhl & Brownell, 2001).

Scientifically, genetic and environmental factors that similarly affect food intake and different types of drug use have been identified. For example, maternal smoking during pregnancy has been shown to increase risk for both nicotine dependence (Buka, Shenassa, & Niaura, 2003) and obesity (Toschke, Ehlin, von Kries, Ekbom, & Montgomery, 2003). A review of relevant studies in nonhuman and human subjects also indicates a strong relationship between preference for sweet foods and alcohol consumption (Kampov-Polevoy, Garbutt, & Janowsky, 1999). Exposure to stressful stimuli has been shown consistently to potentiate both drug and food intake, whereas rodents characterized as highly impulsive show a similarly increased responsivity to reinforcement by either food or cocaine (Anker, Gliddon, & Carroll, 2008; Gluck, 2006; Gluck, Geliebter, & Lorence, 2004; Hagan et al., 2002; Piazza & Le Moal, 1998; Sinha, 2008). Finally, the reinforcing effects of drugs can be modified by particular histories of food intake. Rodents maintained on a high fat diet or given access to a sweetened solution, for example, show a delayed acquisition of stimulant self-administration (Carrol & Lac, 1993; Wellman, Nation, & Davis, 2007). On the other hand, food restriction has been shown to increase cocaine intake in self-administration studies in both rodent and primate species (Carroll, France, & Meisch, 1979; de la Garza & Johanson, 1987; see also Carr, 2007; Carroll, 1998).

In addition to behavioral evidence of a close relationship between mechanisms that control food intake and drug use, overlapping neural circuits have been implicated in obesity and drug addiction (Grigson, 2002; Kelley, Schiltz, & Lawrence, 2005; Volkow, Wise, & Baler, 2017). In this regard, two brain regions are of particular interest for the central role they may play in regulating the intake of abused drugs or preferred foods. First, preclinical and clinical investigations have supported a central role for striatal regions in the mesolimbic dopamine system in the rewarding or reinforcing effects of both abused drugs and calorie-dense foods. For example, microdialysis studies in rodents have shown that access to a preferred oral sucrose solution, like cocaine or other self-administered drugs, increases accumbal dopamine levels (Hajnal, Smith, & Norgren, 2004). Studies in monkeys and human subjects also have shown that striatal D2 receptor density may decrease with chronic cocaine exposure and, as well, may be inversely related to vulnerability to the reinforcing effects of cocaine (Morgan et al., 2002; Nader et al., 2006; Volkow et al., 1990). Analogously, PET imaging studies in obese individuals have revealed that dopamine D2 receptor availability is inversely related to body mass index (BMI; Wang et al., 2001) and, as well, that reduction in striatal D2 receptor density are of similar magnitude to those reported in substance abusers. Taken together, these and other data strongly support the involvement of striatal regions in the reinforcing or rewarding effects of self-administered foods and abused drugs.

A second region of interest, in addition to striatum, has been the hypothalamus—which has been long recognized to play a key role in the regulation of feeding behavior, homeostasis, and control of various physiological processes (Harricharan, Abboussi, & Daniels, 2017). The hypothalamus is a rich source of neuropeptide transmitters—e.g., orexin, leptin, ghrelin, neurotensin—that are known to be associated with the regulation of food intake and satiety. Importantly, the hypothalamus, which projects liberally throughout the brain, densely innervates mesolimbic circuitry, raising the intriguing possibility that satiety mechanisms are intimately involved in reward processing (see Wise, 1997). In support of this view, rats have been shown to respond for intracranial self-stimulation (ICSS) through electrodes implanted in the lateral hypothalamus (LH), in keeping with the view that activation of this region is reinforcing (Olds, 1958; Olds, Travis, & Schwing, 1960). Moreover, both drugs of abuse and food access modulate LH ICSS thresholds (Carr, 1990; Conover & Shizgal, 1994), further supporting the involvement of this region in general reward processes.

A wide range of approaches has been evaluated for the management of both substance abuse and/or food addiction. The following sections are not intended to be an exhaustive review of published literature. Instead, they are meant to highlight the current understanding of how peptide and neurotransmitter systems that regulate feeding behavior have been applied to medication strategies for substance use disorder, and, in some cases, vice versa. In this regard, it must be stressed that eating and food-related disorders (i.e., anorexia, bulimia, overeating, binge-eating, etc.) constitute a spectrum of aberrant behavior, and that the full range of phenotypes are not encompassed within a single definition. Further, the regulation of body weight and food intake is highly complex and involves coordination of multiple hormonal and neurotransmitter systems, many of which are not described below. Finally, the focus on the similarities between drug and food addiction is not to ignore obvious differences between the two classes of behavior—caloric intake being necessary for survival. Notwithstanding these well-deserved caveats, it remains the case that understanding how various mechanisms alter responses to both food and drugs may provide insights regarding key commonalities in relevant regard and reinforcement processes. These insights, in turn, may lead to novel targets for the treatment of addiction disorders.

3. Gut-brain axis peptides in addiction

3.1 Ghrelin

Ghrelin is a peripherally-derived orexigenic hormone generated by gastric oxyntic cells that modulates food intake through two primary mechanisms that have been described as homeostatic and non-homeostatic feeding (Wren et al., 2001; for review, see Howick, Griffin, Cryan, & Shellekens, 2017). While ghrelin is synthesized and secreted in the peripheral nervous system (Sakata & Sakai, 2010), compelling evidence also shows direct actions of ghrelin in the central nervous system, specifically through binding to growth hormone secretagogue receptors (GHSR) in the mediobasal hypothalamus (Mani et al., 2017; Russo, Russo, Pellitteri, & Stanzani, 2017).

One non-homeostatic mechanism by which ghrelin promotes food intake is by increasing levels of dopamine in the ventral tegmental area, a brain region associated with reward processes (Abizaid et al., 2006; Egecioglu et al., 2010; Skibicka, Hansson, Egecioglu, & Dickson, 2012; for review, see Perello & Dickson, 2015). Thus, antagonism and/or deletion of the ghrelin receptor has been shown to decrease intake of alcohol (Jerlhag et al., 2009), attenuate the rewarding and locomotor effects of cocaine and amphetamine (Jerlhag, Egecioglu, Dickson, & Engel, 2010; Wellman, Davis, & Nation, 2005), and suppress the rewarding effects of morphine (Jerabek et al., 2017). Currently, there are no known ghrelin-based medications for the treatment of obesity or substance abuse; however, small molecule ghrelin antagonists (Cameron, Bhattacharya, & Loomis, 2014) and vaccines (Bhat & Sharm, 2017) are currently under development or investigation.

3.2 Leptin

Leptin is an anorectic hormone predominantly generated in adipose tissue (Elmquist, Elias, & Saper, 1999; Schwartz, Woods, Porte, Seeley, & Baskin, 2000). In the 1950s, a subset of mice generated by Jackson Labs grew to be obese and, subsequently, were investigated to explore causal factors in their obesity. As an outcome of studies of these "*ob*" mice, leptin eventually was identified in the mid-1990s as a prominent peptidic regulator of food intake and energy homeostasis (Halaas et al., 1995). Since the discovery of leptin, numerous preclinical studies have illustrated the relationship between leptin and food reward. For example, both Pavlovian and operant-based measures of reward have been used to show that the administration of leptin can block the rewarding effects of a high-fat diet in wildtype and ob/ob mice (Sharma, Hryhorczuk, & Fulton, 2012; Shimizu et al., 2017). Similarly, using functional magnetic resonance techniques (fMRI), regional brain activation studies have shown that neural responses in the ventral striatum to food cues in obese individuals can be directly correlated with plasma leptin levels, suggesting that the regulation of reward pathways may be abnormal in such individuals (Grosshans et al., 2012). In the latter study, the authors hypothesized that the impaired homeostatic feedback mechanism of leptin and neuronal reward pathways might explain why some obese individuals develop addiction-like behaviors (Grosshans et al., 2012). However, this is a speculative view, and it may be that overeating or feeding behavior that results from substrate abnormalities, e.g., leptin dysregulation, should be considered separately from other types of reward-based behavior related to addiction. For instance, the reward-related effects of food in mice have been reported to decrease, rather than increase, following leptin-receptor activation on dopamine neurons (Evans & Anderson, 2017). The further development of leptin as a pharmacotherapeutic target for overeating disorders likely depends on a better understanding of leptin's role in food-based reward processes.

In view of the strong evidence for the role of leptin in feeding behavior and the presumed relationship between leptin and reward processes, it is perhaps unsurprising that some evidence suggests a role for leptin in the abuse-related behavioral effects of drugs. For example, plasma levels of leptin were found to be reduced in heroin users by approximately 25% (Housová, Wilczek, Haluzík, Kremen, & Haluzík, 2005). Additionally, Escobar et al. (2018) recently have reported that the severity of crack-cocaine use may be inversely related to plasma leptin levels, i.e., lower leptin levels were correlated with increased crack-cocaine use. Results from studies in laboratory animals have been consistent with these observations. As discussed previously, leptin has been shown to regulate mesolimbic DA activity (Evans & Anderson, 2017; Hommel et al., 2006). Leptin-dependent mechanisms also have been implicated in the dopaminergic mediation of reinstatement of heroin-seeking behavior that can be induced by food-restriction (Tobin, Newman, Quinn, & Shalev, 2009). In place-conditioning experiments, as well, leptin has been shown to block the development of cocaine conditioned place preference (CPP) whereas the Superactive Mouse Leptin Antagonist, a leptin-receptor blocker, may accentuate the effects of cocaine (Shen, Jiang, Liu, & Ma, 2016; You et al., 2016). Although a great deal more research is needed to understand the role of leptin in addiction processes, findings such as these encourage optimism and support the idea that targeting the leptin receptor may lead to novel candidate medications for the management of substance use disorders.

3.3 Cholecystokinin

Cholecystokinin (CCK) is a gut peptide hormone that stimulates the digestion of fat and protein and that has been associated with satiety. Although CCK is predominantly synthesized by enteroendocrine cells and located in the small intestine, it also can be found in vagal afferent neurons, which has led to a longstanding interest in the role of CCK in gut-brain signaling processes related to feeding behavior (Lieverse, Jansen, Masclee, & Lamers, 1994; Reidelberger et al., 1994; for review, see Pathak, Flatt, & Irwin, 2018).

However, this role is not yet well-delineated, as both activation (Babcock, Livosky, & Avery, 1985) *and* antagonism (Josselyn & Vaccarino, 1996) of CCK receptors have been shown to decrease rates of operant food-maintained responding. CCK also has been suggested to play a role in cocaine-induced changes in reward circuitry (Josselyn, De Cristofaro, & Vaccarino, 1997). In this regard, Beinfeld, Connolly, and Pierce (2002) showed a three- to sixfold increase in CCK levels in the shell of the nucleus accumbens in rats following exposure to intraperitoneal injections of 15 mg/kg cocaine. Furthermore, antagonism of CCK receptors has been reported to attenuate cocaine-induced increases in striatal DA levels (Loonam, Noailles, Yu, Zhu, & Angulo, 2003). Consistent with such results, the CCK antagonist RPR102681 has been shown to both attenuate self-administration of cocaine in rodents (Frata, 1996) and, in a clinical investigation, to reduce cocaine craving in human subjects (Elkashef et al., 2018). These last findings are especially promising and deserve in-depth follow-up. Of note, CCK antagonists have been found to be without effect in opioid self-administration studies (Higgins, Joharchi, Wang, Corrigall, & Sellers, 1994), suggesting that their potential value as candidate medications for substance use disorder may be restricted to psychomotor stimulants like cocaine.

3.4 Cocaine- and amphetamine-regulated transcript peptide

Cocaine- and amphetamine-regulated transcript (CART) is a neuropeptide that is regulated by several gut peptides including leptin (Kristensen et al., 1998; Lee et al., 2013), ghrelin (de Lartigue, Dimaline, Varro, & Dockray, 2007), and CCK (Broberger, Holmberg, Kuhar, & Hökfelt, 1999; de Lartigue et al., 2007; Maletínská et al., 2008; for review, see Lau & Herzog, 2014). CART peptide has been reported to reduce food intake (Aja, Sahandy, Ladenheim, Schwartz, & Moran, 2001; Lau et al., 2018), and CART peptide expression levels are modified in reward circuitry in a rat model of binge eating (Bharne, Borkar, Subhedar, & Kokare, 2015). CART is readily expressed in the mesolimbic dopamine system (Philpot & Smith, 2006) and, consequently, CART modulation of mesolimbic DA has been implicated in food reward processes (Hunter & Kuhar, 2003; Rakosvka et al., 2017).

With respect to substance use disorders, the ability of CART peptide to decrease striatal DA release has been associated with attenuation of abuse-related effects of cocaine (Hurd, Svensson, & Pontén, 1999; Kuhar,

Jaworski, Hubert, Philpot, & Dominguez, 2005; Rakosvka et al., 2017). For example, in cocaine self-administration studies in rats, micro-infusions of CART peptide into the nucleus accumbens, at concentrations that did not alter food-maintained behavior, appeared to decrease cocaine intake (Jaworski, Hansen, Kuhar, & Mark, 2008). While it is somewhat surprising that CART peptide produced selective behavioral effects, such data illustrate why it has been forwarded as a promising target for candidate medications for the management of cocaine use disorder. CART also has been shown to reduce relapse-related reinstatement behavior after cocaine administration (James et al., 2010) and, more recently, to regulate the rewarding properties of the opioid morphine (Upadhya et al., 2012). Taken together, these are promising findings. However, it seems clear that the complex nature of CART's interactions with other peptidic hormones will need to be untangled to fully evaluate its own therapeutic potential for the management of either obesity or substance use disorders.

3.5 Pancreatic peptides (insulin and glucagon)

Insulin and glucagon are both released from pancreatic islet cells and play opposite roles in responding to blood glucose levels. Thus, insulin is secreted in response to increased blood glucose levels and promotes glucose absorption into cells, whereas glucagon is released in response to low blood glucose levels and helps recruit glucose from hepatic storage. The close relationship between insulin resistance and obesity has been recognized for many years (for review, see Kahn & Flier, 2000). Insulin hypersensitivity also has been associated with increased food intake, which can lead to obesity (Guiducci, Iervasi, & Quinones-Galvan, 2014). Recent preclinical studies have demonstrated that insulin receptors on neuropeptide Y neurons, specifically in the paraventricular nucleus of the hypothalamus, can regulate food intake (Loh et al., 2017), suggesting that manipulating blood glucose levels may be useful in managing obesity or other eating disorders. In agreement with this view, GLP-1 agonists that are prescribed for type-II diabetes (e.g., exendin and liraglutide) have been shown to promote weight loss through appetite suppression and, presumably as a consequence, to decrease food consumption (Baggio & Drucker, 2007; McMahon & Wellman, 1998; Verdich et al., 2001). These findings have spurred considerable interest in more closely defining mechanisms through which glucagon-like peptide-1 (GLP-1) may regulate motivational aspects of feeding behavior (for review, see Reddy, Stanwood, & Galli, 2014). Previously, discovery of GLP-1 receptor expression in the VTA and NAc led to the suggestion that GLP-1 in these brain regions, in particular, might play a role in the regulation of food-reward (Alhadeff, Rupprecht, & Hayes, 2012; Dossat, Lilly, Kay, & Williams, 2011; Göke, Larsen, Mikkelsen, & Sheikh, 1995; Gu et al., 2013; Merchenthaler, Lane, & Shughrue, 1999; Rinaman, 2010). Supporting this view, direct injections of the GLP-1 agonist exendin into the VTA in food-deprived rats has been shown to significantly decrease sucrose intake (Alhadeff et al., 2012). Moreover, administration of another GLP-1 agonist, exanitide, has been reported to decrease anticipation of food-reward in humans—illustrated by reduced activation of the right putamen and orbitofrontal cortex in functional imaging studies (van Bloemendaal et al., 2015).

The observations that GLP-1 agonists decrease food-reinforced behavior, presumably through modulation of reward processes, also has led to investigation of these drugs as candidate medications for drug abuse. Studies in rodents indicate that exanitide may block cocaine-induced CPP (Graham, Erreger, Galli, & Standwood, 2013) and reinstatement behavior in cocaine self-administration experiments (Hernandez et al., 2018). Exanitide also has been shown to block cocaine-induced phasic dopamine release events in the NAc core, consistent with the idea that increased levels of dopamine mediate the rewarding effects of cocaine (Fortin & Roitman, 2017). Further, it has been hypothesized that GLP-1 mediated decreases in the rewarding effects of drugs may be associated with insulin release (Reddy et al., 2014), and indeed, insulin also has been demonstrated to regulate reward processes (see Daws et al., 2011). For example, insulin administration into the VTA of rats has been shown to attenuate cocaine induced increases in synaptic DA levels in the NAc (Naef, Seabrook, Hsiao, Li, & Borgland, 2018). While no data regarding the utility of GLP-1 agonists for substance-use disorders in human subjects is available, the promising preclinical data discussed here indicates that further investigation of GLP-1 agonists as candidate medications for substance use disorders is warranted.

3.6 Conclusion

Peptides and hormones associated with the regulation of appetitive behavior offer promising targets for medications aimed at both substance abuse and food-related addictions. Although not a comprehensive list of gut peptides, the several discussed above were chosen to illustrate potential mechanisms by which manipulation of the gut-brain axis can be utilized for the development of both anti-obesity and substance addiction candidate medications. Other peptides, e.g., the orexigenic peptide orexin (Ida et al., 2000), the anorectic peptide Peptide YY (le Roux & Bloom, 2005), and Substance P (Lénárd et al., 2018) provide examples of additional targets within the gut-brain axis that may be fruitful for developing medications to address consummatory behavioral disorders, i.e., overeating and drug addiction.

4. Neurotransmitter systems as modulators of food and drug reward processes

4.1 Opioids

Multiple lines of evidence indicate that opioid ligands with μ-opioid receptor (MOR) activity, e.g., the agonists buprenorphine and methadone, or the antagonist naltrexone can be effective pharmacotherapies that reduce or eliminate the use of illicit opioids (Daniels, Salisbury-Afshar, Hoffberg, Agus, & Fingerhood, 2014; Maire-Claire et al., 2017). Although the mechanism of action is poorly understood, the MOR antagonist naltrexone also is approved by the FDA for the control of alcohol intake. For example, naltrexone has been shown to decrease levels of self-reported craving in individuals undergoing inpatient treatment for alcoholism (Helstrom et al., 2016), and to lower the number of alcoholic beverages consumed by heavy drinkers (O'Malley et al., 2015; see Carmen, Angeles, Munos, & Amate, 2004 for full review of naltrexone's utility in treating alcohol use disorders).

In addition to its identification as a useful target for the management of substance abuse, a great deal of evidence implicate the endogenous opioid system in the regulation of feeding behavior. An early report by McMillan (1971) showed that the MOR antagonist naloxone, which generally is behaviorally silent, enhanced the potency with which the antipsychotic medication chlorpromazine disrupted food-maintained operant behavior. In later studies, naloxone was found to dose-dependently decrease daily food intake in rats (Holtzman, 1974) whereas the opioid agonist β-endorphin was shown to stimulate food intake in rats (Grandison & Guidotti, 1977). Numerous studies have built upon these initial observations to provide a substantive literature regarding opioid mediation of feeding behavior (Bodner & Klein, 2004). Overall, this body of work shows that, via opioid mechanisms in brain regions that have been implicated in feeding processes, opioid agonists increase feeding behavior whereas opioid antagonists only decrease feeding behavior (De Tomasi & Juárez, 2011; Gosnell,

Leving, & Morley, 1986; Recant, Voyles, Luciano, & Pert, 1980). As an extension into the clinical setting, opioid antagonists (e.g., naltrexone) have been investigated in clinical trials both for their ability to prevent weight gain and as candidate weight loss medications. Regarding the prevention of weight gain, clinical studies have shown that naltrexone is quite effective in *preventing* weight gain following discontinuation from tobacco use (King et al., 2012; O'Malley et al., 2006). On the other hand, naltrexone had limited effectiveness in *reducing* weight: it was found to promote only modest weight loss in females, and was without effect in males (Atkinson et al., 1985). Findings such as these have led to the view that, notwithstanding its robust effects in rodent models of obesity (Kurbanov, Currie, Simonson, Borsook, & Elman, 2012), monotherapy with naltrexone is not likely to be an effective weight loss strategy (Lee & Fujioka, 2009). On the other hand, opioid antagonists have fared better when combined with non-opioid pharmacotherapeutics for weight loss. For example, rats treated with a combination of naltrexone and bupropion eat less of a palatable food than groups of rats treated with either drug alone (Wright & Rodgers, 2013). Based on these and other observations (see Clapper et al., 2013; Levy et al., 2018), a naltrexone/bupropion combination therapy marketed as Contrave received FDA approval in 2014 as a weight loss medication (FDA, 2014).

4.2 Acetylcholine

Acetylcholine (ACh) has been shown to regulate both drug- and food-taking behaviors, presumably through modulation of striatal reward systems and activation of cholinergic interneurons in the hypothalamus (Avena & Rada, 2012; Jeong, Lee, & Jo, 2017; Ostlund, Liu, Wassum, & Maidment, 2017). For example, administration of the acetylcholinesterase inhibitor neostigmine directly into the nucleus accumbens (NAc) was shown to significantly decrease food intake in rats without influencing the consumption of water (Mark, Shabani, Dobbs, & Hansen, 2011). Also, activation of muscarinic receptors on cholinergic neurons in the hypothalamus has been shown to regulate both food intake and body weight (Jeong et al., 2017). Despite a great deal of preclinical evidence of cholinergic involvement in feeding behavior, however, there is very little information regarding the capacity of ACh-based ligands to serve as candidate medications for obesity and other food-related disorders. Weight gain during abstinence in nicotine-dependent humans has been well-documented

(Aubin, Farley, Lycett, Lahmek, & Aveyard, 2012), and by extension, supports the hypothesis that cholinergic systems directly influence food intake and body weight. Yet, a recent study showed that varenicline failed to prevent weight gain following the discontinuation of tobacco products (Sun, Duan, Meng, Li, & Jia, 2018). Although varenicline, unlike the full agonist nicotine, is considered a nicotinic partial agonist, findings like these ought to be pursued to better understand the viability of ACh-based medications for the management of obesity, weight gain, and overeating.

A role for cholinergic mechanisms in drug-related reward processes also has been explored. For example, bilateral VTA injections of the nicotinic acetylcholine receptor (nAChR) antagonist mecamylamine have been reported to attenuate self-administration of cocaine in rats (Zhao-Shea et al., 2011), whereas physostigmine injections into the VTA were found to markedly increase heroin reinstatement behavior (Zhou et al., 2007). Consistent with a role for cholinergic mechanisms in such effects, c-fos labeling in the brains of rats has shown that cocaine self-administration can activate cholinergic interneurons in the NAc shell and ventromedial striatum (Berlanga et al., 2003). Despite these somewhat encouraging findings in rodent studies, the effects of mecamylamine on addictive behaviors in the human population have been, for the most part, negligible. Reid, Mickalian, Delucchi, and Berger (1999) showed that mecamylamine may decrease subjective reports of cocaine craving in cocaine-dependent cigarette smokers; however, a role for mecamylamine as a pharmacotherapeutic intervention for cocaine abuse has never materialized. Indeed, notwithstanding its clear nicotinic receptor antagonist actions, mecamylamine has failed as a monotherapy even for smoking cessation and, in clinical trials, was found to increase nicotine intake (Rose, Behm, & Westman, 2001; Rose, Behm, Westman, & Bates, 2003). These latter findings, while consistent with the surmountable antagonist actions of mecamylamine, greatly dampened enthusiasm for its further development as a medication for smoking cessation. It is striking that, in contrast to mecamylamine, the nAChR partial agonist varenicline has been shown to only decrease nicotine intake in rats (Rollema et al., 2007), nonhuman primates (Mello, Fivel, Kohut, & Carroll, 2014), and humans (Ebbert et al., 2015). Of interest, Mello et al. (2014) have shown that varenicline also attenuated the self-administration of nicotine + cocaine mixtures in nonhuman primates, results that are consistent with those observed in a human population of cocaine-dependent subjects (Plebani et al., 2012). These lines of evidence, in conjunction with the reported utility of the opioid buprenorphine for the management of opioid use disorders, support the view that the development of partial agonists rather than full antagonists has been a therapeutically advantageous strategy for developing novel receptor-based medications for substance-use disorders.

4.3 Cannabinoids

Numerous studies have identified a role for the endocannabinoid system in the regulation of food intake and adipogenesis (Lau et al., 2018; Pagano, Rossato, & Vettor, 2008). For example, the cannabinoid (CB) receptor agonist Δ^9-THC is known to promote hyperphagia in humans (Mattes, Engelman, Shaw, & Elsohly, 1994) and rats (Brown, Kassouny, & Cross, 1977; Williams, Rogers, & Kirkham, 1998). Consequently, cannabinoid agonist medications (e.g., dronabinol) are frequently prescribed to stimulate appetite in elderly patients or to counteract chemotherapy-induced nausea and vomiting, and by extension, promote food consumption (Badowski, 2017). Confirming the role of CB receptor mechanisms in such effects, the endogenous cannabinoid anandamide has been shown to increase food consumption in rats through activation of CB1 receptors (Williams & Kirkham, 1999). In keeping with the role of cannabinoid mechanisms in feeding behavior and in contrast to CB receptor agonists, CB1 antagonists have been shown to effectively suppress food intake in both nonhuman and human subjects (Arnone et al., 1997; Colombo et al., 1998; Simiand, Keane, Keane, & Soubrié, 1998). The efficacy of the CB1 inverse-agonist/antagonist rimonabant in this regard led to its clinical introduction as a weight-loss medication. Unfortunately, however, adverse mood and gastro-intestinal effects led to its abrupt withdrawal from the market (Christensen, Kristensen, Bartels, Bliddal, & Astrup, 2007) and the discontinuation of related lines of pharmaceutical development.

Several streams of evidence suggest that CB receptor ligands might be usefully employed as addiction pharmacotherapies. For example, CB1 agonists have been shown to slightly decrease self-administration of heroin in monkeys (Maguire & France, 2016), providing support for the currently popular suggestion that Δ^9-THC may be a useful medication in managing opioid addiction. However, studies in rodents show that antagonists at the CB1 receptor also may attenuate heroin self-administration or heroin relapse-related behaviors (Fattore, Spano, Cossu, Deiana, & Fratta, 2003; He et al., 2019). The similar effects of agonist and antagonist ligands on heroin self-administration are difficult to reconcile as CB receptor-mediated selective actions on heroin self-administration, and necessarily dampen enthusiasm for the development of either CB1 agonist or antagonist medications for the management of opioid addiction. However, the data are considerably more encouraging when considering other types of substance use disorders. Thus, the CB1 inverse agonist/antagonist rimonabant has been shown to decrease self-administration of either Δ^9-THC or nicotine in monkeys (Schindler et al., 2016; Tanda, Munzar, & Goldberg, 2000), and was under consideration for FDA approval as a pharmacotherapy for nicotine cessation. However, as mentioned above, the emergence of clinical data showing significant adverse effects of rimonabant led to its withdrawal from the market as a weight-loss medication and, for the foreseeable future, precludes its application for addiction disorders. More recently, a neutral antagonist at the CB1 receptor, AM4113, also has been shown to attenuate self-administration and reinstatement of nicotine and THC maintained responding in nonhuman primates. Suggesting behavioral selectivity, these effects on drug-maintained responding were obtained in the absence of disruptive effects on food-maintained behavior (Schindler et al., 2016). These findings and similarly positive results in other studies in rodents raise the possibility that neutral antagonists may not produce the adverse effects associated with rimonabant and, consequently, may be better suited as candidate medications for drug abuse. These are enticing data; however, considerably more research is needed to definitively show that the difference between neutral antagonism by drugs like AM4113 and inverse agonism/antagonism by rimonabant can be translated into a significant reduction in side-effect liability.

4.4 Dopamine

Drug abuse has largely, and historically, been associated with modulation of dopamine in striatal brain regions (Volkow et al., 2017). Psychomotor stimulants like methamphetamine and cocaine act directly on dopamine neurons, either through blockade of the DA transporter (DAT) and/or the promotion of vesicular DA release (Nickell, Siripurapu, Vartak, Crooks, & Dwoskin, 2014; Rothman & Baumann, 2003). Other drugs may modulate dopamine activity indirectly through their own receptor-mediated actions. For example, nicotine has been shown to stimulate dopamine (DA) release by directly activating cholinergic receptors on presynaptic nerve terminals, providing input to postsynaptic dopaminergic neurons (Koranda et al., 2014; Leino, Koski, Rannanpää, & Salminen, 2018; Salminen et al., 2004). Similarly, opioids and cannabinoids influence DA release through the activation of, respectively, opioid or cannabinoid receptor-mediated mechanisms (Bloomfield, Ashok, Volkow, & Howes, 2016; Steidl, Wasserman, Blaha, & Yoemans, 2017).

Due to the established connections between drug abuse and DA, non-selective antagonists as well as ligands that selectively block either the D1-family or D2-family subtype of DA receptor, have been examined as candidate medications for the management of substance use disorders. For example, early studies with the nonselective DA receptor antagonist chlorpromazine showed that it could alleviate symptoms of opiate withdrawal in humans (Friedgood & Ripstein, 1955) and, in separate research, decrease self-administration of cocaine in nonhuman primates (Hoffmeister & Goldberg, 1973). However, the debilitating side-effects associated with chlorpromazine or other antipsychotic medications markedly reduced enthusiasm for this type of medicinal use and, after the failure of the D1-selective antagonist ecopipam in human subjects (Astrup et al., 2007), the development of either D1-family or D2-family dopamine antagonists as pharmacotherapy for substance use disorders was relatively dormant. More recently, however, interest in the exploration of dopamine antagonists for the management of substance use disorders has re-emerged, and selective dopamine D3 and D4 receptor blockers have been forwarded for the development of medications for the management of substance use disorders (for review, see Bergman & Rheingold, 2015; Heidbreder & Newman, 2010). In this regard, the D3 antagonist PG01037 has been shown to attenuate the abuse-related effects of cocaine in nonhuman primates (John, Newman, & Nader, 2015), whereas several D3 antagonists have been shown to decrease the reinforcing/rewarding effects of methamphetamine (Chen, Song, Yang, Wu, & Li, 2014), ethanol (Rice, Schonhar, Gaál, Gardner, & Ashby, 2015), and opioids (Boateng et al., 2015; Galaj, Manuszak, Babic, Anantham, & Ranaldi, 2015; You et al., 2017). Importantly, D3 antagonists also have been shown to reduce reward impulsivity in humans (Weber et al., 2016) and to restore deficits in reward processing in drug addicted individuals (Murphy et al., 2017). Recent findings like these have rekindled interest in the development of novel dopamine receptor blockers as candidate medications for substance use disorders. However, despite such encouraging early data, it remains to be determined whether D3 or D4 selectivity confers significant clinical efficacy in the absence of the marked side effect liability that precluded the development of earlier D1- and D2 subtype-selective dopamine antagonists.

DA agonist approaches also have been explored for the development of candidate medications. Inasmuch as the primary mechanism of action of canonical psychomotor stimulants is either blockade of DAT (e.g., cocaine; Ritz, Lamb, Goldberg, & Kuhar, 1988) or the reversal of transport (e.g., methamphetamine; Nickell et al., 2014) leading to increased levels of synaptic DA, it may appear counterintuitive to suggest DA agonists or DAT ligands as potential therapeutics. In this regard, D1-selective ligands, especially partial agonists, previously have been forwarded as candidate medications (with some promising results) but, due to a range of concerns including safety issues, have been largely abandoned. Similarly, D2-selective ligands have been evaluated in nonhuman and human subjects but have yielded only disappointing results (Kohut & Bergman, 2017). On the other hand, a substantive literature does support the viability of DAT ligands as candidate medications for the treatment of psychomotor stimulant abuse (for review, see Stoops & Rush, 2013). In particular, DA releasers appear to be more effective in limiting the abuse of DAT blockers, whereas DAT blockers are thought to be more effective in reducing the abuse-related effects of DA releasers (Stoops & Rush, 2013). For example, in amphetamine-dependent individuals, a 20-week treatment with the DAT blocker methylphenidate decreased positive amphetamine urine samples by 54% (Tihonen et al., 2007), whereas clinical trials of the DA releaser dextroamphetamine produced a highly significant decrease in the number of cocaine-positive urine samples (Grabowski et al., 2001). Thus, there does seem to be a rational basis for the further development of DAT ligands, especially if their own abuse potential can be limited, either pharmacologically or through formulation. In the absence of such developments to reduce abuse potential, the acceptance of novel DAT ligands by the FDA as candidate medications for substance use disorders remains doubtful.

Based upon research data that has accumulated over the past several decades, it is unsurprising that patterns of DA receptor mediated activation of striatal brain regions overlap in response to food and drug cues (Tomasi et al., 2015; Volkow, Wan, Fowler, Tomasi, & Baler, 2012). Additionally, a great deal of evidence supports the involvement of DA mechanisms in these regions in maladaptive feeding behavior. For example, studies in rats have shown that, after the development of obesity, striatal DAT function is blunted (Narayanaswami, Thompson, Cassis, Bardo, & Dwoskin, 2013). Other studies in rodents discussed above have shown that leptin signaling on DA neurons can modulate food-associated reward processes and, by extension, support the hypothesis that DA systems involved in regulation of food consumption may be viable targets for the management of overeating and obesity (Evans & Anderson, 2017). Indeed, amphetamine and amphetamine-like drugs (e.g., phentermine), alone or in combination with other drugs, can serve as effective appetite suppressants (Alfaris, Minnick, Hopkins, Berkowitz, & Wadden, 2015; Freed & Mizel, 1952; Jeffers & Benotsch, 2014; Smith, Meyer, & Trinkley, 2013).

While the DA system can clearly modulate food reward and intake, the development of dopaminergic agonists for the management of obesity and overeating also is complicated by their abuse potential (Volkow et al., 2017). On the other hand, as discussed above with regard to drug use disorders, D3 antagonists also are currently being investigated as candidate medications for food-related disorders. For example, the D3 antagonists SB-277011A and NGB-2904 both have been shown to decrease operant responding for palatable foods in rats (Thanos et al., 2008); however, the effects of D3 antagonists in human populations has been mixed. For example, two imaging studies have been conducted to identify changes in brain activity to food-cues. In one study, the D3 antagonist GSK598809 attenuated neural responses to a food-cue (Mogg et al., 2012) whereas, in the second study, the antagonist had no effect (Dodds et al., 2012). In the absence of additional data that reveal consistent findings, it seems premature to endorse the further development of D3 antagonists as weight-loss pharmacotherapy.

4.5 Serotonin

Several lines of research have delineated the important role of serotonin (5-HT) in feeding behavior. For example, early in vivo microdialysis experiments in rats showed convincingly that 5-HT release in paraventricular and hypothalamic regions can inhibit free-feeding behavior (Hoebel, Hernandez, Schwartz, Mark, & Hunter, 1989). This line of research led to the introduction of the 5-HT releasing agent fenfluramine as an anti-obesity agent, either as a monotherapy or in combination with phentermine (Fen-Phen) (Capriotti, 1998; Pinder, Brogden, Sawyer, Speight, & Avery, 1975). Later investigation of its association with valvular heart disease resulting from 5-HT2B receptor activation revealed an important boundary condition–limited 5-HT2B activity—for the further development of serotonergic pharmacotherapeutics (Elangbam et al., 2008; Rothman & Baumann, 2009; Smith, Waggoner, de las Fuentes, & Davilla-Roman, 2009; Wadden et al., 1998).

In investigations to identify the potential role of distinct 5-HT receptor subtypes in feeding behavior, a drug that directly activates the 2C subtype of 5-HT receptors, Ro 60-0175, was shown to induce hypophagia in rats (Clifton, Lee, & Dourish, 2000). This finding led to the search for selective 5-HT2C ligands for the treatment of obesity and, eventually, to clinical studies showing that the moderately selective 5-HT2C/5-HT2A agonist lorcaserin, which does not have important 5-HT2B activity, could significantly decrease body weight in obese individuals (Aronne et al., 2014; Martin et al., 2011; Smith, Schmidt, Iordanou, & Mustroph, 2008). Importantly, Phase 3 clinical studies with lorcaserin treatment revealed no increase in rates of valvular heart disease compared to a placebo-controlled cohort, further confirming its 5HT2C/2A selectivity (Weissman et al., 2013). These efforts culminated in the approval of lorcaserin, Belviq, as a weight-loss medication by the FDA in 2012. Based on the success of this drug development program, serotonergic systems continue to be actively explored as targets for candidate medications to limit the excessive consummatory behavior that characterizes obesity.

Two areas of research deserve mention regarding the development of serotonin-based candidate medications for substance use disorders, in particular. First, different approaches have been used to increase serotonergic activity. For example, preclinical studies with serotonin-selective reuptake inhibitors (SSRIs) have shown that increases in serotonergic activity can attenuate the rewarding or reinforcing effects of psychomotor stimulants such as amphetamine (Yu, Smith, Smith, & Lyness, 1986) and cocaine (Howell & Byrd, 1995; Kleven & Woolverton, 1993). However, effective doses of SSRIs tend to be relatively high, which leads to undesirable nonspecific behavioral effects that limit the clinical value of this approach. Moreover, beyond a general increase in serotonin levels in suspected target regions, the mechanism that directly mediate reductions in the effects of cocaine or amphetamine after treatment with an SSRI are not well-understood. In another tactic that is based on increasing serotonergic activity, 5-HT releasers have been examined for their ability to modulate the reinforcing effects of psychomotor stimulant drugs. Studies with mixed-action amphetamine analogs that increase synaptic levels of both dopamine and serotonin in rats and monkeys show that increasing 5-HT activity can be inversely correlated with rates of amphetamine or cocaine self-administration (Negus, Mello, Blough, Baumann, & Rothman, 2007; Wee et al., 2005). It is presently unclear whether these results reflect aversive consequences of increased 5-HT release or neurochemical modulation of the rewarding properties that result from increased DA release. Regardless, this line of investigation has generated interesting data but, thus far, has not revealed candidates with a balance of DA and 5-HT activity that can be translated into the management of psychomotor stimulant abuse in a clinical setting.

A second area of serotonin-based drug development research toward medications for substance use disorders is based on the above-discussed capacity of 5-HT2C activation to attenuate food-intake. This earlier work has led to the hypothesis that 5-HT2C agonists (e.g., lorcaserin) might be similarly useful for the management of substance use disorders (for review, see Collins, Gerak, & France, 2018). Indeed, preclinical studies have shown that lorcaserin decreases self-administration of cocaine (Collins, Gerak, Javors, & France, 2016), nicotine (Jacobs, Barkin, Kohut, Bergman, & Kohut, 2017), and heroin (Kohut & Bergman, 2018) in nonhuman primates. Although the generality of lorcaserin's effects across drug classes in these preclinical studies is striking, there is limited information thus far on lorcaserin's effectiveness in human studies. One study in human subjects has reported that, while the positive subjective effects of cocaine were not decreased and perhaps even increased, treatment with lorcaserin delayed self-administration of cocaine and attenuated cocaine "craving," (Pirtle et al., 2019). In another study investigating a mixture of varenicline and lorcaserin as a smoking cessation treatment, lorcaserin was shown to limit weight gain in abstinent smokers but its effectiveness in promoting smoking cessation was unclear (Hurt et al., 2017). Overall, notwithstanding highly consistent preclinical data and some—but not all—promising early clinical results, it remains to be determined whether lorcaserin will be a candidate medication with application across several different types of substance abuse disorders.

4.6 Summary

Overall, it seems clear that the neurobiological overlap between brain reward and satiety systems invites the continued investigation of CNS targets in medication developments for food- and drug-disorders, and that successful medications may find application in the management of both categories of substance use disorder. As a caveat, the pharmacological strategies highlighted in these pages provide a range of research approaches to the development of candidate medications that, while of current interest, is necessarily incomplete. For example, although not discussed here, the modulation of norepinephrine activity with receptor subtype-selective agonists and antagonists previously has been widely researched as a means to block drug-intake and to suppress appetite (Wellman, 2000). Depending on the further development of novel ligands, strong interest in exploiting this system may re-emerge. Other potential CNS targets that deserve mention include neuropeptide Y (Gonçalves, Martins, Baptista, Ambrósio, & Silva, 2016; Parker, Van Heek, & Stamford, 2002) and glutamatergic NMDA receptors (Ezquerra-Romano, Lawn, Krupitsky, & Morgan, 2018). In particular, glutamate activity in specified target regions of the brain has been implicated as a key regulator in drug- and food-motivated behavior (Baptista, Martin-Fardon, & Weiss, 2004; Chaskiel, Paul, Gerstberger, Hübschle, & Konsman, 2016; Cowen, Krstew, & Lawrence, 2007; Eiler, Baez, Yu, & Witkin, 2011; Kalivas, 2009). For this reason, the complex glutamatergic system will continue to present attractive targets for the development of novel candidate medications.

5. Non-pharmacological approaches to the management of substance use disorders

Current thinking suggests that medication approaches for the treatment of addictive behaviors is likely to be most effective when included in comprehensive treatment plans including behavioral therapies (Dakwar & Nunes, 2016; NIDA, 2009). The core tenet of current behavioral approaches is to motivate patients to participate in treatment programs that offer both training of new behavioral repertoires and resources for dealing with cravings, triggers for relapse, and other issues that inevitably challenge abstinence. A number of behavioral therapies including contingency management, cognitive-behavioral therapy, social or peer support programs (e.g., 12-step), and motivational interviewing have demonstrated efficacy in managing addiction disorders involving drugs or food (Dakwar & Nunes, 2016; Dimitrijevic et al., 2015; Hilbert et al., 2012). From this perspective, the role of pharmacotherapy can be viewed as a means of enhancing the efficacy and success rates of such behavioral therapies (Carroll & Onken, 2005).

As a final note, exercise or physical activity has gained favor as another type of behavioral treatment for the treatment of substance use disorders (Lynch, Peterson, Sanchez, Abel, & Smith, 2013). In this regard, exercise has been a recognized effective intervention for addressing obesity for decades (Jakicic & Otto, 2006). A limited number of preclinical and clinical studies provide support for this approach to the treatment of drug addiction (Smith & Lynch, 2011). For example, self-administration studies in rats show that subjects provided access to a running wheel may lower their intake of cocaine (Cosgrove, Hunter, & Carroll, 2002; Smith, Schmidt, et al., 2008) whereas, in methamphetamine users, preliminary evidence indicates that exercise as part of a post-residential treatment care plan may prolong abstinence (Rawson et al., 2015). Clearly, a great deal of work is needed to identify the particular types of conditions under which exercise may be effective (e.g., class of drugs, stage of addiction process, type of exercise, etc.; see Lynch et al., 2013). Nevertheless, the initial foray into this avenue of research appear to be promising and indicate the overall importance of creative approaches to the identification of novel medication strategies for substance-use disorders.

6. Conclusion

Compelling evidence supports the view that mechanisms of food- and drug-based addiction disorders overlap and, on this basis, pharmacotherapeutics that target these mechanisms have been developed as candidate medications. A range of pharmacological systems that mediate gut and/or brain function have shown promise as potential therapeutic interventions for such addiction disorders. It has become increasingly apparent that other compulsive/consummatory behavioral disorders (e.g., gambling, internet addiction, sex addiction) also engage the mechanisms that mediate food- and drug-based addiction. It is reasonable to imagine, then, that pharmacological approaches discussed above also may prove useful in the development of medications for the management of such other behavioral disorders. This perspective already has begun to guide research. For example, dopamine D3 receptor mechanisms which, as discussed earlier, have been suggested to mediate the reinforcing effects of psychomotor stimulant drugs also have been implicated in pathological gambling (Bou Khalil, 2013). The identification of such common mechanisms in different addiction disorders is a critical step toward the discovery of effective solutions to these continuing public health challenges.

Acknowledgment

The preparation of this chapter was supported by DA002519, DA035857 (Bergman, PI), and KO1DA039306 (Kohut, PI).

Conflict of interest statement

The authors have no conflicts of interest to declare.

References

Abizaid, A., Liu, Z. W., Andrews, Z. B., Shanabrough, M., Borok, E., Elsworth, J. D., et al. (2006). Ghrelin modulates the activity and synaptic input organization of midbrain dopamine neurons while promoting appetite. *The Journal of Clinical Investigation, 116*, 3229–3239.

Aja, S., Sahandy, S., Ladenheim, E. E., Schwartz, G. J., & Moran, T. H. (2001). Introcerebroventricular CART peptide reduces food intake and alters motor behavior at a hindbrain site. *American Journal of Physiology Regulatory, Integrative and Comparative Physiology, 281*, R1862–R1867.

Alfaris, N., Minnick, A. M., Hopkins, C. M., Berkowitz, R. I., & Wadden, T. A. (2015). Combination phentermine and topiramate extended release in the management of obesity. *Expert Opinion on Pharmacotherapy, 16*, 1623–1674.

Alhadeff, A. L., Rupprecht, L. E., & Hayes, M. R. (2012). GLP-1 neurons in the nucleus of the solitary tract project directly to the ventral tegmental area and nucleus accumbens to control for food intake. *Endocrinology, 153*, 647–658.

Anker, J. J., Gliddon, L. A., & Carroll, M. E. (2008). Impulsivity on a go/no-go task for intravenous cocaine or food in male and female rats selectively bred for high and low saccharin intake. *Behavioural Pharmacology, 19*, 615–619.

Arnone, M., Maruani, J., Chaperon, F., Thiébot, M. H., Poncelet, M., Soubrié, P., et al. (1997). Selective inhibition of sucrose and ethanol intake by SR 141716, and antagonist of central cannabinoid (CB1) receptors. *Psychopharmacology, 132*, 104–106.

Aronne, L., Shanahan, W., Fain, R., Glicklich, A., Soliman, W., Li, Y., et al. (2014). Safety and efficacy of lorcaserin: A combined analysis of the BLOOM and BLOSSOM trials. *Postgraduate Medicine, 126*, 7–18.

Astrup, A., Greenway, F. L., Ling, W., Pedicone, L., Lachowicz, J., Strader, C. D., et al. (2007). Randomized controlled trials of the D1/D5 antagonist ecopipam for weight loss in obese subjects. *Obesity, 15*, 1717–1731.

Atkinson, R. L., Berke, L. K., Drake, C. R., Bibbs, M. L., Williams, F. L., & Kaiser, D. L. (1985). Effects of long-term therapy with naltrexone on body weight in obesity. *Clinical Pharmacology and Therapeutics, 38*, 419–422.

Aubin, H. J., Farley, A., Lycett, D., Lahmek, P., & Aveyard, P. (2012). Weight gain in smokers after quitting cigarettes: Meta-analysis. *British Medical Journal, 345*, e4439.

Avena, N. M., & Rada, P. V. (2012). Cholinergic modulation of food and drug satiety and withdrawal. *Physiology & Behavior, 106*, 332–336.

Babcock, A. M., Livosky, M., & Avery, D. D. (1985). Cholecystokinin and bombesin suppress operant responding for food reward. *Pharmacology, Biochemistry, and Behavior, 22*, 893–895.

Badowski, M. E. (2017). A review of oral cannabinoids and medical marijuana for the treatment of chemotherapy-induced nausea and vomiting: A focus on pharmacokinetic variability and pharmacodynamics. *Cancer Chemotherapy and Pharmacology, 80*, 441–449.

Baggio, L. L., & Drucker, D. J. (2007). Biology of incretins: GLP-1 and GIP. *Gastroenterology, 132*, 2131–2157.

Baptista, M. A., Martin-Fardon, R., & Weiss, F. (2004). Preferential effects of the metabotropic glutamate 2/3 receptor agonist LY379268 on conditioned reinstatement versus primary reinforcement: comparison between cocaine and a potent conventional reinforcer. *The Journal of Neuroscience, 24*, 4723–4727.

Barry, C. L., McGinty, E. E., Pescosolido, B. A., & Goldman, H. H. (2014). Stigma, discrimination, treatment effectiveness, and policy: Public views about drug addiction and mental illness. *Psychiatric Services*, *65*, 1269–1272.

Beinfeld, M. C., Connolly, K. J., & Pierce, R. C. (2002). Cocaine treatment increases extracellular cholecystokinin (CCK) in the nucleus accumbens shell of awake, freely moving rats, an effect that is enhanced in rats that are behaviorally sensitized to cocaine. *Journal of Neurochemistry*, *81*, 1021–1027.

Bergman, J. (2008). Medications for stimulant abuse: Agonist-based strategies and preclinical evaluation of the mixed-action D_2 partial agonist aripiprazole (abilify). *Experimental and Clinical Psychopharmacology*, *16*, 475–483.

Bergman, J., & Rheingold, C. G. (2015). Dopamine D_4 receptor antagonists for the treatment of cocaine use disorders. *CNS & Neurological Disorders Drug Targets*, *14*, 707–715.

Berlanga, M. L., Olsen, C. M., Chen, V., Ikegami, A., Herring, B. E., Duvauchelle, C. L., et al. (2003). Cholinergic interneurons of the nucleus accumbens and dorsal striatum are activated by the self-administration of cocaine. *Neuroscience*, *120*, 1149–1156.

Bharne, A. P., Borkar, C. D., Subhedar, N. K., & Kokare, D. M. (2015). Differential expression of CART in feeding and reward circuits in binge eating rat model. *Behavioural Brain Research*, *291*, 219–231.

Bhat, S. P., & Sharm, A. (2017). Current drug targets in obesity pharmacotherapy—A review. *Current Drug Targets*, *18*, 983–993.

Bloomfield, M. A., Ashok, A. H., Volkow, N. D., & Howes, O. D. (2016). The effects of Δ^9-tetrahydrocannabinol on the dopamine system. *Nature*, *539*, 369–377.

Boateng, C. A., Bakare, O. M., Zhan, J., Banala, A. K., Burzynski, C., Pommier, E., et al. (2015). High affinity dopamine D3 receptor (D3R)-selective antagonists attenuate heroin self-administration in wild-type but not D3R knockout mice. *Journal of Medicinal Chemistry*, *58*, 6195–6213.

Bodner, R. J., & Klein, G. E. (2004). Endogenous opiates and behavior: 2003. *Peptides*, *25*, 2205–2256.

Bou Khalil, R. (2013). Dopamine D3 receptor antagonists in pathologic gambling. *Journal of Clinical Psychopharmacology*, *33*, 146–148.

Bradberry, C. W., Barrett-Larimore, R. L., Jatlow, P., & Rubino, S. R. (2000). Impact of self-administered cocaine and cocaine cues on extracellular dopamine in mesolimbic and sensorimotor striatum in rhesus monkeys. *The Journal of Neuroscience*, *20*, 3874–3883.

Broberger, C., Holmberg, K., Kuhar, M. J., & Hökfelt, T. (1999). Cocaine- and amphetamine-regulated transcript in the rat vagus nerve: A putative mediator of cholecystokinin-induced satiety. *Proceedings of the National Academy of Sciences of the United States of America*, *96*, 13506–13511.

Brown, J. E., Kassouny, M., & Cross, J. K. (1977). Kinetic studies of food intake and sucrose solution preference in rats treated with low doses of delta9-tetrahydrocannabinol. *Behavioral Biology*, *20*, 104–110.

Brown, R. M., Kupchik, Y. M., & Kalivas, P. W. (2013). The story of glutamate in drug addiction and of N-acetylcysteine as a potential pharmacotherapy. *JAMA Psychiatry*, *70*, 895–897.

Buka, S. L., Shenassa, E. D., & Niaura, R. (2003). Elevated risk of tobacco dependence among offspring of mothers who smoked during pregnancy: A 30-year prospective study. *The American Journal of Psychiatry*, *160*, 1978–1984.

Cameron, K. O., Bhattacharya, S. K., & Loomis, A. K. (2014). Small molecule ghrelin receptor inverse agonists and antagonists. *Journal of Medicinal Chemistry*, *57*, 8671–8691.

Capriotti, T. (1998). In search of a "magic" pill to treat obesity: The rise and fall of "fen-phen". *Medsurg Nursing*, *7*, 52–54.

Carmen, B., Angeles, M., Munos, A., & Amate, J. M. (2004). Efficacy and safety of naltrexone and acamprosate in the treatment of alcohol dependence: A systematic review. *Addiction*, *99*, 811–828.

Carr, K. D. (1990). Effects of antibodies to dynorphin A and beta-endorphin on lateral hypothalamic self-stimulation in ad libitum fed and food-deprived rats. *Brain Research*, *534*, 8–14.

Carr, K. D. (2007). Chronic food restriction: Enhancing effects on drug reward and striatal cell signaling. *Physiology & Behavior*, *91*, 459–572.

Carrol, M. E., & Lac, S. T. (1993). Autoshaping i.v. cocaine self-administration in rats: Effects of nondrug alternative reinforcers on acquisition. *Psychopharmacology*, *110*, 5–12.

Carroll, M. E. (1998). Interactions between food and addiction. In *Drugs of abuse and addiction* (pp. 300–325). CRC Press.

Carroll, M. E., France, C. P., & Meisch, R. A. (1979). Food deprivation increases oral and intravenous drug intake in rats. *Science*, *205*, 319–321.

Carroll, K. M., & Onken, L. S. (2005). Behavioral therapies for drug abuse. *The American Journal of Psychiatry*, *162*, 1451–1460.

Chaskiel, L., Paul, F., Gerstberger, R., Hübschle, T., & Konsman, J. P. (2016). Brainstem metabotropic glutamate receptors reduce food intake and activate dorsal pontine and medullar structures after peripheral bacterial lipopolysaccharide administration. *Neuropharmacology*, *107*, 146–159.

Chen, Y., Song, R., Yang, R. F., Wu, N., & Li, J. (2014). A novel dopamine D3 receptor antagonist YQA14 inhibits methamphetamine self-administration and relapse to drug-seeking behaviour in rats. *European Journal of Pharmacology*, *743*, 126–132.

Christensen, R., Kristensen, P. K., Bartels, E. M., Bliddal, H., & Astrup, A. (2007). Efficacy and safety of the weight-loss drug rimonabant: A meta-analysis of randomized trials. *Lancet*, *370*, 1706–1713.

Clapper, J. R., Athanacio, J., Wittmer, C., Griffin, P. S., D'Souza, L., Parkes, D. G., et al. (2013). Effects of amylin and bupropion/naltrexone on food intake and body weight are interactive in rodent models. *European Journal of Pharmacology*, *698*, 292–298.

Clifton, P. G., Lee, M. D., & Dourish, C. T. (2000). Similarities in the action of Ro 60-0175, a 5-HT2C receptor antagonist and d-fenfluramine on feeding patterns in the rat. *Psychopharmacology*, *152*, 256–267.

Coffin, V. L., Latranyi, M. B., & Chipkin, R. E. (1989). Acute extrapyramidal syndrome in cebus monkeys: Development mediated by dopamine D_2 but not D_1 receptors. *The Journal of Pharmacology and Experimental Therapeutics*, *249*, 769–774.

Collins, G. T., Gerak, L. R., & France, C. P. (2018). The behavioral pharmacology and therapeutic potential of lorcaserin for substance use disorders. *Neuropharmacology*, *142*, 63–71.

Collins, G. T., Gerak, L. R., Javors, M. A., & France, C. P. (2016). Lorcaserin reduces the discriminative stimulus and reinforcing effects of cocaine in rhesus monkeys. *The Journal of Pharmacology and Experimental Therapeutics*, *356*, 85–95.

Colombo, G., Agabio, R., Diaz, G., Lobina, C., Reali, R., & Gessa, G. L. (1998). Appetite suppression and weight loss after the cannabinoid antagonist SR 141716. *Life Sciences*, *63*, PL113–PL114.

Conover, K. L., & Shizgal, P. (1994). Competition and summation between regarding effects of sucrose and lateral hypothalamic stimulation in the rat. *Behavioral Neuroscience*, *108*, 537–548.

Cosgrove, K. P., Hunter, R. G., & Carroll, M. E. (2002). Wheel-running attenuates intravenous cocaine self-administration in rats sex differences. *Pharmacology, Biochemistry, and Behavior*, *73*, 663–671.

Cowen, M. S., Krstew, E., & Lawrence, A. J. (2007). Assessing appetitive and consummatory phases of ethanol self-administration in C57BL/6J mice under operant conditions: Regulation by mGlu5 receptor antagonism. *Psychopharmacology*, *190*, 21–29.

Dagher, A. (2009). The neurobiology of appetite: Hunger as addiction. *International Journal of Obesity, 33*, S30–S33.

Dakwar, E., & Nunes, E. V. (2016). New directions in medication-facilitated behavioral treatment for substance use disorders. *Current Psychiatry Reports, 18*, 64.

Daniels, A. M., Salisbury-Afshar, E., Hoffberg, A., Agus, D., & Fingerhood, M. I. (2014). A novel community-based buprenorphine program: Client description and initial outcomes. *Journal of Addiction Medicine, 8*, 40–46.

Daws, L. C., Avison, M. J., Robertson, S. D., Niswender, K. D., Galli, A., & Saunders, C. (2011). Insulin signaling and addiction. *Neuropharmacology, 61*, 1123–1128.

de la Garza, R., & Johanson, C. E. (1987). The effects of food deprivation on the self-administration of psychoactive drugs. *Drug and Alcohol Dependence, 19*, 17–27.

de Lartigue, G., Dimaline, R., Varro, A., & Dockray, G. J. (2007). Cocaine- and amphetamine-regulated transcript: Stimulation of expression in rat vagal afferent neurons by cholecystokinin and suppressed by ghrelin. *The Journal of Neuroscience, 27*, 2876–2882.

De Tomasi, E. B., & Juárez, J. (2011). Differential effects of chronic naltrexone treatment on food intake patterns and body weight in rats depend on their food deprivation status. *European Journal of Pharmacology, 650*, 261–267.

DePierre, J. A., Puhl, R. M., & Luedicke, J. (2013). A new stigmatized identity? Comparisons of a "food addict" label with other stigmatized health conditions. *Basic and Applied Social Psychology, 35*, 10–21.

Di Chiara, G., Bassareo, V., Fenu, S., De Luca, M. A., Spina, L., Cadoni, C., et al. (2004). Dopamine and drug addiction: The nucleus accumbens shell connection. *Neuropharmacology, 47*, 227–241.

Di Chiara, G., & Imperato, A. (1988). Drugs abused by humans preferentially increase synaptic dopamine concentrations in the mesolimbic system of freely moving rats. *Proceedings of the National Academy of Sciences of the United States of America, 85*, 5274–5278.

DiLeone, R. J., Taylor, J. R., & Picciotto, M. R. (2012). The drive to eat: Comparisons and distinctions between mechanisms of food reward and drug addiction. *Nature Neuroscience, 15*, 1330–1335.

Dimitrijevic, I., Popovic, N., Sabljak, V., Skodric-Trifunovic, V., & Dimitrijevic, N. (2015). Food addiction-diagnosis and treatment. *Psychiatria Danubina, 27*, 101–106.

Dodds, C. M., O'Neill, B., Beaver, J., Makwana, A., Bani, M., Merlo-Pich, E., et al. (2012). Effect of the dopamine D3 receptor antagonist GSK598809 on brain responses to rewarding food images in overweight and obese binge eaters. *Appetite, 59*, 27–33.

Dossat, A. M., Lilly, N., Kay, K., & Williams, D. L. (2011). Glucagon-like peptide 1 receptors in nucleus accumbens affect food intake. *The Journal of Neuroscience, 31*, 144543–144547.

Drevets, W. C., Price, J. C., Kupfer, D. J., Kinahan, P. E., Lopresti, B., Holt, D., et al. (1999). PET measures of amphetamine-induced dopamine release in ventral versus dorsal striatum. *Neuropsychopharmacology, 21*, 694–709.

Ebbert, J. O., Hughes, J. R., West, R. J., Rennard, S. I., Russ, C., McRae, T. D., et al. (2015). Effect of varenicline on smoking cessation through smoking reduction: A randomized clinical trial. *JAMA, 313*, 687–694.

Egecioglu, E., Jerlhag, E., Salomé, N., Skibicka, K. P., Haage, D., Bohlooly-Y, M., et al. (2010). Ghrelin increases intake of rewarding food in rodents. *Addiction Biology, 15*, 304–311.

Eiler, W. J., 2nd, Baez, M., Yu, J., & Witkin, J. M. (2011). mGlu5 receptor deletion reduces relapse to food-seeking and prevents the anti-relapse effects of mGlu5 receptor blockade in mice. *Life Sciences, 89*, 862–867.

Elangbam, C. S., Job, L. E., Zadrozny, L. M., Barton, J. C., Yoon, L. W., Gates, L. D., et al. (2008). 5-Hydroxytryptamine (5HT)-induced valvulopathy: Compositional valvular alterations are associated with 5HT2B receptor and 5HT transporter transcript changes in Sprague-Dawley rats. *Experimental and Toxicologic Pathology, 60*, 253–262.

Elkashef, A., Brašić, J. R., Cantelina, L. R., Jr., Kahn, R., Chiang, N., Ye, W., et al. (2018). A cholecystokinin B receptor antagonist and cocaine interaction, phase I study. *CNS Neuroscience & Therapeutics, 25*, 136–146.

Elmquist, J. K., Elias, C. F., & Saper, C. B. (1999). From lesions to leptin: Hypothalamic control of food intake and body weight. *Neuron, 22*, 221–232.

Escobar, M., Scherer, J. N., Ornell, F., Bristot, G., Soares, C. M., Guimarães, L. S. P., et al. (2018). Leptin levels and its correlation with crack-cocaine use severity: A preliminary study. *Neuroscience Letters, 671*, 56–59.

Evans, M. C., & Anderson, G. M. (2017). Dopamine neuron-restricted leptin receptor signaling reduces some aspects of food reward but exacerbates the obesity of leptin receptor-deficient male mice. *Endocrinology, 158*, 4246–4256.

Ezquerra-Romano, I. I., Lawn, W., Krupitsky, E., & Morgan, C. J. A. (2018). Ketamine for the treatment of addiction: Evidence and potential mechanisms. *Neuropharmacology, 142*, 72–82.

Fattore, L., Spano, M. S., Cossu, G., Deiana, S., & Fratta, W. (2003). Cannabinoid mechanism in reinstatement of heroin-seeking after a long period of abstinence in rats. *The European Journal of Neuroscience, 17*, 1723–1726.

FDA, Food and Drug Administration, NDA 200063, 2014, 1–5, https://www.accessdata.fda.gov/drugsatfda_docs/appletter/2014/200063Orig1s000ltr.pdf.

Fortin, S. M., & Roitman, M. F. (2017). Central GLP-1 receptor activation modulates cocaine-evoked phasic dopamine signaling in the nucleus accumbens core. *Physiology & Behavior, 176*, 17–25.

Frata, W. (1996). *RPR 102681: Effect on intravenous cocaine self-administration in drug-experienced rats*. Basel, Switzerland: RPR Pharma, Inc. Report 96-007.

Freed, S. C., & Mizel, M. (1952). The use of amphetamine combinations for appetite suppression. *Annals of Internal Medicine, 36*, 1492–1497.

Friedgood, C. E., & Ripstein, C. B. (1955). Use of chlorpromazine in the withdrawal of addicting drugs; preliminary report. *The New England Journal of Medicine, 252*, 230–233.

Galaj, E., Manuszak, M., Babic, S., Anantham, S., & Ranaldi, R. (2015). The selective dopamine D3 antagonist, SR 21502, reduces cue-induced reinstatement of heroin seeking and heroin conditioned place preference in rats. *Drug and Alcohol Dependence, 156*, 228–233.

Gerlach, J., Lublin, H., & Peacock, L. (1996). Extrapyramidal symptoms during long-term treatment with antipsychotics: Special focus on clozapine and D_1 and D_2 dopamine antagonists. *Neuropsychopharmacology, 14*, S35–S39.

Gluck, M. E. (2006). Stress response and binge eating disorder. *Appetite, 46*, 26–30.

Gluck, M. E., Geliebter, A., & Lorence, M. (2004). Cortisol stress response is positively correlated with central obesity in obese women with binge eating disorder (BED) before and after cognitive-behavioral treatment. *Annals of the New York Academy of Sciences, 1032*, 202–207.

Göke, R., Larsen, P. J., Mikkelsen, J. D., & Sheikh, S. P. (1995). Distribution of GLP-1 binding sites in the rat brain: Evidence that exendin-4 is a ligand of brain GLP-1 binding sites. *The European Journal of Neuroscience*, 7, 2294–2300.

Gonçalves, J., Martins, J., Baptista, S., Ambrósio, A. F., & Silva, A. P. (2016). Effects of drugs of abuse on the central neuropeptide Y system. *Addiction Biology, 21*, 755–765.

Gordon, E. L., Ariel-Donges, A. H., Bauman, V., & Merlo, L. J. (2018). What is the evidence for "food addiction?" A systematic review. *Nutrients, 10*, 477.

Gosnell, B. A., Leving, A. S., & Morley, J. E. (1986). The stimulation of food intake by selective agonists of mu, kappa and delta opioid receptors. *Life Sciences, 38*, 1081–1088.

Grabowski, J., Rhoades, H., Schmitz, J., Stotts, A., Daruzska, L. A., Creson, D., et al. (2001). Dextroamphetamine for cocaine-dependence treatment: A double-blind randomized clinical trial. *Journal of Clinical Psychopharmacology, 21*, 522–526.

Graham, D. L., Erreger, K., Galli, A., & Standwood, G. D. (2013). GLP-1 analog attenuates cocaine reward. *Molecular Psychiatry*, *18*, 961–962.

Grandison, L., & Guidotti, A. (1977). Stimulation of food intake by muscimol and beta endorphin. *Neuropharmacology*, *16*, 533–536.

Grigson, P. S. (2002). Like drugs for chocolate: Separate rewards modulated by common mechanisms? *Physiology & Behavior*, *76*, 389–395.

Grosshans, M., Vollmert, C., Vollstädt-Klein, S., Tost, H., Leber, S., Bach, P., et al. (2012). Association of leptin with food and cue-induced activation in human reward pathways. *Archives of General Psychiatry*, *69*, 529–537.

Gu, G., Roland, B., Tomaselli, K., Dolman, C. S., Lowe, C., & Heilig, J. S. (2013). Glucagon-like peptide-1 in the rat brain: Distribution of expression and functional implication. *The Journal of Comparative Neurology*, *521*, 2235–2261.

Guiducci, L., Iervasi, G., & Quinones-Galvan, A. (2014). On the paradox insulin resistance/insulin hypersensitivity and obesity: Two tales of the same history. *Expert Review of Cardiovascular Therapy*, *12*, 637–642.

Hagan, M. M., Wauford, P. K., Chandler, P. C., Jarrett, L. A., Rybak, R. J., & Blackburn, K. (2002). A new animal model of binge eating: Key synergistic role of past caloric restriction and stress. *Physiology & Behavior*, *77*, 45–54.

Hajnal, A., Smith, G. P., & Norgren, R. (2004). Oral sucrose stimulation increases accumbens dopamine in the rat. *American Journal of Physiology Regulatory, Integrative and Comparative Physiology*, *286*, R31–R37.

Halaas, J. L., Gajiwala, K. S., Maffei, M., Cohen, S. L., Chait, B. T., Rabinowitz, D., et al. (1995). Weight-reducing effects of the plasma protein encoded by the obese gene. *Science*, *267*, 543–546.

Harricharan, R., Abboussi, O., & Daniels, W. M. U. (2017). Addiction: A dysregulation of satiety and inflammatory processes. *Progress in Brain Research*, *235*, 65–91.

He, X. H., Jordan, C. J., Vemuri, K., Bi, G. H., Gardner, E. L., Makriyannis, A., et al. (2019). Cannabinoid CB_1 receptor neutral antagonist AM4113 inhibits heroin self-administration without depressive side effects in rats. *Acta Pharmacologica Sinica*, *40*, 365–373.

Hebebrand, J., Albayrak, O., Adan, R., Antel, J., Dieguez, C., de Jon, J., et al. (2014). "Eating addiction", rather than "food addiction", better captures addictive-like eating behavior. *Neuroscience and Biobehavioral Reviews*, *47*, 295–306.

Heidbreder, C. A., & Newman, A. H. (2010). Current perspectives on selective dopamine D (3) receptor antagonists as pharmacotherapeutics for addictions and related disorders. *Annals of the New York Academy of Sciences*, *1187*, 4–34.

Helstrom, A. W., Blow, F. C., Slaymaker, V., Kranzler, H. R., Leong, S., & Oslin, D. (2016). Reductions in alcohol craving following naltrexone treatment for heavy drinking. *Alcohol and Alcoholism*, *51*, 562–566.

Hernandez, N. S., Ige, K. Y., Mietlicki-Baase, E. G., Molina-Castro, G. C., Turner, C. A., Hayes, M. R., et al. (2018). Glucagon-like peptide-1 receptor activation in the ventral tegmental area attenuates cocaine seeking in rats. *Neuropsychopharmacology*, *43*, 2000–2008.

Higgins, G. A., Joharchi, N., Wang, Y., Corrigall, W. A., & Sellers, E. M. (1994). The CCKA receptor antagonist devazepide does not modify opioid self-administration or drug discrimination: Comparison with the dopamine antagonist haloperidol. *Brain Research*, *640*, 246–254.

Hilbert, A., Bishop, M. E., Stein, R. I., Tanofsky-Kraff, M., Swenson, A. K., Welch, R. R., et al. (2012). Long-term efficacy of psychological treatments for binge eating disorder. *The British Journal of Psychiatry*, *200*, 232–237.

Hoebel, B. G., Hernandez, L., Schwartz, D. H., Mark, G. P., & Hunter, G. A. (1989). Microdialysis studies of brain norepinephrine, serotonin, and dopamine release during ingestive behavior. *Annals of the New York Academy of Sciences*, *575*, 171–191.

Hoffmeister, F., & Goldberg, S. R. (1973). A comparison of chlorpromazine, imipramine, morphine and d-amphetamine self-administration in cocaine-dependent rhesus monkeys. *The Journal of Pharmacology and Experimental Therapeutics*, *187*, 8–14.

Holtzman, S. G. (1974). Behavioral effects of separate and combined administration of naloxone and d-amphetamine. *The Journal of Pharmacology and Experimental Therapeutics*, *189*, 51–60.

Hommel, J. D., Trinko, R., Sears, R. M., Georgescu, D., Gao, X. B., Thurmon, J. J., et al. (2006). Leptin receptor signaling in midbrain dopamine neurons regulates feeding. *Neuron*, *51*, 801–810.

Housová, J., Wilczek, H., Haluzík, M. M., Kremen, J., & Haluzík, M. (2005). Adipocyte-derived hormones in heroin addictions: The influence of methadone maintenance treatment. *Physiological Reviews*, *54*, 73–78.

Howell, L. L., & Byrd, L. D. (1995). Serotonergic modulation of the behavioral effects of cocaine in the squirrel monkey. *The Journal of Pharmacology and Experimental Therapeutics*, *275*, 1551–1559.

Howick, K., Griffin, B. T., Cryan, J. T., & Shellekens, H. (2017). From belly to brain: Targeting the ghrelin receptor in appetite and food intake regulation. *International Journal of Molecular Sciences*, *18*, pii.E273.

Hunter, R. G., & Kuhar, M. J. (2003). CART peptides as targets for CNS drug development. *Current Drug Targets. CNS and Neurological Disorders*, *2*, 201–205.

Hurd, Y. L., Svensson, P., & Pontén, M. (1999). The role of dopamine, dynorphin, and CART systems in the ventral striatum and amygdala in cocaine abuse. *Annals of the New York Academy of Sciences*, *877*, 499–506.

Hurt, R. T., Croghan, I. T., Schroeder, D. R., Hays, J. T., Choi, D. S., & Ebbert, J. O. (2017). Combination varenicline and lorcaserin for tobacco dependence treatment and weight gain prevention in overweight and obese smokers: A pilot study. *Nicotine & Tobacco Research*, *19*, 994–998.

Ida, T., Nakahara, K., Kuroiwa, T., Fukui, K., Nakazato, M., Murakami, T., et al. (2000). Both corticotropin releasing factor and neuropeptide Y are involved in the effect of orexin (hypocretin) on the food intake in rats. *Neuroscience Letters*, *293*, 119–122.

Ifland, J. R., Preuss, H. G., Marcus, M. T., Rourke, K. M., Taylor, W. C., Burau, K., et al. (2009). Refined food addiction: A classic substance use disorder. *Medical Hypotheses*, *72*, 518–526.

Jacobs, D. S., Barkin, C. E., Kohut, M. R., Bergman, J., & Kohut, S. J. (2017). Effects of lorcaserin (Belviq®) on nicotine- and food-maintained responding in non-human primates. *Drug and Alcohol Dependence*, *181*, 94–101.

Jakicic, J. M., & Otto, A. D. (2006). Treatment and prevention of obesity: What is the role of exercise? *Nutrition Reviews*, *64*, S57–S61.

James, M. H., Charnley, J. L., Jones, E., Levi, E. M., Yeoh, J. W., Flynn, J. R., et al. (2010). Cocaine- and amphetamine-regulated transcript (CART) signaling within the paraventricular thalamus modulates cocaine-seeking behaviour. *PLoS One*, *5*, e12980.

Jaworski, J. N., Hansen, S. T., Kuhar, M. J., & Mark, G. P. (2008). Injection of CART (cocaine- and amphetamine-regulated transcript) peptide into the nucleus accumbens reduces cocaine self-administration in rats. *Behavioural Brain Research*, *191*, 266–271.

Jeffers, A. J., & Benotsch, E. G. (2014). Non-medical use of prescription stimulants for weight loss, disordered eating, and body image. *Eating Behaviors*, *15*, 414–418.

Jeong, J. H., Lee, D. K., & Jo, Y. H. (2017). Cholinergic neurons in the dorsomedial hypothalamus regulate food intake. *Molecular Metabolism*, *6*, 306–312.

Jerabek, P., Havlickova, T., Puskina, N., Charalambous, C., Lapka, M., Kacer, P., et al. (2017). Ghrelin receptor antagonism of morphine-induced conditioned place preference and behavioral and accumbens dopaminergic sensitization in rats. *Neurochemistry International*, *110*, 101–113.

Jerlhag, E., Egecioglu, E., Dickson, S. L., & Engel, J. A. (2010). Ghrelin receptor antagonism attenuates cocaine- and amphetamine-induced locomotor stimulation, accumbal dopamine release, and conditioned placed preference. *Psychopharmacology*, *211*, 415–422.

Jerlhag, E., Egecioglu, E., Landgren, S., Salomé, N., Heilig, M., Moechars, D., et al. (2009). Requirement of central ghrelin signaling for alcohol reward. *Proceedings of the National Academy of Sciences of the United States of America*, *106*, 11318–11323.

John, W. S., Newman, A. H., & Nader, M. A. (2015). Differential effects of the dopamine D3 receptor antagonist PG01037 on cocaine and methamphetamine self-administration in rhesus monkeys. *Neuropharmacology*, *92*, 34–43.

Josselyn, S. A., De Cristofaro, A., & Vaccarino, F. J. (1997). Evidence for CCK(A) receptor involvement in the acquisition of conditioned activity produced by cocaine in rats. *Brain Research*, *763*, 93–102.

Josselyn, S. A., & Vaccarino, F. J. (1996). Acquisition of conditioned reward blocked by intra-accumbens infusion of PD-140548, a CCK_A receptor antagonist. *Pharmacology, Biochemistry, and Behavior*, *55*, 439–444.

Kahn, B. B., & Flier, J. S. (2000). Obesity and insulin resistance. *The Journal of Clinical Investigation*, *106*, 473–481.

Kalivas, P. W. (2009). The glutamate homeostasis hypothesis of addiction. *Nature Reviews. Neuroscience*, *10*, 561–572.

Kampov-Polevoy, A., Garbutt, J. C., & Janowsky, D. S. (1999). Association between preference for sweets and excessive alcohol intake: A review of animal and human studies. *Alcohol and Alcoholism*, *34*, 386–395.

Kelley, A. E., Schiltz, C. A., & Lawrence, A. J. (2005). Neural systems recruited by drug- and food-related cues: Studies of gene activation in corticolimbic regions. *Physiology & Behavior*, *86*, 11–14.

King, A. C., Cao, D., O'Malley, S. S., Kranzler, H. R., Cai, X., deWit, H., et al. (2012). Effects of naltrexone on smoking cessation outcomes and weight gain in nicotine-dependent men and women. *Journal of Clinical Psychopharmacology*, *32*, 630–636.

Kleven, M. S., & Woolverton, W. L. (1993). Effects of three monoamine uptake inhibitors on behavior maintained by cocaine or food presentation in rhesus monkeys. *Drug and Alcohol Dependence*, *31*, 149–158.

Knable, M. B., Heinz, A., Raedler, T., & Weinberger, D. R. (1997). Extrapyramidal side effects with risperidone and haloperidol at comparable D2 receptor occupancy levels. *Psychiatry Research*, *75*, 91–101.

Kohut, S. J., & Bergman, J. (2017). Medication strategies for the management of cocaine use disorder. In V. R. Preedy (Ed.), *The neuroscience of cocaine* (pp. 627–637): Academic Press.

Kohut, S. J., & Bergman, J. (2018). Lorcaserin decreases the reinforcing effects of heroin, but not food, in rhesus monkeys. *European Journal of Pharmacology*, *840*, 28–32.

Koranda, J. L., Cone, J. J., McGehee, D. S., Roitman, M. F., Beeler, J. A., & Zhuang, X. (2014). Nicotinic receptors regulate the dynamic range of dopamine release in vivo. *Journal of Neurophysiology*, *111*, 103–111.

Kosten, T. R., & Baxter, L. E. (2019). Effective management of opioid withdrawal symptoms: A gateway to opioid dependence treatment. *The American Journal on Addictions*, *28*, 55–62.

Kristensen, P., Judge, M. E., Thim, L., Ribel, U., Christjansen, K. N., Wulff, B. S., et al. (1998). Hypothalamic CART is a new anorectic peptide regulated by leptin. *Nature*, *393*, 72–76.

Kuhar, M. J., Jaworski, J. N., Hubert, G. W., Philpot, K. B., & Dominguez, G. (2005). Cocaine- and amphetamine-regulated transcript peptides play a role in drug abuse and are potential therapeutic targets. *The AAPS Journal*, 7, E259–E265.

Kumar, V., Bonifazi, A., Ellenberger, M. P., Keck, T. M., Pommier, E., Rais, R., et al. (2016). Highly selective dopamine D3 receptor (D3R) antagonists and partial agonists based on eticlopride and the D3R crystal structure: New leads for opioids dependence treatment. *Journal of Medicinal Chemistry*, *59*, 7634–7650.

Kurbanov, D. B., Currie, P. J., Simonson, D. C., Borsook, D., & Elman, I. (2012). Effects of naltrexone on food intake and body weight gain in olanzapine-treated rats. *Journal of Psychopharmacology*, *26*, 1244–1251.

Lau, J., Farzi, A., Qi, Y., Heilbronn, R., Mietzsch, M., Shi, Y. C., et al. (2018). CART neurons in the arcuate nucleus and lateral hypothalamic area exert differential controls on energy homeostasis. *Molecular Metabolism*, *7*, 102–118.

Lau, J., & Herzog, H. (2014). CART in the regulation of appetite and energy homeostasis. *Frontiers in Neuroscience*, *8*, 1–25.

le Roux, C. W., & Bloom, S. R. (2005). Peptide YY, appetite and food intake. *The Proceedings of the Nutrition Society*, *64*, 213–216.

Lee, M. W., & Fujioka, K. (2009). Naltrexone for the treatment of obesity: Review and update. *Expert Opinion on Pharmacotherapy*, *10*, 1841–1845.

Lee, S. J., Verma, S., Simonds, S. E., Kirigiti, M. A., Kievit, P., Lindsley, S. R., et al. (2013). Lepting stimulates neuropeptide Y and cocaine amphetamine-regulated transcript coexpressing neuronal activity in the dorsomedial hypothalamus in diet-induced obese mice. *The Journal of Neuroscience*, *33*, 15306–15317.

Leino, S., Koski, S. K., Rannanpää, S., & Salminen, O. (2018). Effects of antidyskinetic nicotine treatment on dopamine release in dorsal and ventral striatum. *Neuroscience Letters*, *672*, 40–45.

Lénárd, L., László, K., Kertes, E., Ollmann, T., Péczely, L., Kovács, A., et al. (2018). Substance P and neurotensin in the limbic system: Their roles in reinforcement and memory consolidation. *Neuroscience and Biobehavioral Reviews*, *85*, 1–20.

Levy, A., Daniels, S., Hudson, R., Horman, T., Flynn, A., Zhou, Y., et al. (2018). Bupropion and naltrexone combination alters high fructose corn syrup self-administration and gene expression in rats. *Neuropharmacology*, *135*, 547–554.

Lieverse, R. J., Jansen, J. B., Masclee, A. M., & Lamers, C. B. (1994). Satiety effects of cholecystokinin in humans. *Gastroenterology*, *106*, 1451–1454.

Loh, K., Zhang, L., Brandon, A., Wang, Q., Begg, D., Qi, Y., et al. (2017). Insulin controls food intake and energy balance via NPY neurons. *Molecular Metabolism*, *6*, 574–584.

Loonam, T. M., Noailles, P. A. H., Yu, J., Zhu, J. P. Q., & Angulo, J. A. (2003). Substance p and cholecystokinin regulate neurochemical responses to cocaine and methamphetamine in the striatum. *Life Sciences*, *73*, 727–739.

Lynch, W. J., Peterson, A. B., Sanchez, V., Abel, J., & Smith, M. A. (2013). Exercise as a novel treatment for drug addiction: A neurobiological and stage-dependent hypothesis. *Neuroscience and Biobehavioral Reviews*, *37*, 1622–1644.

Maguire, D. R., & France, C. R. (2016). Effects of daily delta-9-tetrahydrocannabinol treatment on heroin self-administration in rhesus monkeys. *Behavioural Pharmacology*, *27*, 249–257.

Maire-Claire, C., Jourdaine, C., Lépne, J. P., Belliier, F., Block, V., & Vorspan, F. (2017). Pharmacoepigenomics of opioates and methadone maintenance treatment: Current data and perspectives. *Pharmacogenomics*, *18*, 1359–1372.

Maletínská, L., Maixnerová, J., Matysková, R., Haugvicová, R., Pirník, Z., Kiss, A., et al. (2008). Synergistic effect of CART (cocaine- and amphetamine-regulated transcript) peptide and cholecystokinin on food intake regulation in lean mice. *BMC Neuroscience*, *9*, 101.

Mani, B. K., Osborne-Lawrence, S., Mequinion, M., Lawrence, S., Gautron, L., Andrews, Z. B., et al. (2017). The role of ghrelin-responsive mediobasal hypothalamic neurons in mediating feeding responses to fasting. *Molecular Metabolism*, *6*, 882–896.

Mark, G. P., Shabani, S., Dobbs, L. K., & Hansen, S. T. (2011). Cholinergic modulation of mesolimbic dopamine function and reward. *Physiology & Behavior*, *104*, 76–81.

Martin, C. K., Redman, L. M., Zhang, J., Sanchez, M., Anderson, C. M., Smith, S. R., et al. (2011). Lorcaserin, a 5-HT(2C) receptor agonist, reduces body weight by decreasing energy intake without influencing energy expenditure. *The Journal of Clinical Endocrinology and Metabolism*, *96*, 837–845.

Mattes, R. D., Engelman, K., Shaw, L. M., & Elsohly, M. A. (1994). Cannabinoids and appetite stimulation. *Pharmacology, Biochemistry, and Behavior*, *49*, 187–195.

McMahon, L. R., & Wellman, P. J. (1998). PVN infusion of GLP-1-(7-36) amide suppresses feeding but does not induce aversion or alter locomotion in rats. *The American Journal of Physiology*, *274*, R23–R29.

McMillan, D. E. (1971). Interactions between naloxone and chlorpromazine on behavior under schedule control. *Psychopharmacologia*, *19*, 128–133.

Mello, N. K., Fivel, P. A., Kohut, S. J., & Carroll, F. I. (2014). Effects of chronic varenicline treatment on nicotine, cocaine, and concurrent nicotine + cocaine self-administration. *Neuropsychopharmacology*, *39*, 1222–1231.

Merchenthaler, I., Lane, M., & Shughrue, P. (1999). Distribution of pre-pro-glucagon and glucagon-like peptide-1 receptor messenger RNAs in the rat central nervous system. *The Journal of Comparative Neurology*, *403*, 261–280.

Mogg, K., Bradley, B. P., O'Neill, B., Bani, M., Merlo-Pich, E., Koch, A., et al. (2012). Effect of dopamine D_3 receptor antagonism on approach responses to food cues in overweight and obese individuals. *Behavioural Pharmacology*, *23*, 603–608.

Montoya, I. D. (2012). Advances in the development of biologics to treat drug addictions and overdose. *Addicciones*, *24*, 95–103.

Morgan, D., Grant, K. A., Gage, H. D., Mach, R. H., Kaplan, J. R., Prioleau, O., et al. (2002). Social dominance in monkeys: Dopamine D_2 receptors and cocaine self-administration. *Nature Neuroscience*, *5*, 169–174.

Murphy, A., Nestor, L. J., McGonigle, J., Paterson, L., Boyapati, V., Ersche, K. D., et al. (2017). Acute D3 antagonist GSK598809 selectively enhances neural response during monetary reward anticipation in drug and alcohol dependence. *Neuropsychopharmacology*, *42*, 1049–1057.

Nader, M. A., Morgan, D., Gage, H. D., Nader, S. H., Calhoun, T. L., Buchheimer, N., et al. (2006). PET imaging of dopamine D2 receptors during chronic cocaine self-administration in monkeys. *Nature Neuroscience*, *9*, 1050–1056.

Naef, L., Seabrook, L., Hsiao, J., Li, C., & Borgland, S. L. (2018). Insulin in the ventral tegmental area reduces cocaine-evoked dopamine in the nucleus accumbens in vivo. *The European Journal of Neuroscience*. https://doi.org/10.1111/ejn.14291.

Narayanaswami, V., Thompson, A. C., Cassis, L. A., Bardo, M. T., & Dwoskin, L. P. (2013). Diet-induced obesity: Dopamine transporter function, impulsivity and motivation. *International Journal of Obesity*, *37*, 1095–1103.

National Institute on Drug Abuse (NIDA), Principles of drug addiction treatment. A research-based guide. 2009, NIH Publication No. 12-4180.

Negus, S. S., & Henningfield, J. (2015). Agonist medications for the treatment of cocaine use disorder. *Neuropsychopharmacology*, *40*, 1–11.

Negus, S. S., Mello, N. K., Blough, B. E., Baumann, M. H., & Rothman, R. B. (2007). Monoamine releasers with varying selectivity for dopamine/norepinephrine versus serotonin release as candidate "agonist" medications for cocaine dependence: Studies in assays of cocaine discrimination and cocaine self-administration in rhesus monkeys. *The Journal of Pharmacology and Experimental Therapeutics*, *320*, 627–636.

Newman, A. H., Blaylock, B. L., Nader, M. A., Bergman, J., Sibley, D. R., & Skolnick, P. (2012). Medication discovery for addiction: Translating the dopamine D3 receptor hypothesis. *Biochemical Pharmacology*, *84*, 882–890.

Nickell, J. R., Siripurapu, K. B., Vartak, A., Crooks, P. A., & Dwoskin, L. P. (2014). The vesicular monoamine transporter-2: An important pharmacological target for the

discovery of novel therapeutics to treat methamphetamine abuse. *Advances in Pharmacology, 69*, 71–106.
O'Malley, S. S., Cooney, J. L., Krishnan-Sarin, S., Dubin, J. A., McKee, S. A., Cooney, N. L., et al. (2006). A controlled trial of naltrexone augmentation of nicotine replacement therapy for smoking cessation. *Archives of Internal Medicine, 166*, 667–674.
O'Malley, S. S., Corbin, W. R., Leeman, R. F., DeMartini, K. S., Fucito, L. M., Ikomi, J., et al. (2015). Reduction of alcohol drinking in young adults by naltrexone: A double-blind, placebo-controlled, randomized clinical trial of efficacy and safety. *The Journal of Clinical Psychiatry, 76*, e207–e213.
Olds, J. (1958). Self-stimulation of the brain: Its use to study local effects of hunger, sex, and drugs. *Science, 127*, 315–324.
Olds, J., Travis, R. P., & Schwing, R. C. (1960). Topographic organization of hypothalamic self-stimulation functions. *Journal of Comparative and Physiological Psychology, 53*, 23–32.
Ostlund, S. B., Liu, A. T., Wassum, K. M., & Maidment, N. T. (2017). Modulation of cue-triggered reward seeking by cholinergic signaling in the dorsomedial striatum. *The European Journal of Neuroscience, 45*, 358–364.
Pagano, C., Rossato, M., & Vettor, R. (2008). Endocannabinoids, adipose tissue and lipid metabolism. *Journal of Neuroendocrinology, 1*, 124–129.
Parker, E., Van Heek, M., & Stamford, A. (2002). Neuropeptide Y receptors as targets for anti-obesity drug development: Perspective and current status. *European Journal of Pharmacology, 440*, 173–187.
Pathak, V., Flatt, P. R., & Irwin, N. (2018). Cholecystokinin (CCK) and related adjunct peptide therapies for the treatment of obesity and type 2 diabetes. *Peptides, 100*, 229–235.
Perello, M., & Dickson, S. L. (2015). Ghrelin signaling on food reward: A salient link between the gut and the mesolimbic system. *The Journal of Endocrinology, 27*, 424–434.
Philpot, K., & Smith, Y. (2006). CART peptide and the mesolimbic dopamine system. *Peptides, 27*, 1987–1992.
Piazza, P. V., & Le Moal, M. (1998). The role of stress in drug self-administration. *Trends in Pharmacological Sciences, 19*, 67–74.
Pierce, R. C., & Kumaresan, V. (2006). The mesolimbic dopamine system: The final common pathway for the reinforcing effect of drugs of abuse? *Neuroscience and Biobehavioral Reviews, 30*, 215–238.
Pinder, R. M., Brogden, R. N., Sawyer, P. R., Speight, T. M., & Avery, G. S. (1975). Fenfluramine: A review of its pharmacological properties and therapeutic efficacy in obesity. *Drugs, 10*, 241–323.
Pirtle, J. L., Hickman, M. D., Boinpelly, V. C., Surineni, K., Thakur, H. K., & Grasing, K. W. (2019). The serotonin-2C agonist lorcaserin delays intravenous choice and modifies the subjective and cardiovascular effects of cocaine: A randomized, controlled human laboratory study. *Pharmacology, Biochemistry, and Behavior, 180*, 52–59. https://doi.org/10.1016/j.pbb.2019.02.010.
Plebani, J. G., Lynch, K. G., Yu, Q., Pettinati, H. M., O'Brien, C. P., & Kampman, K. M. (2012). Results of an initial clinical trial of varenicline for the treatment of cocaine dependence. *Drug and Alcohol Dependence, 121*, 163–166.
Puhl, R., & Brownell, K. D. (2001). Bias, discrimination, and obesity. *Obesity Research, 9*, 788–805.
Rakosvka, A., Baranyi, M., Windisch, K., Petkova-Kirova, P., Gagov, H., & Kalfin, R. (2017). Neurochemical evidence that cocaine- and amphetamine-regulated transcript (CART) 55-102 peptide modulates the dopaminergic reward system by decreasing the dopamine release in the mouse nucleus accumbens. *Brain Research Bulletin, 134*, 246–252.

Rawson, R. A., Chudzynski, J., Mooney, L., Gonzales, R., Ang, A., Dickerson, D., et al. (2015). Impact of an exercise intervention of methamphetamine use outcomes post-residential treatment care. *Drug and Alcohol Dependence, 156*, 21–28.
Recant, L., Voyles, N. R., Luciano, M., & Pert, C. B. (1980). Naltrexone reduces weight gain, alters "β-endorphin", and reduces insulin output from pancreatic islets of genetically obese mice. *Peptides, 1*, 309–313.
Reddy, I. A., Stanwood, G., & Galli, A. (2014). Moving beyond energy homeostasis: New roles for glucagon-like peptide-1 in food and drug reward. *Neurochemistry International, 73*, 49–55.
Reid, M. S., Mickalian, J. D., Delucchi, K. L., & Berger, S. P. (1999). A nicotinic antagonist, mecamylamine, reduces cue-induced cocaine craving in cocaine-dependent subjects. *Neuropsychopharmacology, 20*, 297–307.
Reidelberger, R. D., Varga, G., Liehr, R. M., Castellanos, D. A., Rosenquist, G. L., Wong, H. C., et al. (1994). Cholecystokinin suppresses food intake by a nonendocrine mechanism in rats. *The American Journal of Physiology, 267*, R901–R908.
Rice, O. V., Schonhar, C. A., Gaál, J., Gardner, E. L., & Ashby, C. R., Jr. (2015). The selective dopamine D_3 receptor antagonist SB-277011-A significantly decreases binge-like consumption of ethanol in C57BL/6J mice. *Synapse, 69*, 295–298.
Rinaman, L. (2010). Ascending projections from the caudal visceral nucleus of the solitary tract to brain regions involved in food intake and energy expenditure. *Brain Research, 1350*, 18–34.
Ritz, M. C., Lamb, R. J., Goldberg, S. R., & Kuhar, M. J. (1988). Cocaine self-administration appears to be mediated by dopamine uptake inhibition. *Progress in Neuropsychopharmacology and Biological Psychiatry, 12*, 233–239.
Rollema, H., Chambers, L. K., Coe, J. W., Glowa, J., Hurst, R. S., Lebel, L. A., et al. (2007). Pharmacological profile of the alpha4beta2 nicotinic acetylcholine receptor partial agonist varenicline, an effective smoking cessation aid. *Neuropharmacology, 52*, 985–994.
Rose, J. E., Behm, F. M., & Westman, E. C. (2001). Acute effects of nicotine and mecamylamine on tobacco withdrawal symptoms, cigarette reward and ad lib smoking. *Pharmacology, Biochemistry, and Behavior, 68*, 187–197.
Rose, J. E., Behm, F. M., Westman, E. C., & Bates, J. E. (2003). Mecamylamine acutely increases human intravenous nicotine self-administration. *Pharmacology, Biochemistry, and Behavior, 76*, 307–313.
Rothman, R. B., & Baumann, M. H. (2003). Monoamine transporters and psychostimulant drugs. *European Journal of Pharmacology, 479*, 23–40.
Rothman, R. B., & Baumann, M. H. (2009). Serotonergic drugs and valvular heart disease. *Expert Opinion on Drug Safety, 8*, 317–329.
Russo, C., Russo, A., Pellitteri, R., & Stanzani, S. (2017). Hippocampal ghrelin-positive neurons directly project to arcuate hypothalamic and medial amygaloid neuclei. Could they modulate food-intake? *Neuroscience Letters, 653*, 126–131.
Sakata, I., & Sakai, T. (2010). Ghrelin cells in the gastrointestinal tract. *International Journal of Peptide, 2010*, pii: 945056.
Salminen, O., Murphy, K. L., McIntosh, J. M., Drago, J., Marks, M. J., Collins, A. C., et al. (2004). Subunits composition and pharmacology of two classes of striatal presynaptic nicotinic acetylcholine receptors mediating dopamine release in mice. *Molecular Pharmacology, 65*, 1526–1535.
Schindler, C. W., Redhi, G. H., Vemuri, K., Makriyannis, A., Le Foll, B., Bergman, J., et al. (2016). Blockade of nicotine and cannabinoid reinforcement and relapse by a cannabinoid CB1-receptor neutral antagonist AM4113 and inverse agonist rimonabant in squirrel monkeys. *Neuropsychopharmacology, 41*, 2283–2293.
Schwartz, M. W., Woods, S. C., Porte, D., Jr., Seeley, R. J., & Baskin, D. G. (2000). Central nervous system control of food intake. *Nature, 404*, 661–671.

Sharma, S., Hryhorczuk, C., & Fulton, S. (2012). Progressive-ratio responding for palatable high-fat and high-sugar food in mice. *Journal of Visualized Experiments*, *63*, e3754.

Shen, M., Jiang, C., Liu, F., & Ma, L. (2016). Mesolimbic leptin signaling negatively regulates cocaine-conditioned reward. *Translational Psychiatry*, *6*, e972.

Shimizu, Y., Shon, C., Aotani, D., Nomura, H., Hikida, T., Hosoda, K., et al. (2017). Role of leptin in conditioned place preference to high-fat diet in leptin-deficient *ob/ob* mice. *Neuroscience Letters*, *640*, 60–63.

Simiand, J., Keane, M., Keane, P. E., & Soubrié, P. (1998). SR 141716, a CB1 cannabinoid receptor antagonist, selectively reduces sweet food intake in marmoset. *Behavioural Pharmacology*, *9*, 179–181.

Sinha, R. (2008). Chronic stress, drug use, and vulnerability to addiction. *Annals of the New York Academy of Sciences*, *1141*, 105–130.

Skibicka, K. P., Hansson, C., Egecioglu, E., & Dickson, S. L. (2012). Role of ghrelin in food reward: Impact of ghrelin on sucrose self-administration and mesolimbic dopamine and acetylcholine receptor gene expression. *Addiction Biology*, *17*, 95–107.

Smith, M. A., & Lynch, W. J. (2011). Exercise as a potential treatment for drug abuse: Evidence from preclinical studies. *Frontiers in Psychiatry*, *2*, 1–10.

Smith, S. M., Meyer, M., & Trinkley, K. E. (2013). Phentermine/topiramate for the treatment of obesity. *The Annals of Pharmacotherapy*, *47*, 340–349.

Smith, M. A., Schmidt, K. T., Iordanou, J. C., & Mustroph, M. L. (2008). Aerobic exercise decreases the positive-reinforcing effects of cocacine. *Drug and Alcohol Dependence*, *98*, 129–135.

Smith, S. A., Waggoner, A. D., de las Fuentes, L., & Davilla-Roman, R. G. (2009). Role serotonergic pathways in drug-induced valvular heart disease and diagnostic features by echocardiography. *Journal of the American Society of Echocardiography*, *22*, 883–889.

Spanagel, R., & Weiss, F. (1999). The dopamine hypothesis of reward: Past and current status. *TINS*, *22*, 521–527.

Steidl, S., Wasserman, D. I., Blaha, C. D., & Yoemans, J. S. (2017). Opioid-induced rewards, locomotion, and dopamine activation: A proposed model for control by mesopontine and rostromedial tegmental neurons. *Neuroscience and Biobehavioral Reviews*, *83*, 72–82.

Stoops, W. W., & Rush, C. R. (2013). Agonist replacement for stimulant dependence: A review of clinical research. *Current Pharmaceutical Design*, *19*, 7026–7035.

Sun, Y., Duan, W., Meng, X., Li, H., & Jia, C. (2018). Varenicline is associated with a modest limitation in weight gain in smokers after smoking cessation: A meta-analysis. *Journal of Public Health (Oxford, England)*, *40*, e126–e132.

Tanda, G., Munzar, P., & Goldberg, S. R. (2000). Self-administration behavior is maintained by the psychoactive ingredient of marijuana in squirrel monkeys. *Nature Neuroscience*, *3*, 1073–1074.

Thanos, P. K., Michaelides, M., Ho, C. W., Wang, G. J., Newman, A. H., Heidbreder, C. A., et al. (2008). The effects of two highly selective dopamine D3 receptor antagonists (SB-277011A and NGB-2904) on food self-administration in a rodent model of obesity. *Pharmacology, Biochemistry, and Behavior*, *89*, 499–507.

Tihonen, J., Kuoppasalmi, K., Föhr, J., Tuomola, P., Kuikanmäki, O., Vorma, H., et al. (2007). A comparison of aripiprazole, methylphenidate, and placebo for methamphetamine dependence. *The American Journal of Psychiatry*, *164*, 160–162.

Tobin, S., Newman, A. H., Quinn, T., & Shalev, U. (2009). A role for dopamine D1-like receptors in acute food deprivation-induced reinstatement of heroin seeking in rats. *The International Journal of Neuropsychopharmacology*, *12*, 217–226.

Tomasi, D., Wang, G. J., Wang, R., Caparelli, E. C., Logan, J., & Volkow, N. D. (2015). Overlapping patterns of brain activation to food and cocaine cues in cocaine abusers: Association to striatal D2/D3 receptors. *Human Brain Mapping*, *36*, 120–136.

Toschke, A. M., Ehlin, A. G. C., von Kries, R., Ekbom, A., & Montgomery, S. M. (2003). Maternal smoking during pregnancy and appetite control in offspring. *Journal of Perinatal Medicine*, *31*, 251–256.

Upadhya, M. A., Nakhate, K. T., Kokare, D. M., Singh, U., Singru, P. S., & Subhedar, N. K. (2012). CART peptide in the nucleus accumbens shell acts downstream to dopamine and mediates the reward and reinforcement actions of morphine. *Neuropharmacology*, *62*, 1823–1833.

van Bloemendaal, L., Veltman, D. J., Ten Kulve, J. S., Groot, P. F., Ruhé, H. G., Barkof, F., et al. (2015). Brain reward-system activation in response to anticipation and consumption of palatable food is altered by glucagon-like peptide-1 receptor activation in humans. *Diabetes, Obesity & Metabolism*, *17*, 878–886.

Verdich, C., Flint, A., Gutzwiller, J. P., Näslund, E., Beglinger, C., Hellström, P. M., et al. (2001). A meta-analysis of the effect of glucagon-like peptide-1 (7-36) amide on ad libitum energy intake in humans. *The Journal of Clinical Endocrinology and Metabolism*, *86*, 4382–4389.

Volkow, N. D. (2017). Medications for opioid use disorder: Bridging the gap in care. *Lancet*, *391*, 1–3.

Volkow, N. D., Fowler, J. S., Wolf, A. P., Schlyer, D., Shiue, C. Y., Alpert, R., et al. (1990). Effects of chronic cocaine abuse on postsynaptic dopamine receptors. *The American Journal of Psychiatry*, *147*, 719–724.

Volkow, N. D., Wan, G. J., Fowler, F. S., Tomasi, D., & Baler, R. (2012). Food and drug reward: Overlapping circuits in human obesity and addiction. *Current Topics in Behavioral Neurosciences*, *11*, 1–24.

Volkow, N. D., Wang, G. J., Fowler, J. S., Gatley, S. J., Ding, Y. S., Dewek, S. L., et al. (1996). Relationship between psychostimulant-induced "high" and dopamine transporter occupancy. *Proceedings of the National Academy of Sciences of the United States of America*, *93*, 10388–10392.

Volkow, N. D., & Wise, R. A. (2005). How can drug addiction help us understand obesity? *Nature Neuroscience*, *8*, 555–560.

Volkow, N. D., Wise, R. A., & Baler, R. (2017). The dopamine motive system: Implications for drug and food addiction. *Nature Reviews. Neuroscience*, *18*, 741–752.

Wadden, T. A., Berkowitz, R. I., Silvestry, F., Vogt, R. A., St John Sutton, M. G., Stunkard, A. J., et al. (1998). The fen-phen finale: A study of weight loss and valvular heart disease. *Obesity Research*, *6*, 278–284.

Wang, G. J., Volkow, N. D., Logan, J., Pappas, N. R., Wong, C. T., Zhu, W., et al. (2001). Brain dopamine and obesity. *Lancet*, *357*, 354–357.

Weber, S. C., Beck-Schimmer, B., Kajdi, M. E., Müller, D., Tobler, P. N., & Quednow, B. B. (2016). Dopamine D2/D3- and μ-opioid receptor antagonists reduce cue-induced responding and reward impulsivity in humans. *Translational Psychiatry*, *6*, e850.

Wee, S., Anderson, K. G., Baumann, M. H., Rothman, R. B., Blough, B. E., & Woolverton, W. L. (2005). Relationship between the serotonergic activity and reinforcing effects of a series of amphetamine analogs. *The Journal of Pharmacology and Experimental Therapeutics*, *313*, 848–854.

Weissman, N. J., Sanchez, M., Koch, G. G., Smith, S. R., Shanahan, W. R., & Anderson, C. M. (2013). Echocardiographic assessment of cardiac valvular regurgitation with lorcaserin from analysis of 3 phase 3 clinical trials. *Circulation. Cardiovascular Imaging*, *6*, 560–567.

Wellman, P. J. (2000). Norepinephrine and the control of food intake. *Nutrition*, *16*, 837–842.

Wellman, P. J., Davis, K. W., & Nation, J. R. (2005). Augmentation of cocaine hyperactivity in rats by systemic ghrelin. *Regulatory Peptides*, *125*, 151–154.

Wellman, P. J., Nation, J. R., & Davis, K. W. (2007). Impairment of acquisition of cocaine self-administration in rats maintained on a high-fat diet. *Pharmacology, Biochemistry, and Behavior, 88*, 89–93.

Williams, C. M., & Kirkham, T. C. (1999). Anandamide induces overeating: Mediation by central cannabinoid (CB1) receptors. *Psychopharmacology, 143*, 315–317.

Williams, C. M., Rogers, P. J., & Kirkham, T. C. (1998). Hyperphagia in pre-fed rats following oral delta9-THC. *Physiology & Behavior, 65*, 343–346.

Wise, R. A. (1997). Drug self-administration viewed as ingestive behavior. *Appetite, 28*, 1–5.

Wise, R. A., & Rompre, P. P. (1989). Brain dopamine and reward. *Annual Review of Psychology, 40*, 191–225.

Wolfe, W. L., & Maisto, S. A. (2000). The relationship between eating disorders and substance use: Moving beyond co-prevalence research. *Clinical Psychology Review, 20*, 617–631.

Wren, A. M., Seal, L. J., Cohen, M. A., Brynes, A. E., Frost, G. S., Murphy, K. G., et al. (2001). Ghrelin enhances appetite and increases food intake in humans. *The Journal of Clinical Endocrinology and Metabolism, 86*, 5992.

Wright, F. L., & Rodgers, R. J. (2013). Acute behavioural effects of bupropion and naltrexone, alone and in combination, in non-deprived male rats presented with palatable mash. *Psychopharmacology, 228*, 291–307.

Yokel, R. A., & Wise, R. A. (1975). Increased lever pressing for amphetamine after pimozide in rats: Implications for a dopamine theory of reward. *Science, 187*, 547–549.

You, Z. B., Gao, J. T., Bi, G. H., He, Y., Boateng, C., Cao, J., et al. (2017). The novel dopamine D3 receptor antagonists/partial agonists CAB2-015 and BAK4-54 inhibit oxycodone-taking and oxycodone-seeking behavior in rats. *Neuropharmacology, 126*, 190–199.

You, Z. B., Wang, B., Liu, Q. R., Wu, Y., Otvos, L., & Wise, R. A. (2016). Reciprocal inhibitory interactions between the reward-related effects of leptin and cocaine. *Neuropsychopharmacology, 41*, 1024–1033.

Yu, D. S., Smith, F. L., Smith, D. G., & Lyness, W. H. (1986). Fluoxetine-induced attenuation of amphetamine self-administration in rats. *Life Sciences, 39*, 1383–1388.

Zhao-Shea, R., Liu, L., Improgo, M. R., Meyers, E. E., McIntosh, J. M., Grady, S. R., et al. (2011). Nicotine-mediated activation of dopaminergic neurons in distinct regions of the ventral tegmental area. *Neuropsychopharmacology, 36*, 1021–1032.

Zhou, W., Liu, H., Zhang, F., Tang, S., Zhu, H., Lai, M., et al. (2007). Role acetylcholine transmission in nucleus accumbens and ventral tegmental area in heroin-seeking induced by conditioned cues. *Neuroscience, 144*, 1209–1218.

Further reading

Carroll, M. E., Carmona, G. G., & May, S. A. (1991). Modifying drug-reinforced behavior by altering the economic conditions of the drug and a nondrug reinforcer. *Journal of the Experimental Analysis of Behavior, 56*, 361–376.

Elsmore, T. F., Fletcher, G. V., Conrad, D. G., & Sodetz, F. J. (1978). Reduction of heroin intake in baboons by an economic constraint. *Pharmacology, Biochemistry, and Behavior, 13*, 729–731.

Foltin, R. W. (1999). Food and cocaine self-administration by baboons: Effects of alternatives. *Journal of the Experimental Analysis of Behavior, 72*, 215–234.

Lau, B. K., Cota, D., Cristino, L., & Borglan, S. L. (2017). Endocannabinoid modulation of homeostatic and non-homeostatic feeding circuits. *Neuropharmacology, 124*, 38–51.

Lenoir, M., & Ahmed, S. H. (2007). Supply of a nondrug substitute reduces escalated heroin consumption. *Neuropsychopharmacology, 33*, 1–11.

Mutschler, N. H., & Bergman, J. (2002). Effects of chronic administration of the D1 receptor partial agonist SKF 77434 on cocaine self-administration in rhesus monkeys. *Psychopharmacology*, *160*, 362–370.

Smith, B. M., Smith, J. M., Tsai, J. H., Schultz, J. A., Gilson, C. A., Estrada, S. A., et al. (2008). Discovery and structure-activity relationship of (1R)-8-chloro-2,3,4,5-tetrohydro-1-methyl-1H-3-benzazepine (lorcaserin), a selective serotonin 5-HT2C receptor agonist for the treatment of obesity. *Journal of Medicinal Chemistry*, *51*, 305–313.

Votruba, S. B., Horvitz, M. A., & Schoeller, D. A. (2000). The role of exercise in the treatment of obesity. *Nutrition*, *16*, 179–188.

CHAPTER EIGHT

Obsessive compulsive disorder (OCD): Current treatments and a framework for neurotherapeutic research

Erik Z. Woody[a], Kurt Leroy Hoffman[b], Henry Szechtman[c,*]
[a]Department of Psychology, University of Waterloo, Waterloo, ON, Canada
[b]Centro de Investigación en Reproducción Animal (CIRA), Universidad Autónoma de Tlaxcala—CINVESTAV, Tlaxcala, Mexico
[c]Department of Psychiatry and Behavioural Neurosciences, McMaster University, Hamilton, ON, Canada
*Corresponding author: e-mail address: szechtma@mcmaster.ca

Contents

1. Introduction 238
   1.1 Diagnosis and description of OCD 238
   1.2 Current state of research on treatment of OCD: Pharmacotherapy 239
   1.3 Neuromodulatory therapies for OCD 241
   1.4 Psychological treatments for OCD 243
   1.5 Summary 245
2. Toward a new perspective on psychiatric disorder 245
   2.1 The RDoC 245
   2.2 An adaptationist reorientation of the RDoC approach for OCD research 246
   2.3 The security motivation system and OCD 248
   2.4 Revisiting the main themes of the RDoC 250
3. Toward a new perspective on treatment for OCD 253
   3.1 Some key aspects of the SMS for OCD pharmacotherapeutics 253
   3.2 The traditional approach: Discover *magic bullets* 255
   3.3 The *elixir of life* approach: Boost processing power of the brain 257
   3.4 Facilitating relearning: Promote neural plasticity 260
   3.5 Fixing a weak link: Target specific pathways of the SMS network 262
4. Conclusion 262
Conflict of interest 263
References 263

Abstract

We briefly review current approaches to the diagnosis and treatment of OCD, noting their lack of a strong theoretical foundation. In keeping with the Research Domain Criteria project (RDoC) calls for reconceptualizing psychopathology in ways that better

Advances in Pharmacology, Volume 86
ISSN 1054-3589
https://doi.org/10.1016/bs.apha.2019.04.003

link up with normal brain systems, we advance an adaptationist, brain-network perspective on OCD and propose that OCD represents a dysfunction in the stopping dynamics of a normal brain network that evolved to handle potential danger. We then illustrate how this theoretical perspective can be used to organize possibilities for research on neurotherapeutics for OCD and suggest novel directions for future work.

Abbreviations

AM amygdala
BNST bed nucleus of the stria terminalis
CRH corticotropin-releasing hormone
GC glucocorticoids
GPe external segment of the globus pallidus
GPi internal segment of the globus pallidus
HPC hippocampus
LC locus coeruleus
MC motor cortex
MD Thalamus mediodorsal thalamic nucleus
MOPFC medial prefrontal cortex and orbital prefrontal cortex
PMC premotor cortex
PVN paraventricular nucleus
SMA supplementary motor area
SNpc substantia nigra pars compacta
SNr substantia nigra pars reticulata
STN subthalamic nucleus
VA ventroanterior thalamic nucleus
VL ventrolateral thalamic nucleus
VTA ventral tegmental area

1. Introduction

1.1 Diagnosis and description of OCD

For OCD, as for most psychiatric disorders, there is no biological test that identifies the disorder, and the etiology and pathophysiology are unknown. Hence the diagnosis of OCD is based purely on a behavioral profile that defines what constitutes OCD. This is provided in the Diagnostic and Statistical Manual of Mental Disorders, DSM-5 (Chapter 13 in American Psychiatric Association, 2013): "OCD is characterized by the presence of obsessions and/or compulsions. *Obsessions* are recurrent and persistent thoughts, urges, or images that are experienced as intrusive and unwanted, whereas *compulsions* are repetitive behaviors or mental acts that an individual feels driven to perform in response to an obsession or according to rules that must be applied rigidly." Obsessions include concerns about dirt and the spread of disease to self, and of harm to a friend or relative; compulsions include excessive washing and cleaning, generally of hands but sometimes also possessions, and excessive checking, characterized by repeated re-doings of actions related to security or accuracy (Reed, 1985).

Whether or not a person meets the diagnostic criteria for OCD is too coarse a measure of outcome for research on treatment outcome. The most widely used instrument in OCD research studies is the Yale-Brown Obsessive Compulsive Scale (YBOCS; Goodman, Price, Rasmussen, Mazure, Delgado, et al., 1989; Goodman, Price, Rasmussen, Mazure, Fleischmann, et al., 1989), designed as a "measure of the severity of symptoms of obsessive-compulsive disorder that is not influenced by the type of obsessions or compulsions present" (Goodman, Price, Rasmussen, Mazure, Fleischmann, et al., 1989, p. 1006). It quantifies the severity of obsessions and compulsions by tapping aspects such as how much time they occupy and how much they interfere with daily function. Its 10 items yield a total score from 0 to 40, providing a quantitative index.

Although it is sometimes claimed that the OCD diagnostic criteria "are merely descriptive, rather than theory-based or etiologically based" (Abramowitz, 2018, p. 4), unfortunately the OCD profile in DSM-5 is not free of implicit psychological theories. A prominent one is that thoughts drive actions and there is a functional relationship between them. This psychological theory is embodied for example in the definition of compulsion as performed "in response to an obsession" and in the implicit claim that there is a meaningful functional relationship between obsessions and compulsions in that obsessions "in most individuals cause marked anxiety or distress" and compulsions "are aimed at preventing or reducing anxiety or distress" (Chapter 13 in American Psychiatric Association, 2013; Criterion A). Clearly, such diagnostic criteria, rather than being purely descriptive of OCD symptoms, also contain assumptions about the underlying mechanisms, which may seriously hamper alternative lines of inquiry. For this and other reasons, there is growing unease about whether the DSM criteria are a productive foundation for research and increasing interest in alternative approaches, as we address later.

1.2 Current state of research on treatment of OCD: Pharmacotherapy

It was a serendipitous discovery that in depressed patients the tricyclic antidepressant (TCA) clomipramine provided relief also for obsessional symptoms

(Cordoba Fernandez & Lopez Ibor Alino, 1967), which led to extensive investigations of pharmacotherapy for OCD (Ananth, 1986; Philpott, 1976; Yaryura-Tobias & Neziroglu, 1975). Many studies confirmed the effectiveness of clomipramine in OCD—for instance, a large multicenter double-blind clinical trial with over 500 patients showed a reduction of about 40% in YBOCS scores after 10 weeks of treatment compared to only about a 4% reduction for the placebo-treated patients (Clomipramine Collaborative Study Group, 1991).

Clomipramine is a potent inhibitor of serotonin reuptake, and it was found that TCAs without potent effects on serotonin reuptake show little efficacy for OCD (Piccinelli, Pini, Bellantuono, & Wilkinson, 1995). The resulting hypothesis that blockade of serotonin reuptake is essential for a therapeutic effect in OCD was also supported by the finding that selective serotonin-reuptake inhibitors (SSRIs), which have little or no effect on norepinephrine and dopamine reuptake, proved clinically effective, with response rates of 40–60% versus <20% with placebo (Katzman et al., 2014; Soomro, Altman, Rajagopal, & Oakley Browne, 2008); a clinical response was defined as a 25% or more reduction in symptoms measured with the YBOCS. SSRIs are now the clinically recommended first-line of pharmacotherapy for OCD (Fineberg et al., 2015; Katzman et al., 2014; Koran & Simpson, 2013; Pittenger & Bloch, 2014; Skapinakis et al., 2016b). However, although many patients do achieve clinical relief with serotonin-reuptake inhibitor (SRI) pharmacotherapy, there are also many OCD patients who do not (40–60%) (Katzman et al., 2014; Soomro et al., 2008).

These findings from treatment response studies were used to generate hypotheses as to the etiology of OCD (Goodman, Grice, Lapidus, & Coffey, 2014), for example, that OCD reflects a dysfunction in brain serotonergic system (Yaryura-Tobias, Neziroglu, & Bergman, 1976). However, this approach—inferring etiology and pathophysiology from treatment response—is "fraught with problems that have plagued the field of psychiatry for decades … [and] has yielded few new insights or novel treatments" (Goodman et al., 2014, p. 261). The deduction of etiology from findings of treatment effect is a logical fallacy, the "Fallacy of Confirming the Consequence" (Montgomery, 2012). To investigate etiology and pathophysiology requires a basic science discipline where putative causes can be manipulated experimentally (Bolkan, Carvalho Poyraz, & Kellendonk, 2016; Szechtman & Eilam, 2005), as we elaborate later.

The antidepressant drugs used in the treatment of OCD are first-line agents also in the treatment of a wide range of psychiatric disorders

(Katzman et al., 2014), indicating that the serotonergic re-uptake targeted by OCD pharmacotherapy is not for OCD specifically. This suggests that the serotonergic system targeted by these drugs may play a role in the operations of more than one functional network. In addition, the fact that a high percentage of OCD patients do not benefit from intervention with serotonin reuptake inhibitors (Katzman et al., 2014; Pittenger & Bloch, 2014) suggests that more than one neurochemical system mediates OCD symptoms.

The limitations of SSRI monotherapy prompted clinicians to try combining other agents with an SSRI, an approach known as "adjunctive" or "augmentation" therapy. Subsequent meta-analyses supported the efficacy of neuroleptic augmentation (e.g., aripiprazole, haloperidol, or risperidone) in treatment-resistant OCD (Dold, Aigner, Lanzenberger, & Kasper, 2013, 2015; Skapinakis, Papatheodorou, & Mavreas, 2007; Veale et al., 2014). Because the major mode of action for neuroleptics is blockade of dopamine receptors (Seeman, 1980), this raises the hypothesis that the activity of dopamine systems is implicated in some way in the expression of OCD. Further examination of this hypothesis would benefit from a basic science approach that experimentally manipulates the hypothesized causes. Interestingly, preclinical research has shown that repeated injections of the dopamine agonist, quinpirole, can induce in rats a behavioral syndrome that has the features of compulsive symptoms displayed by OCD patients (Szechtman, Sulis, & Eilam, 1998). Thus, this preparation provides an experimental paradigm for investigating a potential role of dopamine in OCD.

1.3 Neuromodulatory therapies for OCD

An older medical intervention for psychiatric disorders is psychosurgery, targeting the anatomy of the brain itself. Some therapeutic success for OCD has been obtained with two surgical procedures: "capsulotomy" and "cingulotomy" (Bari et al., 2018). Capsulotomy involves an ablation in the region of the anterior limb of the internal capsule, and cingulotomy involves a lesion in the region of the cingulate bundle (Neumaier et al., 2017).

Deep brain stimulation (DBS) is another intervention that targets the anatomy of the brain. DBS for refractory OCD has targeted four sites: the junction of the ventral anterior limb of the internal capsule and the adjacent ventral striatum (Greenberg et al., 2010), the bed nucleus of the stria terminalis (BST) (Luyten, Hendrickx, Raymaekers, Gabriels, & Nuttin, 2016), the nucleus accumbens (Denys et al., 2010), and the subthalamic nucleus (STN) (Mallet et al., 2008). These interventions seem to have very good results in some patients, but unsatisfactory ones in others.

One hypothesis why DBS has a therapeutic effect in OCD is that it might create a "functional lesion" by inhibiting the stimulated target region, akin to the therapeutic mechanism first suggested in Parkinson's disease (PD; Benabid, 2003). However, Montgomery and Gale (2008) argued against the functional lesion hypothesis of DBS in PD, instead emphasizing the complexity of physiological effects produced by DBS stimulation and discussing its effects in terms of "systems oscillators theory." Specifically, the effects of DBS are best viewed from a systems perspective rather than as a local functional lesion, with DBS hypothesized to alter the oscillatory characteristics of information flow in a feedback network comprised of basal ganglia-thalamus-cortex (BG–TH–CTX) connections (Montgomery, 2007, 2016, 2017; Montgomery & Gale, 2008; Montgomery & He, 2016; Parent & Hazrati, 1995a, 1995b).

A less invasive type of neurostimulation that has been explored as a possible treatment for OCD is repeated transcranial magnetic stimulation (rTMS; Lefaucheur et al., 2014) Active rTMS has been shown to be superior to sham rTMS for OCD, producing a modest reduction in Y-BOCS scores, and rTMS over the supplementary motor area (SMA) produced greater reduction in Y-BOCS scores than rTMS applied over the dorsolateral prefrontal cortex or orbitofrontal cortex.

One hypothesis for the therapeutic effect of rTMS in reducing OCD symptoms is that it, like psychosurgery and DBS (Bear, Fitzgerald, Rosenfeld, & Bittar, 2010), may alter the functioning of the cortico-striato-thalamo-cortical (CSTC) circuits implicated in OCD. Similar to the foregoing considerations for DBS, "rTMS can interact with spontaneous oscillatory rhythms existing in the cortical circuits activated by the stimulation" (Lefaucheur et al., 2014, p. 2154). In addition, rTMS has been conceptualized as a procedure for manipulating brain plasticity (Hallett, 2007; Pascual-Leone, Amedi, Fregni, & Merabet, 2005); thus, rTMS may foster a neurobiological state enabling new learning to stop performance of compulsions. For this reason, rTMS is often applied during provocation of OCD symptoms (Carmi et al., 2018).

Another type of neurostimulation that has been explored as a possible treatment for OCD is transcranial direct current stimulation (tDCS; Lefaucheur et al., 2017), with the rationale that tDCS can "activate most of the [brain] areas related to OCD" (Senco et al., 2015). A recent review of the results of tDCS administered to a variety of sites (the dorsolateral prefrontal cortex, the orbitofrontal cortex, and the supplementary motor area) found that most studies reported a decrease in Y-BOCS scores (Brunelin et al., 2018). However, further work is clearly necessary, addressing factors such as appropriate stimulation parameters and electrode placements.

1.4 Psychological treatments for OCD

In contrast to the foregoing interventions for OCD, psychotherapy is a non-physical treatment modality. There are two somewhat different forms of psychological intervention for OCD—behavior therapy and cognitive therapy, which ostensibly target different aspects of the disorder, namely behavior patterns and underling cognitions, respectively.

Like the development of pharmacological and neuromodulatory interventions for OCD, psychological treatments for it developed somewhat serendipitously, out of trial and error. Various behavior therapy methods were tested to reduce OCD symptoms, such as desensitization, flooding, aversive conditioning, and relaxation. What ultimately proved efficacious is repeated exposure to the stimuli of particular concern to patients and prevention of their compulsive responses or rituals (Foa, 2010). Research has indicated that the combination of both of these components is more beneficial than either alone (Foa, Steketee, Grayson, Turner, & Latimer, 1984); hence, most behavior therapy protocols involve both components, yielding what is known as "exposure and response prevention" (ERP).

The key working assumption underlying cognitive therapy (CT) is that what drives OCD is thought processes (antecedent cognitions; Tolin, 2009). Accordingly, CT is a method of "cognitive restructuring." Protocols with a sizeable component of "behavioral experiments," which attempt empirically to disconfirm OCD-supportive cognitions, are labeled cognitive behavior therapy (CBT).

Meta-analytic reviews of these psychological interventions for OCD indicate that they are clinically effective, leading to marked reductions in OCD symptoms (Katzman et al., 2014; National Collaborating Centre for Mental Health, 2006; Olatunji, Davis, Powers, & Smits, 2013; Ost, Havnen, Hansen, & Kvale, 2015; Ougrin, 2011; Rosa-Alcazar, Sanchez-Meca, Gomez-Conesa, & Marin-Martinez, 2008; Rosa-Alcazar et al., 2015; Skapinakis et al., 2016a). Despite the differences in focus of ERP and CT, it has been found that they do not differ significantly in effectiveness; moreover, their combination does not seem to yield improvement beyond that shown by either approach separately (Rosa-Alcazar et al., 2008).

These findings suggest that what is effective may be common to both techniques, and it has been speculated that the crucial ingredient may be "interventions that encourage direct behavioral change" (Tolin, 2009, p. 40). However, identifying how various aspects of therapy protocols may affect effectiveness will require challenging, controlled research studies, which mostly remain to be done.

Nonetheless, one intriguing line of research has addressed the effect of the timing of therapy sessions—spaced out in time versus massed or intensive. Evidence suggests "some superiority of the intensive format" (Jonsson, Kristensen, & Arendt, 2015, p. 93). Indeed, it appears that CBT treatment concentrated into a 4-day period—the Bergen 4-day concentrated exposure treatment for OCD—is highly effective and yields treatment gains that are sustained at 1-year follow-up (Hansen, Hagen, Ost, Solem, & Kvale, 2018). Such results may have important implications not only for optimizing the allocation of clinical resources, but also for OCD theory.

It is tempting to regard the success of particular psychotherapeutic approaches as evidence for corresponding theories as applied to OCD. For example, the success of ERP could be interpreted as evidence for a conditioning account in which OCD symptoms were "acquired through classically conditioned fear responses, and maintained through negatively reinforced avoidance responses" (McKay et al., 2015, p. 106). Similarly, the success of CT could be interpreted as evidence for a purely cognitive account in which obsessions and compulsions were produced and maintained by faulty reasoning. Nonetheless, just as etiology cannot be inferred from the success of a pharmacological intervention, the success of a psychotherapeutic approach is not an adequate test of a theory about the disorder. Indeed, very little is known about the mechanisms that may actually underlie the success of psychotherapeutic protocols.

Finally, there has been considerable interest in whether the combination of psychotherapy and pharmacotherapy is more effective than either one alone. Surprisingly, some carefully conducted studies indicate that the answer is no (Foa et al., 2005; Rosa-Alcazar et al., 2008). Although it is possible that combination therapy could be of benefit to severely ill OCD patients (Simpson et al., 2008; Skapinakis et al., 2016a), Wheaton, DeSantis, and Simpson (2016) concluded that "the data do not clearly demonstrate superiority of combination treatment over the most effective psychotherapies" (p. 920). This finding of little or no additive effect may suggest that psychotherapeutic and pharmacological treatments elicit similar underlying changes, which therefore do not complement each other.

1.5 Summary

The diagnosis and description of OCD are based on descriptive phenomenology, as represented by the DSM criteria, which are not founded on knowledge of etiology or pathophysiology. Yet, theoretical preconceptions have tended to sneak into the definition of OCD, such as the assumption that obsessions are the cause of compulsions. In addition, there is growing criticism of the DSM as the foundation for research in psychopathology, because this approach has failed to lead to solid advances in etiology and theory. We pick up this important theme in the next section.

Research shows that several treatments—pharmacological, neuromodulatory, and psychotherapeutic—are effective for OCD, but does not show why they work. It has sometimes been tempting to infer etiology from findings of effective treatment, but this is hazardous (just as it would be faulty to deduce that headache is caused by lack of aspirin). However, the fact that various treatments are effective holds out the promise that there must be some theoretical framework that would explain this effectiveness. More generally, investigating theories of OCD, including etiology and pathophysiology, requires a basic science discipline in which putative causes can be manipulated experimentally.

2. Toward a new perspective on psychiatric disorder

2.1 The RDoC

There is growing realization that reliance on DSM diagnostic criteria as the foundation for research on mental disorders has failed to lead to the development of theory and the discovery of underlying causes (Casey et al., 2013; Cuthbert, 2014; Hyman, 2010; Phillips et al., 2012). DSM-defined psychopathology has generated inconsistent etiological findings and has not served as a useful bridge to advances in neuroscience and genetics (Phillips et al., 2012). Large heterogeneity among people with the same diagnosis and pervasive issues of comorbidity have led critics to argue that DSM diagnoses "have increasingly been shown not to represent valid disease entities" (Cuthbert, 2014, p. 28) and have become an "unintended epistemic prison" (Hyman, 2010, p. 157) impeding research progress (Casey et al., 2013; Hengartner & Lehmann, 2017; Phillips et al., 2012).

A bold alternative to the DSM as the organizing framework for psychopathology is the recently proposed Research Domain Criteria project (RDoC; Cuthbert, 2014). One crucial theme of the RDoC is that research should shift toward a focus on symptoms as problematic patterns of behavior in themselves, rather than broader DSM-like categorical diagnoses, and adopt a more dimensional approach, addressing "the full range of variation, from normal to abnormal" (Casey et al., 2013, p. 812). A second crucial theme of the RDoC is that psychopathology research needs to have a much stronger foundation in neuroscience and genetics. To this end, the RDoC has specified basic types of brain systems to guide and organize psychopathology research: *Negative Valence Systems*, *Positive Valence Systems*, *Cognitive Systems*, *Systems for Social Processes*, and *Arousal/Modulatory Systems*. In addition, each of these brain systems can be studied at a variety of levels, leading to an *RDoC Matrix*, in which the types of brain systems are the rows and the columns are levels of investigation (*Units of Analysis*). At the core of these levels of investigation are *Brain Circuits*, with *Genes*, *Molecules*, and *Cells* as circuit constituents, and with *Physiological Responses*, *Behavior*, and phenomenology (*Self-Reports*) as circuit outputs. In summary, the proposed RDoC approach focuses on the following questions: "What is the normal distribution for a certain trait or characteristic; what is the brain system that primarily implements this function; and, how can we understand, at various levels of mechanism, what accounts for the development of dysregulation or dysfunction in these systems along normal-to-abnormal dimensions?" (Cuthbert, 2014, p. 31).

2.2 An adaptationist reorientation of the RDoC approach for OCD research

How well does the proposed RDoC approach apply to research on OCD? First, the shift toward a dimensional approach fits OCD, because its symptoms are widespread in the general population and reasonably normally distributed in degree (see Szechtman & Woody, 2004, for a review). However, the RDoC approach does not say much about how to make use of this apparent continuity from normal to abnormal. Second, the shift to more focus on underlying brain-systems is exciting for OCD research. However, OCD symptoms involve not just one, but most of the RDoC basic brain systems, namely, Negative Valence Systems (e.g., anxiety), Cognitive Systems (e.g., perception of potential threat, shifts in attention, etc.), Systems for Social Processes (e.g., perception of self and of others), and Arousal/Modulatory Systems (e.g., sustained arousal).

Nonetheless, we may readily reorient the RDoC approach by taking an adaptationist perspective guided by the following well-known statement: "Nothing in biology makes sense except in the light of evolution"

(Dobzhansky, 1973). According to such a perspective, "the architecture of each evolved system should reflect the computational requirements of the adaptive problem that selected for its design" (Sznycer, Cosmides, & Tooby, 2017, p. 56). That is, evolution selected for superordinate brain networks that coordinate brain systems to address particular classes of adaptive problems crucial for survival (Tooby & Cosmides, 1990; Tooby, Cosmides, Sell, Lieberman, & Sznycer, 2008). Rather than being located within any one RDoC-specified brain system, such a functional network "entrains many different 'components,' adjusting their thresholds and parameters, and shuts off others" (Sznycer et al., 2017, p. 57). Adopting this perspective, we propose that OCD is closely tied to a particular class of problems in adaptation, and thus to the functional network of component brain systems recruited through evolution to manage this class of problems.

Most OCD symptoms have a very prominent core theme: concern about preservation of self and others from potential harm, and engagement in precautionary behaviors to ward it off. Behaviors in OCD, such as checking and washing, are pervasive cross-culturally and of considerable evolutionary significance, not only in humans but also in many other animals. These considerations led to the insight that OCD symptoms can be understood as the dysfunctional release of fixed-action patterns preprogrammed through evolution (Fiske & Haslam, 1997; Rapoport, 1989; Wise & Rapoport, 1989).

Because managing risk from potential danger, such as contagion by disease or attack by predators, is essential for survival, it is highly plausible that evolution shaped brain networks for this. Ethologically oriented psychologists have sketched out a motivationally fundamental brain system directed toward the detection and amelioration of potential danger (e.g., Adams, 1979; Bolles & Fanselow, 1980; Gilbert, 1989; Marks & Nesse, 1994; Masterson & Crawford, 1982). Research on how animals manage potential threats (reviewed in Szechtman & Woody, 2004) illuminates the necessary properties of the underlying brain network. First, assessment of potential danger involves the detection and evaluation of uncertain, indirect cues for hidden risks, such as signs a predator may be in the area, which is quite different from perception of actual danger, such as being confronted by a predator. Second, detection of even weak cues suggesting potential danger readily activates a motivational state of vigilance and apprehension, which dissipates slowly even in the absence of further, validating cues. Third, this motivational state drives security-related behaviors, including precautionary actions such as checking, which involve probing and manipulating the environment to obtain further information, and preventative actions such as washing, which counter the potential danger before it eventuates. Fourth, unlike some other types of motivated behavior, security-related behavior is "open-ended" in the sense that the environment does not usually yield any consummatory stimulus to signal goal attainment. That is, even if the behavior pays off, the consequence is a non-event—nothing happens. Instead, it is engagement in the security-related behavior itself that needs to serve as a terminator for the motivational state and hence of the security-related behavior.

2.3 The security motivation system and OCD

Illuminated by this research, Szechtman and Woody (2004) advanced a model of the Security Motivation System (SMS). Fig. 1 shows its proposed functional components and their interconnections. The first functional component, *Appraisal of Potential Danger*, performs a perceptual-cognitive

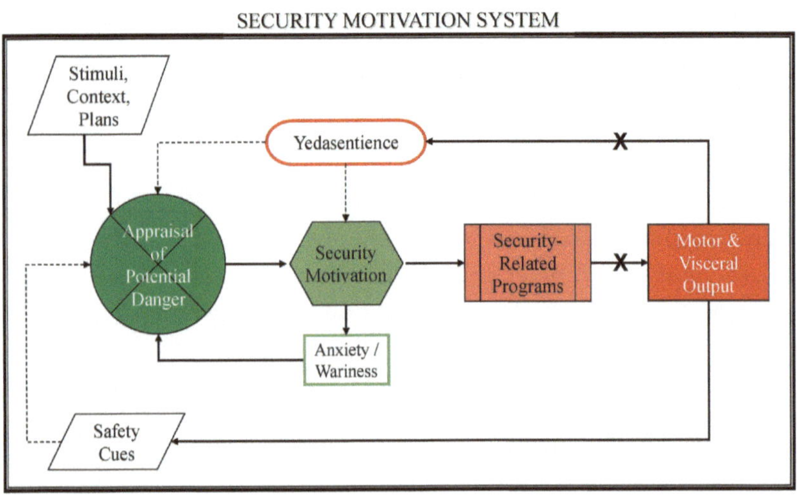

Fig. 1 A conceptual model of the security motivation system and sites of dysfunction producing OCD. Solid arrows indicate excitatory and dashed arrows inhibitory stimulation, respectively. *Yedasentience* output does not act on environmental input but rather on the *Appraisal of Potential Danger* and the *Security Motivation* modules to inhibit their activity. Exposure through motor output to "safety" stimuli provides inhibitory stimulation to *Appraisal of Potential Danger*. Pathways where a disruption of negative feedback could yield OCD are indicated by X. *Reprinted by permission from Woody, E. Z., & Szechtman, H. (2011). Adaptation to potential threat: The evolution, neurobiology, and psychopathology of the security motivation system.* Neuroscience and Biobehavioral Reviews, 35*(4), 1019–1033. doi:10.1016/j.neubiorev.2010.08.003.*

analysis of environmental stimuli to evaluate potential danger to self or others. Upon detecting potential danger, it activates the second component, *Security Motivation*, a motivational state with a protracted half-life. This, in turn, generates two coordinated outputs: *Anxiety*, providing a positive feedback loop to the *Appraisal* component to sustain the appraisal process, and excitation of a third major component, *Security-Related Programs*, which coordinates species-typical motor programs for the protection of self or others, such as checking or washing. Engagement in these behaviors generates the next functional component, *Motor and Visceral Output*. This output provides two possible routes of negative feedback: (1) an internal terminator signal, which Szechtman and Woody termed *Yedasentience*, that provides a sense of task completion and normally inhibits activity of both the *Security Motivation* and *Appraisal* subsystems; and (2) the enhancement of *Safety Cues*, which provides another, slower route for inhibition of the *Appraisal* subsystem.

Szechtman and Woody (2004) proposed that OCD results from a dysfunction in *deactivation* of the above-described biologically primal security motivation system. Specifically, in OCD potential-threat concerns are elicited in the normal way, but once activated, security-related thoughts and actions persist abnormally long because engagement in security-related behaviors is abnormally weak in shutting down the system. In Fig. 1, the X's illustrate how weakening of functional connections would yield OCD. A blockage from *Motor and Visceral Output* to *Yedasentience* would interfere with normal deactivation of the *Security Motivation* and *Appraisal* components. Thus, performance of precautionary behaviors would fail to provide the normal dampening of anxiety and the appraisal of potential danger, and continue for abnormal lengths of time. Alternatively, a blockage from *Species Typical Programs* to *Motor and Visceral Output* would interfere with engagement in the precautionary behaviors that serve as the basis for inhibitory feedback in the SMS. This scenario may correspond to the "pure obsessional" type of OCD (Emmelkamp & Kwee, 1977; Salkovskis & Westbrook, 1989; Steketee, 1993; Stern, 1978).

The SMS theory draws a crucial distinction between the dynamics of starting versus those of stopping in this system. Taylor, McKay, and Abramowitz (2005) critiqued this theory of OCD by arguing that OCD, in essence, is not a dysfunction of termination—that is, a stopping problem—but instead a dysfunction of excitation—that is, a starting problem (Woody & Szechtman, 2005). Subsequent research showed decisively that these critics were wrong: OCD patients differ strongly from normal controls in their stopping dynamics, but not in their starting dynamics (Hinds, Woody, Schmidt, Van Ameringen, & Szechtman, 2015; Hinds, Woody, Van Ameringen, Schmidt, & Szechtman, 2012).

2.4 Revisiting the main themes of the RDoC

This systems-design approach to understanding OCD addresses both main themes of the RDoC project (Cuthbert, 2014). One of these RDoC themes, as discussed earlier, is that psychopathology research should focus on symptoms as patterns of behavior of interest in themselves and take a dimensional view, explicitly linking the normal with the abnormal. In the proposed theoretical framework, psychopathology results from faulty dynamics in an underlying, normal motivational system. Regulatory dysfunction leads to the exaggeration of normal patterns, because when these behaviors are less appropriately regulated, they appear in simpler, but magnified form (Teitelbaum, 2012; Teitelbaum & Pellis, 1992). This linkage between normal and pathology means that the study of normal behavior informs psychopathology; likewise, the study of psychopathology, in turn, informs normal functioning, because some of its properties appear in a simpler or starker form (Jaspers, 1963).

A second main theme of the RDoC project is that psychopathology research should be solidly anchored in neuroscience; however, we noted earlier that OCD symptoms could not plausibly be located in any one RDoC-targeted basic brain system. Instead, our theoretical specification of the functional components of the SMS network, as in Fig. 1, suggests a network recruiting and organizing multiple brain systems. Fig. 2 presents our hypotheses about the brain circuits involved in this network, and Fig. 3 presents our hypotheses about the associated physiological pathways. Note that the indicated connections involve important feedback loops (Kendler, 2008). The set of interlocking hypotheses represented by Figs. 2 and 3 make use of knowledge from basic neuroscience about the brain systems that could perform these component processes (Szechtman & Woody, 2004; Woody & Szechtman, 2011)—for example, the cascading functional loops in Fig. 2 are partly based on the cortico-striato-pallido-thalamo-cortical connections pioneered by Alexander, DeLong, and Strick (1986).

Finally, in keeping with the RDoC goal of fostering novel research directions, this adaptationist, systems-design approach has important implications for the role of animal models in preclinical research on OCD. Research using animal models, rather than attempting to imitate the

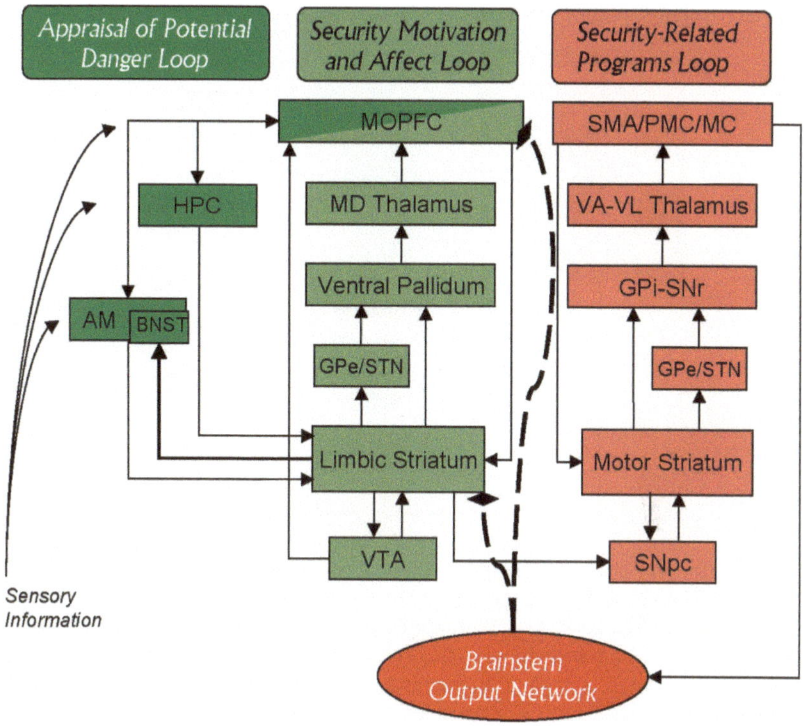

Fig. 2 A neural circuit model of the security motivation system. Each of the four distinct subcircuits (loops) subserves one of the functional components in Fig. 1 and identified by corresponding colors. The dashed line indicates possible sites of yedasentience feedback inhibition. *Abbreviations*: AM, amygdala; BNST, bed nucleus of the stria terminalis; GPe, external segment of the globus pallidus; GPi, internal segment of the globus pallidus; HPC, hippocampus; MC, motor cortex; MD, Thalamus, mediodorsal thalamic nucleus; MOPFC, medial prefrontal cortex and orbital prefrontal cortex; PMC, premotor cortex; SMA, supplementary motor area; SNpc, substantia nigra pars compacta; SNr, substantia nigra pars reticulata; STN, subthalamic nucleus; VA, ventroanterior thalamic nucleus; VL, ventrolateral thalamic nucleus; VTA, ventral tegmental area. *Reprinted by permission from Woody, E. Z., & Szechtman, H. (2011). Adaptation to potential threat: The evolution, neurobiology, and psychopathology of the security motivation system.* Neuroscience and Biobehavioral Reviews, 35*(4), 1019–1033. doi:10.1016/j.neubiorev.2010.08.003.*

descriptive phenomenology of psychiatric disorders, should move toward the experimental investigation of *theories* of psychiatric disorders (Davis & Isles, 2014; Hyman, 2010; Kendler, 2008; Nestler & Hyman, 2010). In keeping with the RDoC theme of multiple levels of investigation, the functioning of a network like the SMS is affected by multiple types of factors, including genetics, learning, environmental conditions, and drugs,

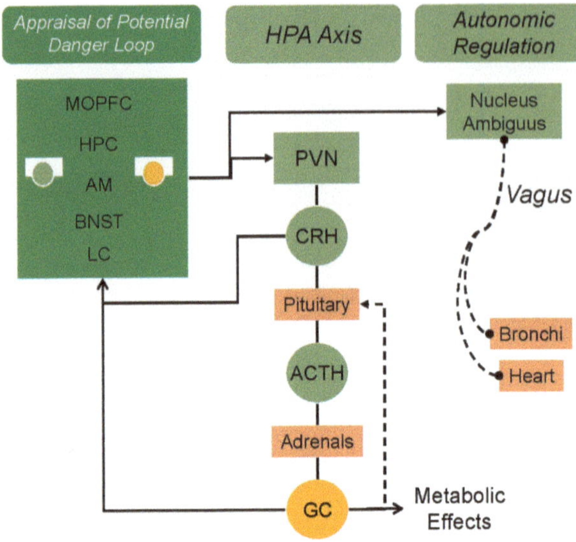

Fig. 3 The physiological network associated with security motivation. The *Appraisal of Potential Danger Loop* of Fig. 2 connects with the *HPA Axis*, which has both input from and output to the Appraisal Loop. Within the Appraisal Loop there are receptors for CRH and GC, denoted by the respective circles in white rectangles, by which HPA can modulate it; CHR also acts as a neurotransmitter within the Appraisal Loop. Finally, the Appraisal Loop affects *Autonomic Regulation*, by which the myelinated vagus modulates the bronchi and heart. *Abbreviations*: AM, amygdala; BNST, bed nucleus of the stria terminalis; CRH, corticotropin-releasing hormone; GC, glucocorticoids; HPC, hippocampus; LC, locus coeruleus; MOPFC, medial prefrontal cortex and orbital prefrontal cortex; PVN, paraventricular nucleus. *Reprinted by permission from Woody, E. Z., & Szechtman, H. (2011). Adaptation to potential threat: The evolution, neurobiology, and psychopathology of the security motivation system.* Neuroscience and Biobehavioral Reviews, 35*(4), 1019–1033. doi:10.1016/j.neubiorev.2010.08.003.*

which operate at multiple levels, including neuroanatomy, component circuits and programs, and neurochemistry. Animal research is important to investigate the basic mechanisms by which this functional network operates, to trace the dynamics of its normal functioning, to observe the effects of environmental conditions and learning on it, and to study its plasticity, including hypotheses about how to boost aspects of the system to improve its dynamics in the case of dysfunction. Moreover, findings from animal research can be translated into insightful programs of research with humans, as shown in some of our own work (e.g., Hinds et al., 2015, 2012), demonstrating the power of a comparative approach across species.

3. Toward a new perspective on treatment for OCD

3.1 Some key aspects of the SMS for OCD pharmacotherapeutics

The previous section has addressed the need to revise our conception of psychiatric disorder, and hence our approach to research on OCD. From this need to reconceptualize disorder, it follows that there is a corresponding need to revise our conception of the role of pharmacological intervention. To illustrate, in this section we use the SMS theory as a framework for developing some ideas about research on pharmacological treatment of OCD. Specifically, we address how to conceptualize what is needed and where to look for new possibilities.

Let's first briefly summarize some key aspects of the SMS theory of OCD that will provide a framework for our discussion of the role of pharmacological intervention in OCD. First, underlying OCD is hypothesized to be a special motivational system, which in most individuals is normal and adaptive in managing the detection of and response to potential danger. Because this is a normal system present and operating in everyone, we need to be careful in distinguishing what specific aspects of this system are pathological in OCD.

In particular, activation of security motivation in the face of cues for potential danger is normal, as is the subsequent engagement in protective and precautionary behaviors. For example, consider research in non-clinical samples linking hormonal changes with putative OCD symptoms. In a study by Dillon and Brooks (1992), healthy women self-reported an increase in "unusual" cleaning behaviors, including excessive cleaning and cleaning of things that were not typically cleaned, during the luteal phase of the menstrual cycle. Fleischman and Fessler (2011) reported that healthy women experienced a luteal phase increase in behaviors related to self-cleanliness, grooming, and protection from germs. Pregnancy and childbirth have also been associated with behaviors reminiscent of OCD symptoms in individuals not previously diagnosed with OCD, such as intrusive thoughts about some horrible accident happening to the infant, contamination or illness, or thoughts about intentionally harming the baby (Abramowitz, Nelson, Rygwall, & Khandker, 2007; Leckman et al., 1999). In some cases, these thoughts were accompanied by repeatedly checking the baby even though they "knew everything was fine" (Abramowitz et al., 2007; Leckman et al., 1999). These observations may be interesting findings, but from the perspective of the SMS theory, they are not akin to OCD, because they merely involve variants of normal SMS activation and the behavioral responses it evokes.

According to the SMS theory of OCD, it is not the activation of security motivation and the resulting protective behavior that is the crucial fault in OCD; instead, it is the termination or stopping process. In the regulatory networks that govern motivational processes, activation and termination dynamics are quite distinct (Park & van Leeuwen, 2014). The hypothesis that the crucial defect is difficulty in stopping—that is, terminating SMS activation (Hinds et al., 2012)—may be an important clue to guide research on possible pharmacological treatments, as we discuss later.

Although changes that increase the tendency of the SMS to become activated do not cause OCD, they could nonetheless make pre-existing OCD worse. This is because the stopping deficit in OCD comes into play whenever the system has been activated. For example, Guglielmi et al. (2014) found that about 38% women diagnosed with OCD reported an exacerbation of existing symptoms during the week prior to menses, and around 40% experienced a worsening of symptoms during pregnancy or shortly after childbirth.

Thus, activation dynamics could be relevant for pharmacological research in a secondary way, because activation of the SMS is a necessary precondition for the stopping deficit in OCD to become problematic. In summary, the core deficit in OCD is stopping, so this may be the main place to look for pharmacological interventions; nonetheless, starting is not irrelevant, because reducing the likelihood of activation may effectively bypass the stopping deficit.

A further key aspect of the SMS theory of OCD is that the SMS is hypothesized to be a network coordinating activity across multiple brain systems, with information flowing through feedback loops, which also involve autonomic regulation and the HPA axis (Woody & Szechtman, 2011). This systemic approach is in accord with the recent shift in neuroscience from a relatively narrow localizationist perspective to a perspective that considers an entire functional network (e.g., Boes et al., 2015; Darby, Laganiere, Pascual-Leone, Prasad, & Fox, 2017; Shine & Poldrack, 2018). Such brain networks, rather than consisting of straightforward additive mechanisms, are likely to include "multiple nonlinear interactions and causal loops" (Kendler, 2008, p. 695). As West (2017) has argued, "A typical complex system is composed of myriad individual constituents or agents that once aggregated take on collective characteristics that are usually not manifested in, nor could easily be predicted from, the properties of the individual components themselves" (p. 21). This perspective draws our attention to the functional integrity of information flow throughout the network, and, in particular, to the prospects for enhancing or restoring it in OCD. Because of the complexity of the system, there are likely many factors that could influence the nature of this information flow, although it is also possible that because of the self-correcting qualities of feedback loops, the effect of any one influence may be limited.

With the foregoing points as a guiding framework, we now turn to a consideration of alternative ways to conceptualize potential targets for pharmacological intervention in OCD. These alternatives sketch out very different approaches to looking for a pharmacological agent to treat OCD.

3.2 The traditional approach: Discover *magic bullets*

There is an extensive literature addressing the very wide range of factors that appear to affect the expression of OCD and OCD-like behaviors. These influences include biological vulnerability factors (e.g., genetics and biological sex), chemical agents (e.g., serotonin, dopamine, glutamate, and GABA modulators), endogenous processes (e.g., oxidative stress, neuroinflammation, etc.), and tonic states (e.g., age, altered immune responses, reproductive state, etc.). Our impression is that underlying much of this body of work is the hope that somewhere among all these findings may lurk the clue or set of clues that will lead to an agent with a strong and specific, corrective effect on OCD—a "magic bullet," so to speak. However, this hope may be misguided, as should become evident from a consideration below of the historical roots of the "magic bullet" concept.

There is something paradoxical in Paul Ehrlich, the 1908 Nobel Laureate, calling the compounds he developed for the treatment of syphilis, "magic bullets" (Bosch & Rosich, 2008). It is paradoxical because the route to these compounds was not "magic" but exemplary basic science research which revealed that the "biological effect of a chemical compound depends on its chemical composition and the cell on which it acts" (Strebhardt & Ullrich, 2008, p. 473). Ehrlich was struck by the observation that different dyes selectively stained a different biological component of an organism; for instance, methylene blue, a phenothiazine dye, preferentially stained bacterial microorganisms and cell nuclei, and "in living tissue, … methylene blue selectively stained certain nerve fibers – sensory, olfactory and in the medulla oblongata" (Witkop, 1982, p. 149). In further pursuit of this seminal observation of selective histochemical staining, Ehrlich developed the side-chain (receptor) theory and the concept that the biological or pharmacological effect of a chemical substance is exerted by specific "chemical groups" in the molecule, a concept that evolved into what today is termed "pharmacophore" (Guner & Bowen, 2014). In analogy with the dual-action theory of dyes, where one chemical moiety is responsible for anchoring (binding) the dyestuff to the fabric or tissue and another chemical grouping (chromophore) is responsible for imparting coloring of the stain, Ehrlich conceptualized that molecules such as bacterial toxins have two chemically differentiated parts in their molecule. One part of the toxin molecule is a chemical group (called *haptophore*) which causes the molecule to bind selectively to receptors on certain cells. Upon being attached to these certain receptors, the other part of the molecule, a chemical group called *toxophore*, exerts then its characteristic biologic effect on those cells. For the bacterial toxin molecules attached to receptors of the host cells, the biologic effect of the toxophore would involve "poisoning" the cells of the host. Ehrlich applied this concept to search for and design drugs for the treatment of infectious diseases as well as cancerous tumors. The search strategy was for compounds that attach selectively to specific microorganisms (such as the bacteria which result in syphilis) and where the biologic effect of the toxophore would be to poison the foreign bacteria. Moreover, to the extent that it was possible to construct the drug as to be highly selective for the pathogen without having affinity for host receptors, there would be no toxicity to the cells of the infected host. The antisyphilitic compound, Salvarsan, was one of the first such rationally discovered and designed therapeutic drugs (Guner & Bowen, 2014; Witkop, 1982).

Although Ehrlich advocated more generally that medicinal chemists must "learn to take aim in a chemical way" (Witkop, 1982, p. 151), such attacks can work well principally if the "enemy" is a bacteria, parasite, or virus that has a unique chemical signature, absent in the host. In those circumstances a "bullet" with seemingly truly "magical" properties is plausible, as a drug could be synthesized which would target the infectious enemy, so to speak, but would not strike the indigenous cells of the host itself. Unfortunately, for psychiatric disorders that are not caused by an infectious agent but reflect instead some dynamic disturbance in the operation of a normal system, the quest for a "magic bullet" is probably inappropriate: It seems extremely unlikely that the disturbed normal system would have a unique chemical signature, absent in the intact normal brain systems. This is because all brain systems are constructed from the same pool of elemental constituents—it is the pattern of connectivity that gives each system a different functional property.

Even without there being any infection, a normal system can become "out-of-tune" and the ensuing discordance in system dynamics may produce symptoms characteristic of a psychiatric disorder, as we hypothesize is the case in OCD. In those situations, with no apparent malicious "enemy" to eliminate, the pharmacological strategy for a therapeutic effect should focus instead on targets that could rebalance the dysfunctional system back toward normal operation. We next consider some alternative ways to conceptualize how to do this.

3.3 The *elixir of life* approach: Boost processing power of the brain

While the "magic bullets" approach prizes specificity—drugs that target only an invading "enemy" without damaging the host—the strategy we call the *elixir of life* approach is, by contrast, non-specific. Here, rather than a direct effect on a faulty element itself, the aim of pharmacotherapy is a global enhancement of brain processing.

We call this the *elixir of life* approach, as alongside the quest for "magic bullets" to cure all ills, there is a long-standing tradition to find the *Elixir of Life*, a "magical" substance or liquid that gives eternal life (Wikipedia Contributors, 2018). The focus of this quest is not a potion that can repair the damage already inflicted. Rather, the focus is on an intervention that will boost the workings of the healthy body—enhance bodily normal processes, making life enduring and resilient to potential harms. In today's terminology, it can be said that the target of the *elixir of life* is the "infrastructure" of a healthy body—all the biological facilities needed for the body, and the brain in particular, to operate well, enabling the various specialized systems to better carry out their specific functions.

From the perspective of OCD as a disturbance in SMS dynamics, it is a reasonable therapeutic option to evaluate whether SMS function is brought back toward normal operation with some boost to "infrastructure" facilities. This is a reasonable therapeutic option as it is possible for SMS to become out-of-balance not because of a fault in the security motivation system itself but rather because the SMS is not reliably receiving some infrastructure input to operate properly. By boosting infrastructure, an oversupply of needed inputs may be present and given this surfeit, the vulnerable neural constituents can perform properly, bringing to normal the operation of security motivation.

Clearly, boosting infrastructure facilities is a "non-specific" intervention as the enhanced supply of vital ingredients helps not only a compromised SMS but is of potential value to all brain systems. However, it is not necessarily the case that every brain system would function at a superior level after the infrastructure boost as some systems could already operate at maximum efficiency. In those cases an infrastructure boost merely provides an oversupply of materials, without operational utility.

It may be of value to illustrate the logic of the proposed approach by analogy with efforts to regulate the economy. There are many tools to stimulate the economy, without identifying what is the core problem or fixing the problem directly. For instance, cutting taxes or lowering the interest rate may be used even though neither one is the cause of the poorly functional economy. Yet these interventions, which target the infrastructure of economic activity, may raise economic growth though clearly not by aiding every component of the economic system or even the ones that were in trouble.

The following is an example of boosting the biological infrastructure of relevance to OCD. Perhaps surprisingly, some current treatments for OCD can be interpreted as in fact boosting infrastructure facilities.

In a recent PET study using $[^{11}C]$-α-methyl-L-tryptophan as a tracer for serotonin synthesis, the authors observed that 10 of 16 OCD patients who responded well to a 12 week course of treatment with either the SSRI sertraline or CBT showed a "brain-wide, rather than localized, enhancement of central 5-HT synthesis capacity" (Lissemore et al., 2018). From these and additional observations, the authors suggested that "increases in 5-HT synthesis capacity with effective treatment support a *compensatory*, rather than pathological, role of 5-HT neurotransmission in OCD" (Lissemore et al., 2018). Stated in another way, the neurobiological change associated with a shift away from OCD and toward normal function was not specific to any particular brain region but available to the entire brain, as befits boosting the operation of an infrastructure facility. Indeed, brain serotonin systems have a hallmark property of an infrastructure facility in that a set of neurons concentrated in a relatively small region of the brain (*nuclei raphes lineares*) can have a widespread impact by virtue of innervating almost the entire CNS (Charnay & Leger, 2010; Fidalgo, Ivanov, & Wood, 2013; Jacobs & Azmitia, 1992). The fact that treatments which target serotonin neurotransmission are effective not only for OCD but also for a number of psychiatric disorders (Katzman et al., 2014) further supports the notion of an infrastructure boost as the therapeutic mechanism. Moreover, it had been commented that "serotonin is an enigma. It is at once implicated in virtually everything, but responsible for nothing" (Jacobs & Fornal, 1995, p. 461). However, this characterization of serotonin is not an enigma but an apt description of an infrastructure facility.

From the perspective of OCD as a disturbance in SMS dynamics, what could be the nature of the infrastructure support provided by serotonin signal transduction? One reasonable possibility is that the monoamine systems (serotonin, dopamine and norepinephrine) constitute a network managing brain "arousal" (Pfaff, 2006), where arousal is a label for the category of neurobiological processes needed for operational efficiency by neurons and neural circuits to perform their specialized functions, including analysis of stimuli, integrating various inputs, computing appropriate outputs and coordinating motor behavior. The arousal infrastructure involves quite complex molecular, biochemical, endocrine and genetic mechanisms and includes the provision of energy, nutrients, and removal of waste products, all of which are impacted by serotonin (Azmitia, 2001; Charnay & Leger, 2010; Fidalgo et al., 2013). Accordingly, out-of-tune SMS dynamics may shift toward normal operation by benefiting from a boost in the management of arousal as provided by a regulated injection of serotonin activity.

Not only serotonin but also dopamine systems have a neuroanatomy indicative of an infrastructure facility (a circumscribed location of neurons yet relatively widespread innervation). As noted before, drugs targeting dopamine neurotransmission may augment effectiveness of SSRI treatment in OCD (Dold et al., 2015; Veale et al., 2014). From the perspective advanced here this clinical observation indicates that another tool impacting arousal is modulation of dopamine activity. However, it seems unlikely that both serotonin and dopamine do the same job. More likely, they each play different but complementary regulatory roles in managing arousal. One notion proposed often for dopamine and serotonin is that the former acts to instigate arousal and approach while the latter promotes deactivation of arousal, with the two systems operating in fine balance and in a coordinated manner (Alex & Pehek, 2007; Di Giovanni, Di Matteo, Pierucci, & Esposito, 2008; Kapur & Remington, 1996; Soubrie, 1986; Szechtman & Woody, 2004), a notion supported by studies with animal models of OCD (Alkhatib, Dvorkin-Gheva, & Szechtman, 2013; Johnson & Szechtman, 2016; Tucci, Dvorkin-Gheva, Johnson, et al., 2014; Tucci, Dvorkin-Gheva, Sharma, et al., 2014). Accordingly, out-of-tune SMS dynamics may shift toward normal operation when supplied with an appropriate level of arousal as provided by interventions that adjust the balance of dopamine and serotonin activity.

Although in the clinic OCD pharmacotherapy does not include agents that target specifically norepinephrine, this possibility should be investigated since norepinephrine pathways are also part of the arousal network (Pfaff, 2006). A rational approach for such an endeavor should entail basic science research to identify the particular jobs that serotonin, dopamine and norepinephrine perform in management of arousal.

Not only drugs but a broad range of methods should be considered for an infrastructure boost, ranging from nutrition, hormones and electrical brain stimulation to exercise and behavioral interventions that foster a positive attitude and reduce stress, for example.

3.4 Facilitating relearning: Promote neural plasticity

As noted in the first section of this article, psychotherapy can ameliorate OCD. From the perspective of OCD as a disturbance in SMS dynamics, this effectiveness demonstrates that the operation of the SMS can be nudged toward normal processing by means of psychological intervention. Although the specific mechanisms underlying the effectiveness of psychotherapy have not yet been identified, nevertheless it must be the case that the intervention process includes acquisition of new information and reorganization of the knowledge network used by the SMS—that is, a process of learning or relearning.

Thus, another important approach to OCD pharmacotherapy can be drugs that facilitate new learning, for example, by enhancing neural plasticity. Pharmacological treatment might help patients become more open to new ways to perceive and behave with regard to potential dangers, promoting the restoration of the normal operation of the SMS. This approach is quite different from, for example, the prescription of an antibiotic for an infection, in which the drug alone may be effective without any further effort or action taken by the patient. Instead, it would be essential that circumstances in which new learning can take place accompany administration of the drug. In short, pharmacological intervention may act directly on signal transduction processes to engage synaptic plasticity, and thereby, given appropriate opportunities for new learning, enable the needed shift in how problems of potential danger are processed.

Along these lines, recently several studies have examined the possibility that drugs that are cognitive enhancers, such as D-cycloserine (DCS), may augment the effectiveness of ERP (Sulkowski et al., 2014). The rationale is that the cognitive enhancer would augment learning and memory processes elicited by psychotherapy. Although some findings for OCD are promising (de Leeuw, van Megen, Kahn, & Westenberg, 2017), meta-analyses indicate rather mixed results, with future research needed to address the role of therapy characteristics in drug-augmented outcomes (Mataix-Cols et al., 2017; McGuire, Wu, Piacentini, McCracken, & Storch, 2017).

The SMS theory of OCD may provide a useful perspective on the kinds of learning that occur in psychotherapy that could be augmented by cognitive enhancers. Specifically, some kinds of learning focus on the input side of the SMS—that is, the appraisal of potential danger. A likely effect of ERP is to reduce the OCD patient's sensitivity to cues for potential danger, so that the system is less readily activated, thus bypassing the main underlying dysfunction in shutting down the system (Woody & Szechtman, 2005). Accordingly, one effect of cognitive enhancers would be to promote this kind of desensitization process. However, another important kind of learning focuses on the output side of the SMS—that is, engagement in preventative behavior and its negative feedback effect, through a sense of task completion, to shut down activation of the SMS. This is an avenue for the effect of cognitive enhancers that would be quite distinct from promoting desensitization.

In ERP, the patient's relearning is typically guided by instructions not to engage in security-related responses when faced with cues for potential danger. In a sense, output is suppressed; however, this circumstance clearly does not approach what is normal for the SMS. The normal process in the SMS is for activation of the system to lead to the performance of security-related behaviors, and in the normal case the individual has typically learned some behavior or set of behaviors that afford the sense of task completion to shut down the system. Thus, the de-emphasis on behavioral output in ERP is quite unlike how the SMS operates normally. A closer approximation to normal functioning of the SMS would be for OCD patients to learn security-related behaviors that are more moderate or less extended in time, but that come to be associated with yedasentience, or the feeling of task completion. Cognitive enhancers could be of particular benefit for such learning.

In addition to cognitive-enhancer drugs, there are other important possibilities for interventions that could increase plasticity and foster relearning. These include immune modulation (Yirmiya & Goshen, 2011), glutamate drugs, and rTMS. In using these augmentation methods, it will be important to conceptualize clearly what kind of learning is being promoted, as described above.

3.5 Fixing a weak link: Target specific pathways of the SMS network

We noted earlier that for most instances of OCD the discovery of a "magic bullet" seems unlikely; nonetheless, this does not rule out other approaches that may be relatively specific in their effect. In particular, the SMS theory of OCD hypothesizes specifically that it is the system-termination or stopping dynamics that are the crucial defect in OCD. Thus, a promising place to look may be drugs that enhance or otherwise modulate the negative-feedback loop, associated with yedasentience, that plays a crucial role in shutting down SMS activation.

To proceed along these lines, we need basic science research to elucidate the neurobiological mechanism of yedasentience. Because a major function of the SMS, in the face of cues for potential danger, is to prepare the organism for the possibility of imminent danger by priming the neurobiology of systems that handle imminent danger (Woody & Szechtman, 2011). A sensible conjecture, then, would be that the SMS shares some of the neurobiology of these imminent-danger systems. For example, consider the potential threat of infection, for which imminent danger is handled by the immune system. It would make sense that the SMS, as part of its operational mechanisms, would utilize immune-signal transduction pathways. Indeed, these immune-system pathways include their own stop signals, both to limit inadvertent activation of immune responses and to shut down the immune system once it has been activated. Part of the stop mechanism for the SMS may be the same, conceivably, for example, making use of the recently identified "checkpoints" that arrest immune-cell activity (Graeber, 2018; Wei, Duffy, & Allison, 2018).

4. Conclusion

As we have pointed out, many of the treatments for OCD arose somewhat serendipitously, without a strong theoretical rationale. Perhaps this is not surprising, given the lack of a good theory of OCD. However, as the RDoC project has emphasized, there are important limitations to a basically atheoretical approach in the search for better treatments, as well as in uncovering the neurobiology of the disorder. Using the SMS theory of OCD, this article has illustrated the advantages of a more theoretically driven approach, which helps to clarify underlying processes and points in potentially productive directions for the development of treatments.

Conflict of interest

The authors have no conflicts of interest to declare.

References

Abramowitz, J. S. (2018). Presidential address: Are the obsessive-compulsive related disorders related to obsessive-compulsive disorder? A critical look at DSM-5's new category. *Behavior Therapy*, *49*(1), 1–11. https://doi.org/10.1016/j.beth.2017.06.002.

Abramowitz, J. S., Nelson, C. A., Rygwall, R., & Khandker, M. (2007). The cognitive mediation of obsessive-compulsive symptoms: A longitudinal study. *Journal of Anxiety Disorders*, *21*(1), 91–104. https://doi.org/10.1016/j.janxdis.2006.05.003.

Adams, D. B. (1979). Brain mechanisms for offense, defense, and submission. *The Behavioral and Brain Sciences*, *2*(2), 201–213. https://doi.org/10.1017/S0140525x00061926.

Alex, K. D., & Pehek, E. A. (2007). Pharmacologic mechanisms of serotonergic regulation of dopamine neurotransmission. *Pharmacology and Therapeutics*, *113*(2), 296–320. https://doi.org/10.1016/j.pharmthera.2006.08.004.

Alexander, G. E., DeLong, M. R., & Strick, P. L. (1986). Parallel organization of functionally segregated circuits linking basal ganglia and cortex. *Annual Review of Neuroscience*, *9*, 357–381. https://doi.org/10.1146/annurev.ne.09.030186.002041.

Alkhatib, A. H., Dvorkin-Gheva, A., & Szechtman, H. (2013). Quinpirole and 8-OH-DPAT induce compulsive checking behavior in male rats by acting on different functional parts of an OCD neurocircuit. *Behavioural Pharmacology*, *24*(1), 65–73. https://doi.org/10.1097/FBP.0b013e32835d5b7a.

American Psychiatric Association. (2013). *Diagnostic and statistical manual of mental disorders (DSM-5®)*. Arlington, VA: American Psychiatric Pub.

Ananth, J. (1986). Clomipramine: An antiobsessive drug. *Canadian Journal of Psychiatry. Revue Canadienne de Psychiatrie*, *31*(3), 253–258.

Azmitia, E. C. (2001). Modern views on an ancient chemical: Serotonin effects on cell proliferation, maturation, and apoptosis. *Brain Research Bulletin*, *56*(5), 413–424.

Bari, A. A., Mikell, C. B., Abosch, A., Ben-Haim, S., Buchanan, R. J., Burton, A. W., et al. (2018). Charting the road forward in psychiatric neurosurgery: Proceedings of the 2016 American Society for stereotactic and functional neurosurgery workshop on neuromodulation for psychiatric disorders. *Journal of Neurology, Neurosurgery, and Psychiatry*, *89*(8), 886–896. https://doi.org/10.1136/jnnp-2017-317082.

Bear, R. E., Fitzgerald, P., Rosenfeld, J. V., & Bittar, R. G. (2010). Neurosurgery for obsessive-compulsive disorder: Contemporary approaches. *Journal of Clinical Neuroscience*, *17*(1), 1–5. https://doi.org/10.1016/j.jocn.2009.02.043.

Benabid, A. L. (2003). Deep brain stimulation for Parkinson's disease. *Current Opinion in Neurobiology*, *13*(6), 696–706.

Boes, A. D., Prasad, S., Liu, H., Liu, Q., Pascual-Leone, A., Caviness, V. S., Jr., et al. (2015). Network localization of neurological symptoms from focal brain lesions. *Brain*, *138*(Pt 10), 3061–3075. https://doi.org/10.1093/brain/awv228.

Bolkan, S. S., Carvalho Poyraz, F., & Kellendonk, C. (2016). Using human brain imaging studies as a guide toward animal models of schizophrenia. *Neuroscience*, *321*, 77–98. https://doi.org/10.1016/j.neuroscience.2015.05.055.

Bolles, R. C., & Fanselow, M. S. (1980). A perceptual-defensive-recuperative model of fear and pain. *The Behavioral and Brain Sciences*, *3*(2), 291–301. https://doi.org/10.1017/S0140525x0000491x.

Bosch, F., & Rosich, L. (2008). The contributions of Paul Ehrlich to pharmacology: A tribute on the occasion of the centenary of his nobel prize. *Pharmacology*, *82*(3), 171–179. https://doi.org/10.1159/000149583.

Brunelin, J., Mondino, M., Bation, R., Palm, U., Saoud, M., & Poulet, E. (2018). Transcranial direct current stimulation for obsessive-compulsive disorder: A systematic review. *Brain Sciences*, *8*(2), 37. https://doi.org/10.3390/brainsci8020037.

Carmi, L., Alyagon, U., Barnea-Ygael, N., Zohar, J., Dar, R., & Zangen, A. (2018). Clinical and electrophysiological outcomes of deep TMS over the medial prefrontal and anterior cingulate cortices in OCD patients. *Brain Stimulation*, *11*(1), 158–165. https://doi.org/10.1016/j.brs.2017.09.004.

Casey, B. J., Craddock, N., Cuthbert, B. N., Hyman, S. E., Lee, F. S., & Ressler, K. J. (2013). DSM-5 and RDoC: Progress in psychiatry research? *Nature Reviews. Neuroscience*, *14*(11), 810–814. https://doi.org/10.1038/nrn3621.

Charnay, Y., & Leger, L. (2010). Brain serotonergic circuitries. *Dialogues in Clinical Neuroscience*, *12*(4), 471–487.

Clomipramine Collaborative Study Group. (1991). Clomipramine in the treatment of patients with obsessive-compulsive disorder. The clomipramine collaborative study group. *Archives of General Psychiatry*, *48*(8), 730–738. https://doi.org/10.1001/archpsyc.1991.01810320054008.

Cordoba Fernandez, E., & Lopez Ibor Alino, J. J. (1967). Monochlorimipramine in psychiatric patients resistant to other forms of treatment. *Acta Luso-Espanolas Neurologia y Psiquiatrica*, *26*, 119–147.

Cuthbert, B. N. (2014). The RDoC framework: Facilitating transition from ICD/DSM to dimensional approaches that integrate neuroscience and psychopathology. *World Psychiatry*, *13*(1), 28–35. https://doi.org/10.1002/wps.20087.

Darby, R. R., Laganiere, S., Pascual-Leone, A., Prasad, S., & Fox, M. D. (2017). Finding the imposter: Brain connectivity of lesions causing delusional misidentifications. *Brain*, *140*(2), 497–507. https://doi.org/10.1093/brain/aww288.

Davis, B. A., & Isles, A. R. (2014). Modelling the genetic contribution to mental illness: A timely end for the psychiatric rodent? *European Journal of Neuroscience*, *39*(11), 1933–1942. https://doi.org/10.1111/ejn.12607.

de Leeuw, A. S., van Megen, H. J., Kahn, R. S., & Westenberg, H. G. (2017). D-Cycloserine addition to exposure sessions in the treatment of patients with obsessive-compulsive disorder. *European Psychiatry*, *40*, 38–44. https://doi.org/10.1016/j.eurpsy.2016.06.011.

Denys, D., Mantione, M., Figee, M., van den Munckhof, P., Koerselman, F., Westenberg, H., et al. (2010). Deep brain stimulation of the nucleus accumbens for treatment-refractory obsessive-compulsive disorder. *Archives of General Psychiatry*, *67*(10), 1061–1068. https://doi.org/10.1001/archgenpsychiatry.2010.122.

Di Giovanni, G., Di Matteo, V., Pierucci, M., & Esposito, E. (2008). Serotonin-dopamine interaction: Electrophysiological evidence. In G. DiGiovanni, V. DiMatteo, & E. Esposito (Eds.), *Vol. 172. Serotonin-dopamine interaction: Experimental evidence and therapeutic relevance* (pp. 45–71). Amsterdam: Elsevier Science Bv.

Dillon, K. M., & Brooks, D. (1992). Unusual cleaning behavior in the luteal phase. *Psychological Reports*, *70*(1), 35–39. https://doi.org/10.2466/pr0.1992.70.1.35.

Dobzhansky, T. (1973). Nothing in biology makes sense except in the light of evolution. *The American Biology Teacher*, *35*(3), 125–129. https://doi.org/10.2307/4444260.

Dold, M., Aigner, M., Lanzenberger, R., & Kasper, S. (2013). Antipsychotic augmentation of serotonin reuptake inhibitors in treatment-resistant obsessive-compulsive disorder: A meta-analysis of double-blind, randomized, placebo-controlled trials. *International Journal of Neuropsychopharmacology*, *16*(3), 557–574. https://doi.org/10.1017/S1461145712000740.

Dold, M., Aigner, M., Lanzenberger, R., & Kasper, S. (2015). Antipsychotic augmentation of serotonin reuptake inhibitors in treatment-resistant obsessive-compulsive disorder: An update meta-analysis of double-blind, randomized, placebo-controlled trials. *International Journal of Neuropsychopharmacology*, *18*(9). https://doi.org/10.1093/ijnp/pyv047. pyv047.

Emmelkamp, P. M., & Kwee, K. G. (1977). Obsessional ruminations: A comparison between thought-stopping and prolonged exposure in imagination. *Behaviour Research and Therapy*, *15*(5), 441–444.

Fidalgo, S., Ivanov, D. K., & Wood, S. H. (2013). Serotonin: From top to bottom. *Biogerontology*, *14*(1), 21–45. https://doi.org/10.1007/s10522-012-9406-3.

Fineberg, N. A., Reghunandanan, S., Simpson, H. B., Phillips, K. A., Richter, M. A., Matthews, K., et al. (2015). Obsessive-compulsive disorder (OCD): Practical strategies for pharmacological and somatic treatment in adults. *Psychiatry Research*, *227*(1), 114–125. https://doi.org/10.1016/j.psychres.2014.12.003.

Fiske, A. P., & Haslam, N. (1997). Is obsessive-compulsive disorder a pathology of the human disposition to perform socially meaningful rituals? Evidence of similar content. *Journal of Nervous and Mental Disease*, *185*(4), 211–222.

Fleischman, D. S., & Fessler, D. M. (2011). Progesterone's effects on the psychology of disease avoidance: Support for the compensatory behavioral prophylaxis hypothesis. *Hormones and Behavior*, *59*(2), 271–275. https://doi.org/10.1016/j.yhbeh.2010.11.014.

Foa, E. B. (2010). Cognitive behavioral therapy of obsessive-compulsive disorder. *Dialogues in Clinical Neuroscience*, *12*(2), 199–207.

Foa, E. B., Liebowitz, M. R., Kozak, M. J., Davies, S., Campeas, R., Franklin, M. E., et al. (2005). Randomized, placebo-controlled trial of exposure and ritual prevention, clomipramine, and their combination in the treatment of obsessive-compulsive disorder. *American Journal of Psychiatry*, *162*(1), 151–161. https://doi.org/10.1176/appi.ajp.162.1.151.

Foa, E. B., Steketee, G., Grayson, J. B., Turner, R. M., & Latimer, P. R. (1984). Deliberate exposure and blocking of obsessive-compulsive rituals: Immediate and long-term effects. *Behavior Therapy*, *15*(5), 450–472. https://doi.org/10.1016/S0005-7894(84)80049-0.

Gilbert, P. (1989). *Human nature and suffering*. Hove and London: Lawrence Erlbaum.

Goodman, W. K., Grice, D. E., Lapidus, K. A., & Coffey, B. J. (2014). Obsessive-compulsive disorder. *Psychiatric Clinics of North America*, *37*(3), 257–267. https://doi.org/10.1016/j.psc.2014.06.004.

Goodman, W. K., Price, L. H., Rasmussen, S. A., Mazure, C., Delgado, P., Heninger, G. R., et al. (1989). The yale-brown obsessive compulsive scale. II. Validity. *Archives of General Psychiatry*, *46*(11), 1012–1016.

Goodman, W. K., Price, L. H., Rasmussen, S. A., Mazure, C., Fleischmann, R. L., Hill, C. L., et al. (1989). The yale-brown obsessive compulsive scale. I. Development, use, and reliability. *Archives of General Psychiatry*, *46*(11), 1006–1011.

Graeber, C. (2018). *The breakthrough: Immunotherapy and the race to cure cancer*. Grand Central Publishing.

Greenberg, B. D., Gabriels, L. A., Malone, D. A., Jr., Rezai, A. R., Friehs, G. M., Okun, M. S., et al. (2010). Deep brain stimulation of the ventral internal capsule/ventral striatum for obsessive-compulsive disorder: Worldwide experience. *Molecular Psychiatry*, *15*(1), 64–79. https://doi.org/10.1038/mp.2008.55.

Guglielmi, V., Vulink, N. C., Denys, D., Wang, Y., Samuels, J. F., & Nestadt, G. (2014). Obsessive-compulsive disorder and female reproductive cycle events: Results from the OCD and reproduction collaborative study. *Depression and Anxiety*, *31*(12), 979–987. https://doi.org/10.1002/da.22234.

Guner, O. F., & Bowen, J. P. (2014). Setting the record straight: The origin of the pharmacophore concept. *Journal of Chemical Information and Modeling*, *54*(5), 1269–1283. https://doi.org/10.1021/ci5000533.

Hallett, M. (2007). Transcranial magnetic stimulation: A primer. *Neuron*, *55*(2), 187–199. https://doi.org/10.1016/j.neuron.2007.06.026.

Hansen, B., Hagen, K., Ost, L. G., Solem, S., & Kvale, G. (2018). The Bergen 4-day OCD treatment delivered in a group setting: 12-month follow-up. *Frontiers in Psychology*, *9*(639), 639. https://doi.org/10.3389/fpsyg.2018.00639.

Hengartner, M. P., & Lehmann, S. N. (2017). Why psychiatric research must abandon traditional diagnostic classification and adopt a fully dimensional scope: Two solutions to a persistent problem. *Frontiers in Psychiatry*, *8*, 101. https://doi.org/10.3389/fpsyt.2017.00101.

Hinds, A. L., Woody, E. Z., Schmidt, L. A., Van Ameringen, M., & Szechtman, H. (2015). In the wake of a possible mistake: Security motivation, checking behavior, and OCD. *Journal of Behavior Therapy and Experimental Psychiatry*, *49*(Pt B), 133–140. https://doi.org/10.1016/j.jbtep.2015.03.016.

Hinds, A. L., Woody, E. Z., Van Ameringen, M., Schmidt, L. A., & Szechtman, H. (2012). When too much is not enough: Obsessive-compulsive disorder as a pathology of stopping, rather than starting. *PLoS One*, 7(1), e30586. https://doi.org/10.1371/journal.pone.0030586.

Hyman, S. E. (2010). The diagnosis of mental disorders: The problem of reification. *Annual Review of Clinical Psychology*, *6*, 155–179. https://doi.org/10.1146/annurev.clinpsy.3.022806.091532.

Jacobs, B. L., & Azmitia, E. C. (1992). Structure and function of the brain serotonin system. *Physiological Reviews*, *72*(1), 165–229.

Jacobs, B. L., & Fornal, C. A. (1995). Serotonin and behavior: A general hypothesis. In F. E. Bloom & D. J. Kupfer (Eds.), *Psychopharmacology: The fourth generation of progress* (pp. 461–470). New York: Raven Press.

Jaspers, K. (1963). In J. Hoenig & M. W. Hamilton (Eds.), *General psychopathology*. Chicago, IL: University of Chicago Press. Translated from the German by.

Johnson, E. F., & Szechtman, H. (2016). A dose-response study of separate and combined effects of the serotonin agonist 8-OH-DPAT and the dopamine agonist quinpirole on locomotor sensitization, cross-sensitization, and conditioned activity. *Behavioural Pharmacology*, *27*(5), 439–450. https://doi.org/10.1097/FBP.0000000000000219.

Jonsson, H., Kristensen, M., & Arendt, M. (2015). Intensive cognitive behavioural therapy for obsessive-compulsive disorder: A systematic review and meta-analysis. *Journal of Obsessive-Compulsive and Related Disorders*, *6*, 83–96. https://doi.org/10.1016/j.jocrd.2015.04.004.

Kapur, S., & Remington, G. (1996). Serotonin-dopamine interaction and its relevance to schizophrenia. *American Journal of Psychiatry*, *153*(4), 466–476. https://doi.org/10.1176/ajp.153.4.466.

Katzman, M. A., Bleau, P., Blier, P., Chokka, P., Kjernisted, K., Van Ameringen, M., et al. (2014). Canadian clinical practice guidelines for the management of anxiety, posttraumatic stress and obsessive-compulsive disorders. *BMC Psychiatry*, *14*(Suppl 1), S1. https://doi.org/10.1186/1471-244X-14-S1-S1. 1.

Kendler, K. S. (2008). Explanatory models for psychiatric illness. *American Journal of Psychiatry*, *165*(6), 695–702. https://doi.org/10.1176/appi.ajp.2008.07071061.

Koran, L. M., & Simpson, H. B. (2013). *Guideline watch (2013): Practice guideline for the treatment of patients with obsessive-compulsive disorder*. American Psychiatric Association.

Leckman, J. F., Mayes, L. C., Feldman, R., Evans, D. W., King, R. A., & Cohen, D. J. (1999). Early parental preoccupations and behaviors and their possible relationship to the symptoms of obsessive-compulsive disorder. *Acta Psychiatrica Scandinavica. Supplementum*, *396*, 1–26.

Lefaucheur, J. P., Andre-Obadia, N., Antal, A., Ayache, S. S., Baeken, C., Benninger, D. H., et al. (2014). Evidence-based guidelines on the therapeutic use of repetitive transcranial magnetic stimulation (rTMS). *Clinical Neurophysiology*, *125*(11), 2150–2206. https://doi.org/10.1016/j.clinph.2014.05.021.

Lefaucheur, J. P., Antal, A., Ayache, S. S., Benninger, D. H., Brunelin, J., Cogiamanian, F., et al. (2017). Evidence-based guidelines on the therapeutic use of transcranial direct current stimulation (tDCS). *Clinical Neurophysiology*, *128*(1), 56–92. https://doi.org/10.1016/j.clinph.2016.10.087.

Lissemore, J. I., Sookman, D., Gravel, P., Berney, A., Barsoum, A., Diksic, M., et al. (2018). Brain serotonin synthesis capacity in obsessive-compulsive disorder: Effects of cognitive behavioral therapy and sertraline. *Translational Psychiatry*, *8*(1), 82. https://doi.org/10.1038/s41398-018-0128-4.

Luyten, L., Hendrickx, S., Raymaekers, S., Gabriels, L., & Nuttin, B. (2016). Electrical stimulation in the bed nucleus of the stria terminalis alleviates severe obsessive-compulsive disorder. *Molecular Psychiatry*, *21*(9), 1272–1280. https://doi.org/10.1038/mp.2015.124.

Mallet, L., Polosan, M., Jaafari, N., Baup, N., Welter, M. L., Fontaine, D., et al. (2008). Subthalamic nucleus stimulation in severe obsessive-compulsive disorder. *New England Journal of Medicine*, *359*(20), 2121–2134. https://doi.org/10.1056/NEJMoa0708514.

Marks, I. M., & Nesse, R. M. (1994). Fear and fitness: An evolutionary analysis of anxiety disorders. *Ethology and Sociobiology*, *15*(5–6), 247–261. https://doi.org/10.1016/0162-3095(94)90002-7.

Masterson, F. A., & Crawford, M. (1982). The defense motivation system—A theory of avoidance-behavior. *Behavioral and Brain Sciences*, *5*(4), 661–675. https://doi.org/10.1017/S0140525x00014114.

Mataix-Cols, D., Fernandez de la Cruz, L., Monzani, B., Rosenfield, D., Andersson, E., Perez-Vigil, A., et al. (2017). D-Cycloserine augmentation of exposure-based cognitive behavior therapy for anxiety, obsessive-compulsive, and posttraumatic stress disorders: A systematic review and meta-analysis of individual participant data. *JAMA Psychiatry*, *74*(5), 501–510. https://doi.org/10.1001/jamapsychiatry.2016.3955.

McGuire, J. F., Wu, M. S., Piacentini, J., McCracken, J. T., & Storch, E. A. (2017). A meta-analysis of D-Cycloserine in exposure-based treatment: Moderators of treatment efficacy, response, and diagnostic remission. *Journal of Clinical Psychiatry*, *78*(2), 196–206. https://doi.org/10.4088/JCP.15r10334.

McKay, D., Sookman, D., Neziroglu, F., Wilhelm, S., Stein, D. J., Kyrios, M., et al. (2015). Efficacy of cognitive-behavioral therapy for obsessive-compulsive disorder. *Psychiatry Research*, *227*(1), 104–113. https://doi.org/10.1016/j.psychres.2015.02.004.

Montgomery, E. B., Jr. (2007). Basal ganglia physiology and pathophysiology: A reappraisal. *Parkinsonism & Related Disorders*, *13*(8), 455–465. https://doi.org/10.1016/j.parkreldis.2007.07.020.

Montgomery, E. B., Jr. (2012). The epistemology of deep brain stimulation and neuronal pathophysiology. *Frontiers in Integrative Neuroscience*, *6*, 78. https://doi.org/10.3389/fnint.2012.00078.

Montgomery, E. B., Jr. (2016). Modeling and theories of pathophysiology and physiology of the basal ganglia-thalamic-cortical system: Critical analysis. *Frontiers in Human Neuroscience*, *10*, 469. https://doi.org/10.3389/fnhum.2016.00469.

Montgomery, E. B., Jr. (2017). *Deep brain stimulation programming: Mechanisms, principles, and practice,* kindle edition (2nd ed.). New York, NY: Oxford University Press.

Montgomery, E. B., Jr., & Gale, J. T. (2008). Mechanisms of action of deep brain stimulation (DBS). *Neuroscience and Biobehavioral Reviews*, *32*(3), 388–407. https://doi.org/10.1016/j.neubiorev.2007.06.003.

Montgomery, E. B., Jr., & He, H. (2016). Deep brain stimulation frequency—A divining rod for new and novel concepts of nervous system function and therapy. *Brain Sciences*, *6*(3), E34. https://doi.org/10.3390/brainsci6030034.

National Collaborating Centre for Mental Health. (2006). National Institute for health and clinical excellence: Guidance. In *In obsessive-compulsive disorder: Core interventions in the treatment of obsessive-compulsive disorder and body dysmorphic disorder.* Leicester, UK: The British Psychological Society & The Royal College of Psychiatrists.

Nestler, E. J., & Hyman, S. E. (2010). Animal models of neuropsychiatric disorders. *Nature Neuroscience*, *13*(10), 1161–1169. https://doi.org/10.1038/nn.2647.

Neumaier, F., Paterno, M., Alpdogan, S., Tevoufouet, E. E., Schneider, T., Hescheler, J., et al. (2017). Surgical approaches in psychiatry: A survey of the world literature on psychosurgery. *World Neurosurgery*, *97*, 603–634.e608. https://doi.org/10.1016/j.wneu.2016.10.008.

Olatunji, B. O., Davis, M. L., Powers, M. B., & Smits, J. A. (2013). Cognitive-behavioral therapy for obsessive-compulsive disorder: A meta-analysis of treatment outcome and moderators. *Journal of Psychiatric Research*, *47*(1), 33–41. https://doi.org/10.1016/j.jpsychires.2012.08.020.

Ost, L. G., Havnen, A., Hansen, B., & Kvale, G. (2015). Cognitive behavioral treatments of obsessive-compulsive disorder. A systematic review and meta-analysis of studies published 1993–2014. *Clinical Psychology Review*, *40*, 156–169. https://doi.org/10.1016/j.cpr.2015.06.003.

Ougrin, D. (2011). Efficacy of exposure versus cognitive therapy in anxiety disorders: Systematic review and meta-analysis. *BMC Psychiatry*, *11*, 200. https://doi.org/10.1186/1471-244X-11-200.

Parent, A., & Hazrati, L. N. (1995a). Functional anatomy of the basal ganglia. I. The cortico-basal ganglia-thalamo-cortical loop. *Brain Research: Brain Research Reviews*, *20*(1), 91–127.

Parent, A., & Hazrati, L. N. (1995b). Functional anatomy of the basal ganglia. II. The place of subthalamic nucleus and external pallidum in basal ganglia circuitry. *Brain Research: Brain Research Reviews*, *20*(1), 128–154.

Park, J. H., & van Leeuwen, F. (2014). The asymmetric behavioral homeostasis hypothesis: Unidirectional flexibility of fundamental motivational processes. *Review of General Psychology*, *18*(2), 89–100. https://doi.org/10.1037/gpr0000004.

Pascual-Leone, A., Amedi, A., Fregni, F., & Merabet, L. B. (2005). The plastic human brain cortex. *Annual Review of Neuroscience*, *28*(1), 377–401. https://doi.org/10.1146/annurev.neuro.27.070203.144216.

Pfaff, D. W. (2006). *Brain arousal and information theory: Neural and genetic mechanisms*. Cambridge, Mass: Harvard University Press.

Phillips, J., Frances, A., Cerullo, M. A., Chardavoyne, J., Decker, H. S., First, M. B., et al. (2012). The six most essential questions in psychiatric diagnosis: A pluralogue part 3: Issues of utility and alternative approaches in psychiatric diagnosis. *Philosophy, Ethics, and Humanities in Medicine*, 7, 9. https://doi.org/10.1186/1747-5341-7-9.

Philpott, R. (1976). The assessment of drugs in obsessional states. *British Journal of Clinical Pharmacology*, *3*(1 Suppl 1), 91–95. https://doi.org/10.1111/j.1365-2125.1976.tb03721.x.

Piccinelli, M., Pini, S., Bellantuono, C., & Wilkinson, G. (1995). Efficacy of drug treatment in obsessive-compulsive disorder. A meta-analytic review. *British Journal of Psychiatry*, *166*(4), 424–443.

Pittenger, C., & Bloch, M. H. (2014). Pharmacological treatment of obsessive-compulsive disorder. *Psychiatric Clinics of North America*, *37*(3), 375–391. https://doi.org/10.1016/j.psc.2014.05.006.

Rapoport, J. L. (1989). The biology of obsessions and compulsions. *Scientific American*, *260*(3), 82–89.

Reed, G. F. (1985). *Obsessional experience and compulsive behaviour: A cognitive-structural approach*. Orlando, Florida: Academic Press, Inc.

Rosa-Alcazar, A. I., Sanchez-Meca, J., Gomez-Conesa, A., & Marin-Martinez, F. (2008). Psychological treatment of obsessive-compulsive disorder: A meta-analysis. *Clinical Psychology Review*, *28*(8), 1310–1325. https://doi.org/10.1016/j.cpr.2008.07.001.

Rosa-Alcazar, A. I., Sanchez-Meca, J., Rosa-Alcazar, A., Iniesta-Sepulveda, M., Olivares-Rodriguez, J., & Parada-Navas, J. L. (2015). Psychological treatment of obsessive-compulsive disorder in children and adolescents: A meta-analysis. *Spanish Journal of Psychology*, *18*, E20. https://doi.org/10.1017/sjp.2015.22.

Salkovskis, P. M., & Westbrook, D. (1989). Behaviour therapy and obsessional ruminations: Can failure be turned into success? *Behaviour Research and Therapy, 27*(2), 149–160. https://doi.org/10.1016/0005-7967(89)90073-9.

Seeman, P. (1980). Brain dopamine receptors. *Pharmacological Reviews, 32*(3), 229–313.

Senco, N. M., Huang, Y., D'Urso, G., Parra, L. C., Bikson, M., Mantovani, A., et al. (2015). Transcranial direct current stimulation in obsessive-compulsive disorder: Emerging clinical evidence and considerations for optimal montage of electrodes. *Expert Review of Medical Devices, 12*(4), 381–391. https://doi.org/10.1586/17434440.2015.1037832.

Shine, J. M., & Poldrack, R. A. (2018). Principles of dynamic network reconfiguration across diverse brain states. *Neuroimage, 180*(Pt B), 396–405. https://doi.org/10.1016/j.neuroimage.2017.08.010.

Simpson, H. B., Foa, E. B., Liebowitz, M. R., Ledley, D. R., Huppert, J. D., Cahill, S., et al. (2008). A randomized, controlled trial of cognitive-behavioral therapy for augmenting pharmacotherapy in obsessive-compulsive disorder. *American Journal of Psychiatry, 165*(5), 621–630. https://doi.org/10.1176/appi.ajp.2007.07091440.

Skapinakis, P., Caldwell, D., Hollingworth, W., Bryden, P., Fineberg, N., Salkovskis, P., et al. (2016b). A systematic review of the clinical effectiveness and cost-effectiveness of pharmacological and psychological interventions for the management of obsessive-compulsive disorder in children/adolescents and adults. *Health Technology Assessment, 20*(43), 1–392. https://doi.org/10.3310/hta20430.

Skapinakis, P., Caldwell, D. M., Hollingworth, W., Bryden, P., Fineberg, N. A., Salkovskis, P., et al. (2016a). Pharmacological and psychotherapeutic interventions for management of obsessive-compulsive disorder in adults: A systematic review and network meta-analysis. *Lancet Psychiatry, 3*(8), 730–739. https://doi.org/10.1016/S2215-0366(16)30069-4.

Skapinakis, P., Papatheodorou, T., & Mavreas, V. (2007). Antipsychotic augmentation of serotonergic antidepressants in treatment-resistant obsessive-compulsive disorder: A meta-analysis of the randomized controlled trials. *European Neuropsychopharmacology, 17*(2), 79–93. https://doi.org/10.1016/j.euroneuro.2006.07.002.

Soomro, G. M., Altman, D. G., Rajagopal, S., & Oakley Browne, M. (2008). Selective serotonin re-uptake inhibitors (SSRIs) versus placebo for obsessive compulsive disorder (OCD). *Cochrane Database of Systematic Reviews,* (1), Art. No.: CD001765. https://doi.org/10.1002/14651858.CD001765.pub3.

Soubrie, P. (1986). Reconciling the role of central serotonin neurons in human and animal behavior. *The Behavioral and Brain Sciences, 9*, 319–364.

Steketee, G. S. (1993). *Treatment of obsessive compulsive disorder*. New York: Guilford Press.

Stern, R. S. (1978). Obsessive thoughts: The problem of therapy. *British Journal of Psychiatry, 133*, 200–205.

Strebhardt, K., & Ullrich, A. (2008). Paul Ehrlich's magic bullet concept: 100 years of progress. *Nature Reviews. Cancer, 8*(6), 473–480. https://doi.org/10.1038/nrc2394.

Sulkowski, M. L., Geller, D. A., Lewin, A. B., Murphy, T. K., Mittelman, A., Brown, A., et al. (2014). The future of D-Cycloserine and other cognitive modifiers in obsessive-compulsive and related disorders. *Current Psychiatry Reviews, 10*(4), 317–324. https://doi.org/10.2174/157340051066140619224942.

Szechtman, H., & Eilam, D. (2005). Psychiatric models. In I. Q. Whishaw & B. Kolb (Eds.), *The behavior of the laboratory rat: A handbook with tests* (pp. 462–474). New York: Oxford University Press. [Reprinted from: IN FILE].

Szechtman, H., Sulis, W., & Eilam, D. (1998). Quinpirole induces compulsive checking behavior in rats: A potential animal model of obsessive-compulsive disorder (OCD). *Behavioral Neuroscience, 112*(6), 1475–1485. https://doi.org/10.1037/0735-7044.112.6.1475.

Szechtman, H., & Woody, E. (2004). Obsessive-compulsive disorder as a disturbance of security motivation. *Psychological Review, 111*(1), 111–127. https://doi.org/10.1037/0033-295X.111.1.111.

Sznycer, D., Cosmides, L., & Tooby, J. (2017). Adaptationism carves emotions at their functional joints. *Psychological Inquiry, 28*(1), 56–62. https://doi.org/10.1080/1047840x.2017.1256132.

Taylor, S., McKay, D., & Abramowitz, J. S. (2005). Is obsessive-compulsive disorder a disturbance of security motivation? Comment on Szechtman and Woody (2004). *Psychological Review, 112*(3), 650–657. https://doi.org/10.1037/0033-295x.112.3.650.

Teitelbaum, P. (2012). Some useful insights for graduate students beginning their research in physiological psychology: Anecdotes and attitudes. *Behavioural Brain Research, 231*(2), 234–249. https://doi.org/10.1016/j.bbr.2012.01.030.

Teitelbaum, P., & Pellis, S. M. (1992). Toward a synthetic physiological psychology. *Psychological Science, 3*(1), 4–20. https://doi.org/10.1111/j.1467-9280.1992.tb00249.x.

Tolin, D. F. (2009). Alphabet soup: ERP, CT, and ACT for OCD. *Cognitive and Behavioral Practice, 16*(1), 40–48. https://doi.org/10.1016/j.cbpra.2008.07.001.

Tooby, J., & Cosmides, L. (1990). The past explains the present: Emotional adaptations and the structure of ancestral environments. *Ethology and Sociobiology, 11*, 375–424.

Tooby, J., Cosmides, L., Sell, A., Lieberman, D., & Sznycer, D. (2008). Internal regulatory variables and the design of human motivation: A computational and evolutionary approach. In A. Elliot (Ed.), *Handbook of approach and avoidance motivation* (pp. 251–271). Mahwah, N.J: Lawrence Erlbaum Associates.

Tucci, M. C., Dvorkin-Gheva, A., Johnson, E., Cheon, P., Taji, L., Agarwal, A., et al. (2014). Performance of compulsive behavior in rats is not a unitary phenomenon—validation of separate functional components in compulsive checking behavior. *European Journal of Neuroscience, 40*(6), 2971–2979. https://doi.org/10.1111/ejn.12652.

Tucci, M. C., Dvorkin-Gheva, A., Sharma, R., Taji, L., Cheon, P., Peel, J., et al. (2014). Separate mechanisms for development and performance of compulsive checking in the quinpirole sensitization rat model of obsessive-compulsive disorder (OCD). *Psychopharmacology, 231*(18), 3707–3718. https://doi.org/10.1007/s00213-014-3505-6.

Veale, D., Miles, S., Smallcombe, N., Ghezai, H., Goldacre, B., & Hodsoll, J. (2014). Atypical antipsychotic augmentation in SSRI treatment refractory obsessive-compulsive disorder: A systematic review and meta-analysis. *BMC Psychiatry, 14*, 317. https://doi.org/10.1186/s12888-014-0317-5.

Wei, S. C., Duffy, C. R., & Allison, J. P. (2018). Fundamental mechanisms of immune checkpoint blockade therapy. *Cancer Discovery, 8*(9), 1069–1086. https://doi.org/10.1158/2159-8290.CD-18-0367.

West, G. B. (2017). *Scale: The universal laws of growth, innovation, sustainability, and the pace of life in organisms, cities, economies, and companies.* New York: Penguin Press.

Wheaton, M. G., DeSantis, S. M., & Simpson, H. B. (2016). Network meta-analyses and treatment recommendations for obsessive-compulsive disorder. *Lancet Psychiatry, 3*(10), 920. https://doi.org/10.1016/S2215-0366(16)30280-2.

Wikipedia contributors. (2018). *Elixir of life. In Wikipedia, the free encyclopedia.* Retrieved fromhttps://en.wikipedia.org/w/index.php?title=Elixir_of_life&oldid=874244664.

Wise, S., & Rapoport, J. L. (1989). Obsessive compulsive disorder—Is it a basal ganglia dysfunction? In J. Rapoport (Ed.), *Obsessive compulsive disorder in children and adolescence* (pp. 327–344). Washington, DC: American Psychiatric Press.

Witkop, B. (1982). Paul Ehrlich: His ideas and his legacy. In C. G. Bernhard, E. Crawford, & P. Sörbom (Eds.), *Science, Technology & Society in the time of Alfred Nobel: Nobel symposium 52 held at Björkborn, Karlskoga, Sweden, 17–22 August 1981* (pp. 146–166). Amsterdam: Pergamon.

Woody, E. Z., & Szechtman, H. (2005). Motivation, time course, and heterogeneity in obsessive-compulsive disorder: Response to Taylor, McKay, and Abramowitz (2005). *Psychological Review, 112*(3), 658–661. https://doi.org/10.1037/0033-295x.112.3.658.

Woody, E. Z., & Szechtman, H. (2011). Adaptation to potential threat: The evolution, neurobiology, and psychopathology of the security motivation system. *Neuroscience and Biobehavioral Reviews, 35*(4), 1019–1033. https://doi.org/10.1016/j.neubiorev.2010.08.003.

Yaryura-Tobias, J. A., & Neziroglu, F. (1975). The action of chlorimipramine in obsessive-compulsive neurosis: A pilot study. *Current Therapeutic Research, Clinical and Experimental, 17*(1), 111–116.

Yaryura-Tobias, J. A., Neziroglu, F., & Bergman, L. (1976). Chlorimipramine, for obsessive-compulsive neurosis: An organic approach. *Current Therapeutic Research, 20*(4, Pt 2), 541–548.

Yirmiya, R., & Goshen, I. (2011). Immune modulation of learning, memory, neural plasticity and neurogenesis. *Brain, Behavior, and Immunity, 25*(2), 181–213. https://doi.org/10.1016/j.bbi.2010.10.015.

CHAPTER NINE

Positive allosteric modulators of the dopamine D1 receptor: A new mechanism for the treatment of neuropsychiatric disorders☆

Kjell A. Svensson[a,*], Junliang Hao[b], Robert F. Bruns[b]

[a]Neuroscience Discovery, Lilly Research Laboratories, Eli Lilly & Co, Lilly Corporate Center, Indianapolis, IN, United States

[b]Discovery Chemistry and Research Technologies, Lilly Research Laboratories, Eli Lilly & Co, Lilly Corporate Center, Indianapolis, IN, United States

*Corresponding author: e-mail address: svensson_kjell_a@lilly.com

Contents

1. Introduction 275
2. D1 PAM pharmacology 276
   2.1 Initial discovery of tetrahydroisoquinoline (THIQ) based D1 PAMs 276
   2.2 In vitro properties of D1 PAMs 278
   2.3 In vivo behavioral profile of D1 PAMs 283
   2.4 In vivo neurochemical effects of D1 PAMs 290
3. Potential therapeutic applications of D1 PAMs 293
   3.1 Schizophrenia 295
   3.2 Parkinson's disease 296
   3.3 Alzheimer's disease 298
   3.4 Major depressive disorder 298
   3.5 Other therapeutic opportunities for D1 PAMs 299
4. Conclusion 300
Acknowledgment 300
Conflicts of interest 300
References 300

Abstract

The dopamine D1 receptor plays an important role in motor activity, reward, and cognition. Efforts to develop D1 agonists have been mixed due to poor drug-like properties, tachyphylaxis, and inverted U-shaped dose-response curves. Recently, positive allosteric modulators (PAMs) for the dopamine D1 receptor were discovered and initial

☆Major portions of this work have been presented previously (Bruns et al., 2018; Meltzer et al., 2019; Svensson et al., 2017; Wang et al., 2018).

Advances in Pharmacology, Volume 86
ISSN 1054-3589
https://doi.org/10.1016/bs.apha.2019.06.001

pharmacological profiling has suggested that several of the above issues could be addressed with this mechanism. This paper presents an overview of key findings for DETQ (2-(2,6-dichlorophenyl)-1-((1S,3R)-3-(hydroxymethyl)-5-(2-hydroxypropan-2-yl)-1-methyl-3,4-dihydroisoquinolin-2(1H)-yl)ethan-1-one), which is currently the only D1 PAM for which published in vivo data is available. In vitro studies showed selective potentiation of the human D1 receptor without significant allosteric agonist effects. Due to a species difference in affinity for DETQ, transgenic mice expressing the human D1 receptor (hD1 mice) were used in vivo. In contrast to D1 agonists, DETQ increased locomotor activity over a wide dose-range without inverted U-shaped dose response or tachyphylaxis. DETQ also reversed hypo-activity in mice with dopamine depletion due to reserpine pretreatment, suggesting potential for treatment of motor symptoms in Parkinson's disease. Potential pro-cognitive effects were supported by improved performance in the novel object recognition task, enhanced release of cortical acetylcholine and histamine, and increased phosphorylation of the AMPA receptor (GluR1) and the transcription factor CREB. In addition, DETQ enhanced wakefulness in EEG studies and decreased immobility in the forced-swim test. Together, these results provide support for potential utility of D1 PAMs in the treatment of several neuropsychiatric disorders. LY3154207, a close analog of DETQ, is currently in phase 2 clinical trials.

Abbreviations

ACh	acetylcholine
cAMP	cyclic adenosine monophosphate
CIAS	cognitive impairment associated with schizophrenia
CREB	cyclic AMP response element binding protein
DETQ	2-(2,6-dichlorophenyl)-1-((1S,3R)-3-(hydroxymethyl)-5-(2-hydroxypropan-2-yl)-1-methyl-3,4-dihydroisoquinolin-2(1H)-yl)ethan-1-one
DPTQ	2-(2,6-dichlorophenyl)-1-((1S,3R)-3-(hydroxymethyl)-5-(2-hydroxy-2-methylpropan-1-yl)-1-methyl-3,4-dihydroisoquinolin-2(1H)-yl)ethan-1-one
GluR1	ionotropic glutamate receptor 1
GPCR	G-protein coupled receptor
hD1	human D1 receptor
hD1 mouse	human D1 knock-in mouse
LMA	locomotor activity
LY3154207	2-(2,6-dichlorophenyl)-1-((1S,3R)-3-(hydroxymethyl)-5-(3-hydroxy-3-methylbutan-1-yl)-1-methyl-3,4-dihydroisoquinolin-2(1H)-yl)ethan-1-one
NOR	novel object recognition
PAM	positive allosteric modulator
PCP	phencyclidine
pCREB	phosphorylated CREB
PD	Parkinson's disease
pGluR1	phosphorylated GluR1
tCREB	total CREB
tGluR1	total GluR1
THIQ	tetrahydroisoquinoline

1. Introduction

The neurotransmitter dopamine plays a key role in several important central functions including cognition, motor activity, vigilance, mood, and reward. Examples of currently used therapeutics working through the dopamine system include dopamine agonists for Parkinson's disease, dopamine releasers (amphetamine-like) for attention deficit hyperactivity disorders and narcolepsy, dopamine reuptake inhibitors for depression, and dopamine receptor antagonists for schizophrenia and bipolar disorders (Iversen & Iversen, 2007). There are five known mammalian dopamine receptor subtypes (Beaulieu & Gainetdinov, 2011). Of these, the D1 and D5 subtypes are closely related, belonging to the D1-like subgroup that couples positively to adenylate cyclase through the G-proteins G_s and G_{olf} (Zhuong, Belluscio, & Hen, 2000). The second subgroup consists of the D2-like receptor subtypes, D2, D3, and D4, that couple negatively to adenylate cyclase via G_i. The D1 and D2 receptors are the most abundant subtypes in the brain with at least a 10-fold higher expression than the D3, D4, and D5. The highest expression of dopamine D1 and D2 receptors is seen in the basal forebrain, in particular, in the nigro-striatal pathway from the substantia nigra to the caudate-putamen and the meso-limbic pathway from the ventral tegmental area (VTA) to the olfactory bulb and the ventral striatum/nucleus accumbens (Beaulieu & Gainetdinov, 2011). In addition, the D1 receptor subtype shows relatively high expression in meso-cortical projections to the prefrontal cortex and other cortical areas of importance for cognitive functions. Of particular interest is the importance of the D1 receptor subtype for higher cognitive functions including working memory, attention, and executive function (Arnsten, 2013; Goldman-Rakic, Castner, Svensson, Siever, & Williams, 2004). Based on the expression of D1 receptors in the mammalian brain, D1 agonists have been a target for drug discovery efforts to develop improved therapies for movement disorders such as Parkinson's disease and for cognitive disorders such as cognitive impairment associated with schizophrenia (CIAS) and various forms of dementia including Alzheimer's disease. In particular, the urgent need to find more effective treatments for cognitive impairment across neuropsychiatric disorders has focused attention on developing selective D1 agonists (Arnsten, Girgis, Gray, & Mailman, 2017; Hall, Provins, & Valade, 2019).

Beyond movement disorders and cognition, there are several additional therapeutic opportunities associated with central dopamine D1 receptor activation. These include treatments for depression and other mood related symptoms such as apathy and negative symptoms of schizophrenia, as well as narcolepsy and excessive daytime sleepiness (Bruns et al., 2018).

However, despite promising preclinical validation, efforts to develop novel D1 agonists have largely been unsuccessful due to poor drug-like properties including inverted U-shaped dose-response on cognition and other endpoints, rapid tolerance development, poor metabolic stability, and tolerability issues including hypotension and dyskinesias (Arnsten et al., 2017). This is in part related to early efforts focusing on catechol-like molecules that suffered from low bioavailability and poor safety profiles and in some cases rapid tolerance development (Hall et al., 2019). It should be noted that, because of these issues, recent efforts with D1 agonists have focused on non-catechol molecules with selectivity for specific downstream signaling pathways (Davoren et al., 2018; Gray, Allen, et al., 2018; Hall et al., 2019); several of these compounds showed encouraging preclinical data and have progressed to clinical development (Gray, Zhang, et al., 2018; Papapetropoulos, Liu, Duvvuri, Thayer, & Gray, 2018), including phase 2 in Parkinson's disease. Future clinical results will determine whether this approach is successful.

As an alternative to the D1 agonist approach, the current review describes positive allosteric modulation of the D1 receptor as a strategy for amplifying the D1 system. Based on promising preclinical results described below, a compound embodying this mechanism has been advanced to a phase 2 clinical trial in Lewy Body dementias, including Parkinson's disease dementia (Hembre et al., 2018).

2. D1 PAM pharmacology

2.1 Initial discovery of tetrahydroisoquinoline (THIQ) based D1 PAMs

In 2002, Lilly scientists initiated an effort to develop a novel approach to activate central D1 receptors: a dopamine D1 potentiator (or positive allosteric modulator, PAM). The identification of novel allosteric mechanisms as new targets for GPCR related drug discovery had gained momentum over the previous decade (Bruns & Fergus, 1990; Christopoulos & Kenakin, 2002; Nemeth et al., 1998), and in light of the lack of progress in the D1 agonist area, this approach seemed attractive. The underlying hypothesis

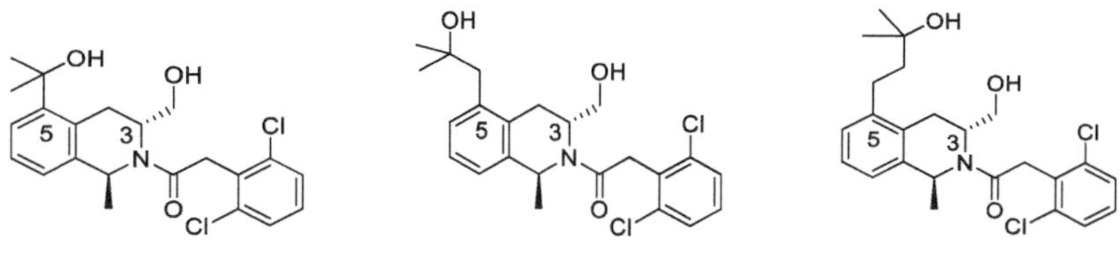

Fig. 1 Chemical structures of several THIQ-based D1 PAMs.

was that the activity of a PAM would be dependent on endogenous dopaminergic tone, thereby offering a more physiological approach that could provide a better therapeutic margin, possibly avoiding the inverted U-shaped dose response and rapid tolerance development seen with D1 agonists. Also, previous results with GPCR PAMs (Bruns & Fergus, 1990) offered hope that a PAM approach could deliver a high degree of selectivity between the D1 receptor and the other four dopamine receptors. Finally, a D1 PAM would presumably not be a catechol, and therefore would lack the specific pharmacokinetic liabilities of this structural group.

High-throughput screening of over 400,000 compounds using a PAM-mode cAMP assay in HEK293 cells expressing the human D1 receptor identified a single validated hit (Hall et al., 2019; Hembre et al., 2018).

A subsequent drug discovery program focused on improving functional potency along with properties important for in vivo activity such as solubility and metabolic stability, eventually resulted in compounds with robust activity in vivo (Fig. 1).

Although other chemical series with D1 PAM activity have been described, these have not yet reported agents having in vivo activity (Lewis et al., 2015; Luderman et al., 2018), or have not been described outside of the patent literature (Shiraki, Tobe, Kawakami, Moritomo, & Ohmiya, 2015). The current review will therefore focus mainly on the THIQ series.

Of the three compounds in Fig. 1, DETQ and DPTQ have been used as pharmacological tools, while LY3154207 is a clinical candidate currently in Phase 2 trials. DETQ was the subject of initial publications by the Lilly group (Bruns et al., 2018; Svensson et al., 2017; Wang et al., 2018), whereas the other two THIQs have yet to be profiled in detail in the scientific literature. For this reason, DETQ will serve as a prototypical D1 PAM throughout this review. The remainder of this article will consist of: (1) description of the in vitro profile of DETQ, followed by a brief summary of the in vitro profiles of the non-THIQ D1 PAMs; (2) in vivo profile of DETQ; (3) discussion of potential therapeutic applications for D1 PAMs.

2.2 In vitro properties of D1 PAMs

2.2.1 In vitro profile of DETQ as a prototypical D1 PAM

In vitro studies using HEK-293 cells expressing the human dopamine D1 receptor revealed that DETQ increased cAMP with an EC_{50} of 5.8nM when tested in the presence of an EC_{20} concentration of dopamine (Fig. 2). With increasing concentrations of DETQ, the response reached the same maximum as that observed with high concentrations of dopamine. Interestingly, in the absence of dopamine, there was only a small (12%) increase in cAMP and the EC_{50} was shifted fivefold to the right, indicating an overall loss of potency of 43-fold in the absence of dopamine (Svensson et al., 2017). This result suggests that allosteric agonist activity of the THIQ-based D1 PAMs should be minimal at realistic doses, a prediction that has been confirmed in animal studies (Bruns et al., 2018).

In the same study, curve shift experiments in HEK-293 cells revealed that DETQ produced a 21-fold leftward shift in the concentration-response curve for the increase in cAMP caused by dopamine. DETQ was also found to potentiate the dopamine-induced displacement of the D1 receptor antagonist ^{3}H-SCH23390 at the human D1 (hD1) receptor, without being able to displace the D1 antagonist in the absence of dopamine. These results suggest that DETQ acts by shifting the D1 receptor into an activated conformation that has a higher affinity for dopamine (Svensson et al., 2017; Wang et al., 2018).

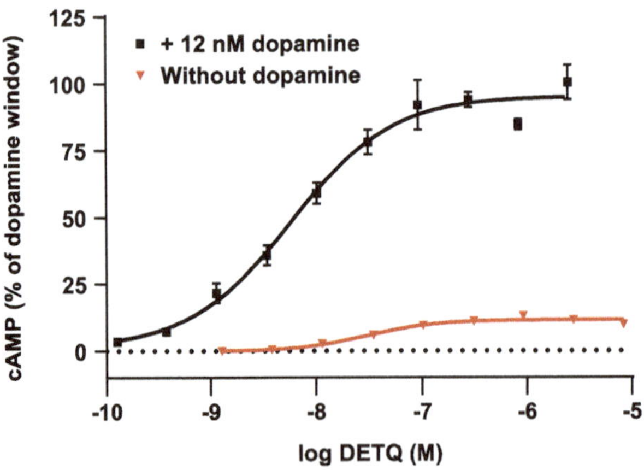

Fig. 2 Increase in cAMP by DETQ in the presence and absence of an EC_{20} concentration of dopamine in HEK293 cells expressing the human D1 receptor. *From Svensson, K. A., Heinz, B. A., Schaus, J. M., Beck, J. P., Hao, J., Krushinski, J. H., et al. (2017). An allosteric potentiator of the dopamine D1 receptor increases locomotor activity in human D1 knock-in mice without causing stereotypy or tachyphylaxis.* The Journal of Pharmacology and Experimental Therapeutics, 360*(1), 117–128. doi:10.1124/jpet.116.236372.*

Relative to the human D1 receptor, DETQ was found to be 28-fold less potent at the rat D1 receptor, and a similar loss of potency was noted for the mouse (Fig. 3). In addition, DETQ was found to be a partial PAM at the rodent D1 receptors (Svensson et al., 2017). This species difference was noted for the rodent line only, as DETQ had potencies in both the dog and rhesus monkey similar to its potency at the human D1 receptor (Fig. 3) (Svensson et al., 2017; Wang et al., 2018).

DETQ was found to be inactive as a PAM at the human D5 receptor at concentrations up to 25 μM. This result was surprising, inasmuch as agonists with meaningful selectivity for the D1 receptor compared to the D5 have never been reported. However, extreme selectivity has been reported for PAMs at other GPCRs (Bruns & Fergus, 1990; Epping-Jordan, Le Poul, & Rocher, 2007), and this may be due to PAM sites existing at locations that have been weakly conserved during evolution. In addition, no significant cross-reactivity was observed at closely related GPCRs (including D2, β2, and 5-HT6 receptors) or other targets at concentrations up to 10 μM (Svensson et al., 2017). The high selectivity for the D1 receptor suggests that new compounds with profiles like DETQ offer suitable tools to further explore the functional role of the D1 receptor and also the potential of selectively targeting the D1 receptor for therapeutic indications.

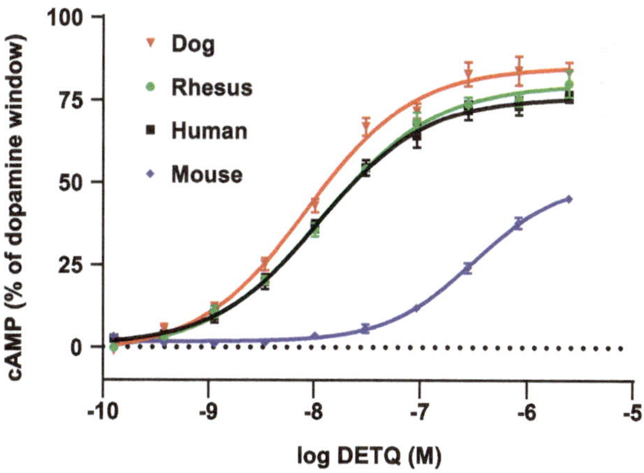

Fig. 3 Species differences in affinity for DETQ. Human, dog, rhesus, and mouse D1 receptors were transiently expressed in HEK293 cells. *From Svensson, K. A., Heinz, B. A., Schaus, J. M., Beck, J. P., Hao, J., Krushinski, J. H., et al. (2017). An allosteric potentiator of the dopamine D1 receptor increases locomotor activity in human D1 knock-in mice without causing stereotypy or tachyphylaxis.* The Journal of Pharmacology and Experimental Therapeutics, 360*(1), 117–128. doi:10.1124/jpet.116.236372.*

During the early testing of D1 PAM leads in wild-type rodents, we consistently failed to see behavioral or neurochemical effects using systemic or intracranial dosing, a result that is consistent with the human-rodent species difference described above. Subsequent molecular pharmacology studies, including work using receptor chimeras and site directed mutagenesis, revealed a key human Arg130 to rodent Gln130 mutation in the second intracellular loop, ICL2 (Fig. 4). This mutation was found to be deleterious for the potency of the THIQ-based D1 PAMs (Beadle et al., 2014; Wang et al., 2018) as well as for two other D1 PAM compounds with structural resemblance to the THIQ series (Lewis et al., 2015; Luderman et al., 2018). In agreement with the species-related differences described above,

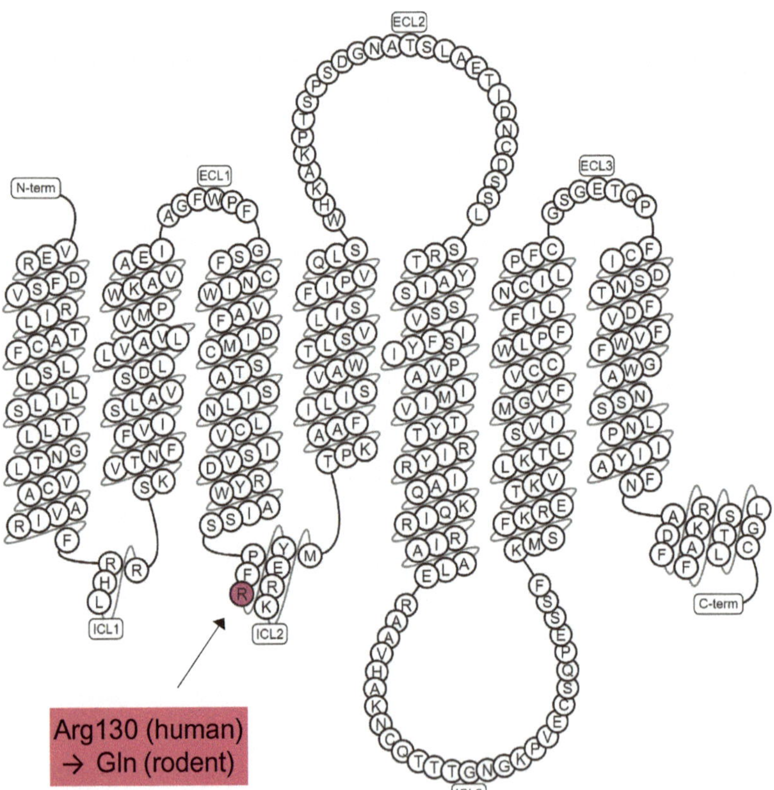

Fig. 4 The human dopamine D1 receptor with the putative binding pocket for THIQ-based D1 PAMs highlighted at intracellular loop 2 (ICL2). The critical arginine-to-glutamine mutation at position 130 seen in rodents is depicted. The "snake diagram" was generated by the diagram function at https://GPCRdb.org (Munk et al., 2016).

the mutation of arginine-130 to glutamine occurred in a common ancestor of the rodent line and is seen in all rodents but not in non-rodent species (www.uniprot.org).

The human versus rodent preference for the THIQ series triggered work to generate a humanized dopamine D1 receptor mouse in collaboration with Artemis (Taconic Biosciences). The availability of the new humanized dopamine D1 knock-in mouse model, together with improved compounds with better drug-like properties, allowed us for the first time to show in vivo activity in this series. This development gave a significant boost to the drug discovery project and allowed identification of the pharmacological tool DETQ (Svensson et al., 2017) and the clinical candidate LY3154207 (Beadle et al., 2014; Hembre et al., 2018). We were also able to verify predicted advantages of the allosteric mechanism by performing side by side comparisons with D1 agonists (Bruns et al., 2018; Svensson et al., 2017). To our knowledge, this was the first selective D1 PAM series to show drug-like properties that allowed progression to clinical testing. [A D1 PAM from Astellas is reported to be in clinical trials, but the exact structure of this compound has not yet been made public (Hall et al., 2019; Shiraki et al., 2015).]

2.2.2 Non-THIQ D1 PAMs

Novel D1 PAMs of diverse structural types (Fig. 5) have been reported by groups from Bristol-Myers Squibb (Lewis et al., 2015), the National Institutes of Health (Luderman et al., 2018), and Astellas (Shiraki et al., 2015). Functional affinities for potentiation of dopamine range from mid-nanomolar to low micromolar (Table 1). Interestingly, two of the PAMs, Compound B and MLS1082, have lower activity at rodent D1 receptors and are sensitive to the R130Q mutation, indicating that they bind to the same site in intracellular loop 2 as the Lilly THIQs. In contrast, MLS6585 (also known as CID 2886111) is unaffected by the R130Q mutation, suggesting that it operates through a different site. This is confirmed by experiments combining two PAMs. Receptor theory predicts that if two allosteric modulators bind to the same site, the maximum response to both together will be the same as for each separately, and this is observed for the two ICL2 binders, Compound B and MLS1082 (Luderman et al., 2018). In contrast, combining MLS6585 with DETQ, MLS1082, or Compound B causes a much greater response than the maximum for either compound alone (Luderman et al., 2018; Wang et al., 2018), as expected if the two

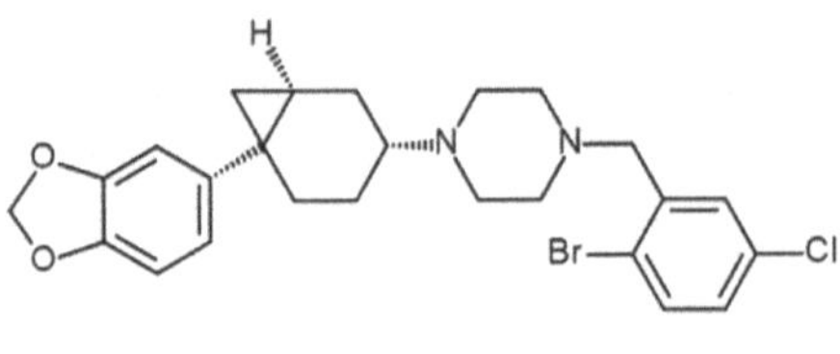

Compound A

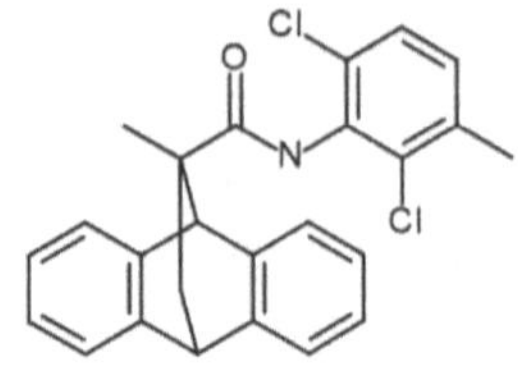

Compound B

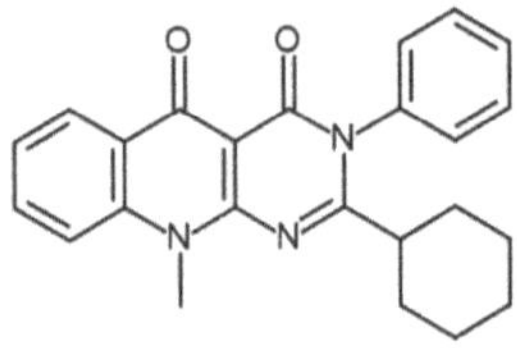

MLS1082

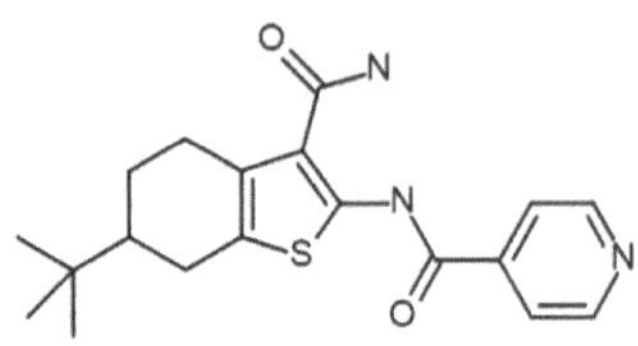

MLS6585

Fig. 5 Chemical structures of non-THIQ D1 PAMs.

Table 1 In vitro activity of THIQ and non-THIQ D1 PAMs.

Compound	**EC_{50} (nM)**	**Max (%)**	**ICL2 binder?**
DETQ	14.2	92	Yes
DPTQ	76	83	Yes
LY3154207	3.7	84	Yes
Compound A	210		No
Compound B	30		Yes
MLS1082	Low μM		Yes
MLS6585	1740	97	No
Astellas	460		Unknown

Values are for stimulation of cAMP accumulation in the presence of an EC_{20} concentration of dopamine, except for the Astellas compound, for which the concentration required for a twofold leftward shift of the dopamine curve is given. An EC_{50} value for MLS1082 has not been published, but it is less potent than MLS6585 (Luderman et al., 2018), implying an EC_{50} in the low μM range. Data for DETQ and MLS6585 are averages from Figs. 2, 3, and 7 in (Wang et al., 2018); for DPTQ from (Hembre et al., 2018); for LY3154207 from (Beadle et al., 2014); for Compounds A and B from (Lewis et al., 2015); and for Astellas example 1 from (Shiraki et al., 2015). "ICL2 binder" refers to whether the compound binds to the intracellular loop 2 binding site inferred from site-directed mutagenesis (Lewis et al., 2015; Luderman et al., 2018; Wang et al., 2018).

compounds bound to different sites but stabilized the same activated conformation of the D1 receptor.

The phenomenon of biased signaling involves the ability of certain ligands to selectively activate one downstream pathway relative to another. For GPCRs, the two main pathways are the G-protein pathway and the β-arrestin pathway. DETQ, MLS1082, and MLS6585 each activate the β-arrestin pathway with activity roughly equal to that seen for the G-protein pathway (Luderman et al., 2018; Wang et al., 2018), consistent with the null hypothesis of unbiased signaling. The two Bristol-Myers Squibb compounds and the Astellas series lack published data on activity at the β-arrestin pathway.

Probe dependence is the observation of different activity of an allosteric molecule for modulation of different ligands. Striking probe dependence has been seen for certain compounds acting at muscarinic and chemokine receptors (Kenakin, 2012; Valant, Felder, Sexton, & Christopoulos, 2012). In contrast, MLS1082 and MLS6585 (Luderman et al., 2018) and compounds from the THIQ series (unpublished observation) robustly potentiate a range of D1 full and partial agonists, indicating that these modulators show little or no probe dependence.

The >1000-fold loss of activity for DETQ at the D5 receptor compared to D1 is due to an A139M mutation in the human D5 receptor (Wang et al., 2018). In contrast to DETQ, MLS1082 and MLS6585 are nearly as active at the D5 receptor as at the D1 (Luderman et al., 2018). This result is not surprising for MLS6585, given that this compound doesn't bind to the ICL2 site; in the case of ML1082, it suggests a different binding mode from DETQ, one in which the niche containing A139 remains unoccupied.

Of the non-THIQ PAMs, MLS1082 and MLS6585 probably lack the in vitro potency needed for in vivo activity (Table 1). On the other hand, Compound B has relatively good in vitro potency (EC_{50} 30 nM), but the large, hydrophobic ethanoanthracene group likely confers unacceptable pharmacokinetic properties. The claimed activity of Astellas example 1 at 0.1 mg/kg in vivo (Shiraki et al., 2015) is puzzling, given the modest EC_{50} of 460 nM. Further investigation is need to understand this result (Hall et al., 2019).

2.3 In vivo behavioral profile of D1 PAMs

Due to the significant species difference in potency of the THIQ-based D1 PAMs like DETQ, the human D1 knock-in (hD1) mouse was generated in collaboration with Artemis (Taconic Biosciences) (Svensson et al., 2017).

The transgenic model was generated using gene replacement in which the mouse D1 gene was deleted and replaced with the human D1 counterpart using the C57Bl/6NTac as background strain. After successful breeding of the homozygotes, characterization of the hD1 mice revealed no obvious behavioral differences from wild-type animals. In vitro autoradiography binding studies using the D1 antagonist ligand ^{3}H-SCH23390 showed that the distribution of the D1 receptors in the brain was similar in the hD1 and wild-type animals, although the D1 receptor expression level was about 50% lower in the hD1 animals. Additional studies revealed no significant genotypic differences in response to dopamine agonists and antagonists using both behavioral and neurochemical analyses, and a study examining ^{3}H-SCH23390 binding with and without GTP suggested that the D1 receptor coupling to G_s in the hD1 mouse was normal (unpublished observations). Based on these studies, the hD1 mouse model was considered to be a relevant model for further in vivo evaluation of D1 PAMs. An overview of the in vivo behavioral profile of the D1 PAM DETQ is described below and exemplifies in general the profiles of THIQ-based D1 PAMs.

When dosed to hD1 mice habituated to the environment for 60min, DETQ produced a dose-related increase in forward locomotion and rearing behavior (Fig. 6). The behavioral activation was blocked by the D1 receptor antagonist SCH23390 and no significant behavioral activation was seen in wild-type mice (Svensson et al., 2017). This result suggests that the effects of DETQ are dependent on action of endogenous dopamine at the human

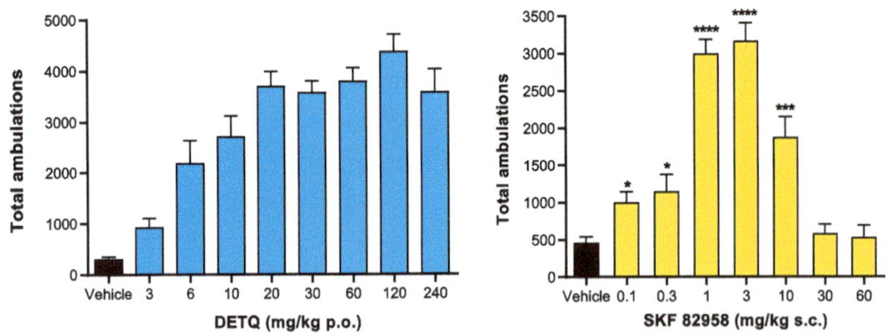

Fig. 6 Locomotor response to DETQ and the D1 agonist SKF82958 in habituated hD1 mice. LMA responses were recorded for 60min after dosing, $n = 8–32$. *From Svensson, K. A., Heinz, B. A., Schaus, J. M., Beck, J. P., Hao, J., Krushinski, J. H., et al. (2017). An allosteric potentiator of the dopamine D1 receptor increases locomotor activity in human D1 knock-in mice without causing stereotypy or tachyphylaxis.* The Journal of Pharmacology and Experimental Therapeutics, 360*(1), 117–128. https://doi.org/10.1124/jpet.116.236372.*

D1 receptor. Interestingly, and in contrast to orthosteric D1 agonists like SKF82958 (Fig. 6), the behavioral activation induced by DETQ reached a plateau around 20 mg/kg, p.o., and this was maintained even at the highest dose tested. This behavioral profile was seen even though the unbound brain concentrations continued to increase over the entire dose range. The lack of an inverted U-shaped dose-response curve is a clear differentiation versus orthosteric D1 agonists (and also psychostimulants) and is likely related to lack of intense stereotyped behavior including sniffing and grooming behavior at higher doses (Svensson et al., 2017). This unique profile of D1 PAMs could relate to a selective potentiation/modulation of released dopamine at the D1 receptors. Importantly, by amplifying the effectiveness of specific dopamine circuits, a D1 PAM could provide a needed boost to a hypoactive/deficient system while allowing normal feedback loops to remain in control. The latter properties may help prevent overstimulation and impaired function, implying that D1 PAMs could provide treatment that is in general better tolerated over a wider dose-range.

In addition to the above, some D1 agonists, particularly long-acting compounds such as A-77636, are known to induce rapid tolerance development based on behavioral and neurochemical measures. This is related to a down-regulation or internalization of the D1 receptor, resulting in loss of function (Gulwadi et al., 2001). In contrast to D1 agonists like A-77636, where tolerance to increases in locomotor activity developed already on day 2 (Fig. 7), DETQ retained behavioral activation upon repeat dosing

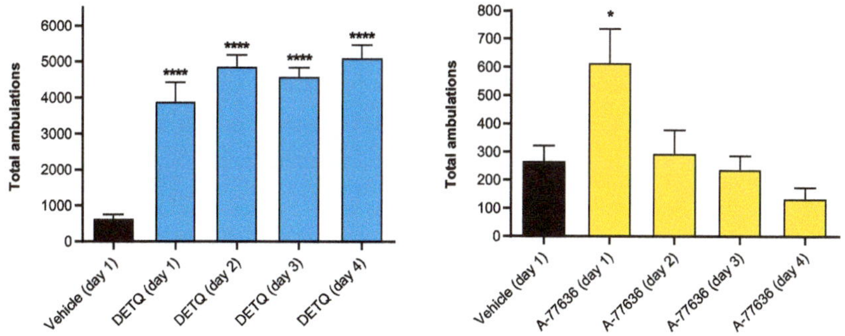

Fig. 7 LMA responses to A-77636 and DETQ after repeated daily dosing ($n = 7–8$ per group). A-77636 was dosed at 10 mg/kg SC and DETQ at 30 mg/kg PO. *From Svensson, K. A., Heinz, B. A., Schaus, J. M., Beck, J. P., Hao, J., Krushinski, J. H., et al. (2017). An allosteric potentiator of the dopamine D1 receptor increases locomotor activity in human D1 knock-in mice without causing stereotypy or tachyphylaxis.* The Journal of Pharmacology and Experimental Therapeutics, 360*(1), 117–128. https://doi.org/10.1124/jpet.116.236372.*

up to 4 days. Unpublished observations show retained efficacy for at least 14 days in this model. This is another distinct profile difference between orthosteric dopamine D1 agonists and D1 PAMs that could offer therapeutic advantages. Recent progress with the development of non-catechol based partial D1 agonists may however offer some improvements regarding tolerance development (Gray, Allen, et al., 2018).

2.3.1 Models of movement disorders

The alkaloid reserpine can induce depletion of biogenic amines through an irreversible blockade of neurotransmitter reuptake into vesicles. About 60 years ago, it was shown that it is the depletion of brain dopamine levels that is primarily responsible for the development of hypomotility and akinesia, and these symptoms could be reversed by exogenous L-DOPA administration (Carlsson, Lindqvist, & Magnusson, 1957). Subsequent work also identified dopamine as a key neurotransmitter in its own right (Carlsson, Lindqvist, Magnusson, & Waldeck, 1958). These findings led to the introduction of L-DOPA, which revolutionized the treatment of Parkinson's disease (PD) in the mid-1960s. Reserpine has since served as an in vivo screening model for development of novel therapies for PD motor symptoms.

A low dose of reserpine produces a partial (30%) reduction in striatal dopamine levels, and this results in decreased exploratory locomotion when animals are exposed to a novel environment, but not akinesia or catalepsy (Fig. 8). DETQ showed a dose-dependent and complete reversal of the hypokinesia, which suggests that D1 PAMs could have efficacy in improving motor symptoms in earlier stages of PD when some striatal dopamine terminals are intact. This could potentially delay the need for initiating levodopa therapy. In a separate study, we administered a high dose of reserpine (2.5 mg/kg, SC, 18 h before). Here we observed a strong akinesia/immobility with a 95% decrease in striatal dopamine levels. In this experiment, DETQ alone failed to significantly reverse the akinesia; however, when combined with lower doses of L-DOPA, DETQ acted in a supra-additive fashion to reverse the akinesia (Bruns et al., 2018). These studies show that DETQ is dependent on synaptic dopamine to trigger a behavioral response (i.e., lack of significant agonist properties). Also, the results suggest that D1 PAMs could be beneficial for the treatment of motor symptoms also in the later stages of PD, where there is an opportunity to

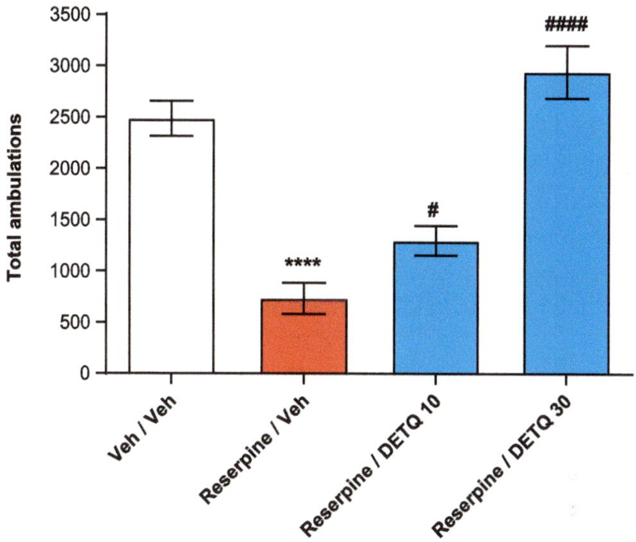

Fig. 8 Effects of DETQ on the suppression of locomotor activity induced by a low dose (0.3 mg/kg, SC, 18 h before) of reserpine ($n = 6$/group). *From Bruns, R. F., Mitchell, S. N., Wafford, K. A., Harper, A. J., Shanks, E. A., Carter, G., et al. (2018). Preclinical profile of a dopamine D1 potentiator suggests therapeutic utility in neurological and psychiatric disorders.* Neuropharmacology, 128, *351–365. https://doi.org/10.1016/j.neuropharm.2017.10.032.*

lower the L-DOPA dose or improve the maximal effect of L-DOPA (Bruns et al., 2018). Ongoing and future clinical investigations with D1 PAMs in PD will address these questions.

2.3.2 Models of cognitive disorders

Further behavioral testing of the D1 PAM DETQ in hD1 mice support a potential role of this new mechanism in the treatment of cognitive impairment. In the spontaneous alternation model, DETQ was dosed to hD1 mice exploring a Y-shaped maze for 15 min. The animals normally use spatial cues to alternate between arms (about 55% alternation between arms for control), a behavior that optimizes exploratory efficiency. DETQ showed a dose-dependent increase in motor activity (distance traveled) while not affecting the alternation between arms over the dose range tested (Bruns et al., 2018). This suggests that animals maintained ability to use spatial cues even as activity was increased. In contrast, the D1 agonist SKF82958 at the doses tested did not significantly alter the active exploratory behavior in the Y-maze but reduced alternation at higher doses (Bruns et al., 2018). The effects on alternation seen with the D1 agonist could be related to interfering repetitive grooming behavior observed at these doses.

The novel object recognition (NOR) model is a simple procedure that reflects an animal's ability to recognize and explore a novel object in preference to a familiar object (Ennaceur & Delacour, 1988). This behavior reflects components of curiosity, working memory, attention, and episodic memory, and involves the hippocampus, temporal lobe and frontal cortex. Working and object recognition memory deficits are present in both Alzheimer's and PD as well as schizophrenia (Castner & Goldman-Rakic, 2004).

Sub-chronic treatment of mice with the NMDA receptor antagonist phencyclidine (PCP) produces a prolonged deficit of NOR (Horiguchi et al., 2013). This deficit has been shown to be rescued by D1 agonists like SKF38393 and SKF82958 (Horiguchi et al., 2013; Meltzer et al., 2019). However, D1 agonists may produce an inverted U-shaped dose response due to overstimulation at higher doses (Horiguchi et al., 2013).

A recent study explored the effects of DETQ in the NOR task in hD1 and wild-type mice (Meltzer et al., 2019). Overall, the exploration time and ability to discriminate between a familiar and novel object did not differ between the two genotypes. Animals exposed to sub-chronic treatment with PCP (10 mg/kg, ip, BID for 7 days) followed by a 7-day drug free period displayed a highly significant deficit in NOR. This deficit was dose-dependently and fully reversed by DETQ in hD1 mice (Fig. 9) but not in wild-type animals, and the effects of DETQ were also blocked by the D1 antagonist SCH23390 (Meltzer et al., 2019).

In contrast to what has been reported for D1 agonists, there was no evidence of an inverted U-shaped dose response at the dose range explored of DETQ. In addition, the effects of DETQ in this model were sustained after 7 days of repeated daily dosing. In the same report, the cholinesterase inhibitor rivastigmine was found to reverse the PCP-induced deficit at a dose of 1.0 mg/kg, IP but not at the lower doses of 0.03 and 0.3 mg/kg (Meltzer et al., 2019). Interestingly, a combination of low doses of DETQ and rivastigmine resulted in a synergistic effect with full reversal of the NOR deficit (Fig. 9). A similar positive interaction between DETQ and rivastigmine was also seen in the in vivo microdialysis assay measuring hippocampal acetylcholine release (see below).

Together, these studies provide behavioral support for potential pro-cognitive effects of D1 PAMs as stand-alone treatment or in combination with a cholinesterase inhibitor.

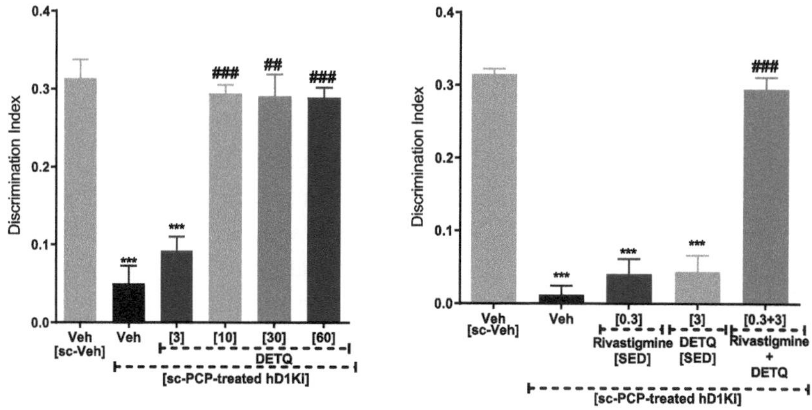

Fig. 9 Left: Effects of DETQ (3–60 mg/kg, IP) on reversal of deficit in novel object recognition memory in sub-chronic PCP treated hD1 mice. Right: Rivastigmine (0.3 mg/kg, IP) and DETQ (3 mg/kg, IP) act synergistically to reverse the PCP-induced deficits. *From Meltzer, H., Rajagopal, L., Matrisciano, F., Hao, J., Svensson, K., & Huang, M. (2019). The allosteric dopamine D1 receptor potentiator, DETQ, ameliorates sub-chronic phencyclidine-induced object recognition memory deficits and enhances cortical acetylcholine efflux in male humanized D1 receptor knock-in mice.* Behavioural Brain Research, 361, *139–150. https://doi.org/10.1016/j.bbr.2018.12.006.*

2.3.3 Models of other neuropsychiatric disorders

D1 agonists have been shown to increase wakefulness in animals (Isaac & Berridge, 2003) and a D1 antagonist promotes sleep in humans (Eder, Zdravkovic, & Wildschiødtz, 2003). We tested the effects of DETQ on sleep-wake activity in freely moving hD1 mice with implanted cortical EEG electrodes (Bruns et al., 2018). DETQ showed a dose-dependent increase in wakefulness and increased the time to fall asleep measured during a 7 h period following dosing. In the same study SKF82958 was also wake promoting, whereas the D1 antagonist SCH39166 decreased the time to fall asleep when compared to vehicle treated animals.

D1 agonists are known to be active in the forced-swim (behavioral despair) test in rodents. This test has historically been used as a screen to identify compounds that could display antidepressant-like properties (Nikulina, Skrinskaya, & Popova, 1991; Petit-Demouliere, Chenu, & Bourin, 2005). A potential caveat is that behavioral activating compounds are expected to be active in this test. Nevertheless, this test does offer predictive validity (Petit-Demouliere et al., 2005). When tested in hD1 mice, DETQ showed a dose-dependent decrease in immobility time with a maximal response similar to that of the tricyclic antidepressant imipramine (Bruns et al., 2018).

In order to explore the effects of D1 PAM in a non-rodent species, we considered the spontaneous eye-blink model in the rhesus monkey. It has previously been shown that D1 agonists increase eye-blink rate in this model (Jutkiewicz & Bergman, 2004). In addition, PD patients have reduced spontaneous eye-blink rate (Deuschl & Goddemeier, 1998; Karson, Lewitt, Calne, & Wyatt, 1982). Although there are many neurotransmitter systems involved in eye-blink rate, this model could be used as a pharmacodynamic marker for central dopamine D1 receptor activation. DETQ was dosed in a cumulative fashion at 3 and 10 mg/kg, IM and the spontaneous eye-blink rate was increased about twofold for the subsequent 60 min. In the same study, a dose dependent increase was seen with the D1 agonist SKF82958, with a stronger maximum response than that seen with DETQ (Bruns et al., 2018)

2.4 In vivo neurochemical effects of D1 PAMs

Dopamine D1 receptor agonists and dopamine-releasing compounds are known to increase the release of neurotransmitters such as acetylcholine (ACh) and histamine in multiple brain areas including the prefrontal cortex, the striatum and the hippocampus (Damsma, Tham, Robertson, & Fibiger, 1990; Day & Fibiger, 1993; Ishizuka, Sakamoto, Sakurai, & Yamatodani, 2003). The mechanism for D1 activation-induced cortical ACh release is not fully understood but may include activation of D1 receptors on pyramidal cortical neurons or inhibition of local GABAergic interneurons (see Meltzer et al., 2019 for a discussion). Although activation of the dopamine D5 receptor has been suggested to be responsible for this effect (Hersi, Kitaichi, Srivastava, Gaudreau, & Quirion, 2000; Laplante, Sibley, & Quirion, 2004), our results with D1 PAMs (see Figs. 10 and 11) suggest that the effects are specific to the D1 receptor. In addition to ACh, the neurotransmitter histamine is also implicated in cognition, and the central cholinergic and histaminergic projections are tightly connected (Alvarez, 2009). Histamine release in rodents is also known to accompany various forms of arousal, including behaviorally activating drugs, handling-induced stress, and circadian changes in basal activity (Fell et al., 2011; Horner, Johnson, Schmidt, & Rollema, 2007; Westerink et al., 2002).

We recently showed that systemic dosing of DETQ to freely moving hD1 mice produced a robust increase in extracellular levels of cortical ACh measured in the prefrontal cortex (Fig. 10) and hippocampus

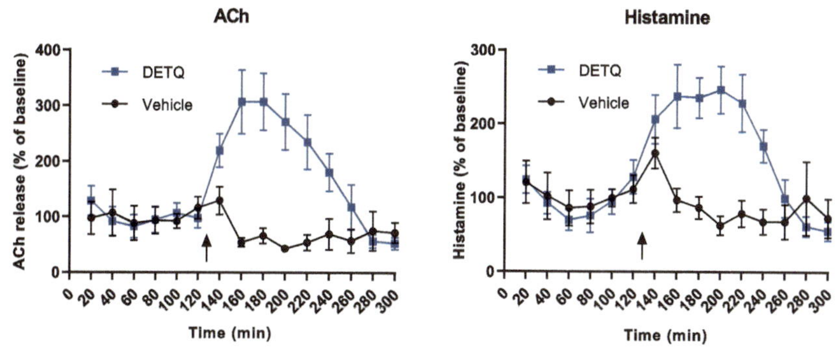

Fig. 10 Effects of DETQ (30 mg/kg, PO) on the release of ACh and histamine in the prefrontal cortex in freely moving hD1 mice ($N = 8$/group). *From Bruns, R. F., Mitchell, S. N., Wafford, K. A., Harper, A. J., Shanks, E. A., Carter, G., et al. (2018). Preclinical profile of a dopamine D1 potentiator suggests therapeutic utility in neurological and psychiatric disorders.* Neuropharmacology, 128, *351–365. https://doi.org/10.1016/j.neuropharm.2017.10.032.*

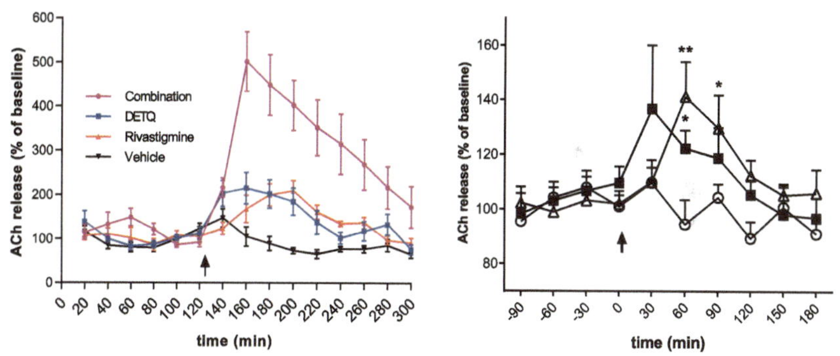

Fig. 11 Left: Effects of DETQ (30 mg/kg, PO) and rivastigmine (0.3 mg/kg, PO) on extracellular levels of ACh in the hippocampus of freely moving hD1 mice (n = 7/group), Right: open circles: vehicle, solid squares: DETQ (30 mg/kg, IP acute dosing), and open triangles: DETQ 30 mg/kg, IP after 7 days of repeat dosing. *From Bruns, R. F., Mitchell, S. N., Wafford, K. A., Harper, A. J., Shanks, E. A., Carter, G., et al. (2018). Preclinical profile of a dopamine D1 potentiator suggests therapeutic utility in neurological and psychiatric disorders.* Neuropharmacology, 128, *351–365. doi:10.1016/j.neuropharm.2017.10.032 (left) and Meltzer, H., Rajagopal, L., Matrisciano, F., Hao, J., Svensson, K., & Huang, M. (2019). The allosteric dopamine D1 receptor potentiator, DETQ, ameliorates subchronic phencyclidine-induced object recognition memory deficits and enhances cortical acetylcholine efflux in male humanized D1 receptor knock-in mice.* Behavioural Brain Research, 361, *139–150. https://doi.org/10.1016/j.bbr.2018.12.006 (right).*

(Fig. 11). The magnitude of the effects of DETQ on ACh release appeared similar to what was observed for the D1 agonist SKF38393 (Meltzer et al., 2019) and the acetylcholinesterase inhibitor rivastigmine (Fig. 11).

Importantly, the time course for increases in extracellular ACh paralleled measured levels of DETQ in the dialysates (Figs. 10 and 11), suggesting a central action of the D1 PAM. Furthermore, and in support of several behavioral findings described above, there was no tolerance development regarding the increases in cortical ACh release after 7 days of repeat dosing with DETQ (Meltzer et al., 2019). Interestingly, when DETQ was co-dosed with the acetylcholinesterase inhibitor rivastigmine (0.3 mg/kg, PO) there was evidence for an additive increase in extracellular acetylcholine, and based on drug exposure analyses of dialysates, this effect was not related to a pharmacokinetic interaction between DETQ and rivastigmine (Fig. 11). Together with the observations that DETQ and rivastigmine had a positive interaction on performance on the novel object recognition task (Fig. 9), these results support an opportunity for adjunct treatment using D1 PAMs in addition to standard of care to improve cognition in neurodegenerative disorders.

Similar to what was observed for ACh release, extracellular levels of histamine and the histamine metabolite tele-methylhistamine were increased in the prefrontal cortex after oral dosing with DETQ (Fig. 10). In support of this, we found that DETQ (10 mg/kg, PO) increased striatal levels of both tele-methylhistamine and the terminal histamine metabolite tele-methyl-imidazolacetic acid post mortem (Bruns et al., 2018).

While the primary acute effects of DETQ on neurotransmitter release appear to involve increases in synaptic ACh and histamine, we have recently observed that 7-day repeat dosing with DETQ results in decreased extracellular levels of both GABA and glutamate in the hippocampus (Meltzer et al., 2019). Because of the significance of these neurotransmitters for the excitatory/inhibitory balance in the hippocampus, additional studies are needed to explore the functional relevance of these findings (Abekawa, Ohmori, Ito, & Koyama, 2000).

As discussed above, activation of brain D1 receptors plays an important role in maintaining higher cognitive functions. Here, a key component is the close association between D1 receptor activation and insertion of glutamate (AMPA and NMDA) receptors in synapses. A dopamine D1 receptor mediated increase of cAMP leads to activation of protein kinase A, which then phosphorylates key substrates including AMPA receptors (such as GluR1) and the transcription factor cyclic AMP response element binding protein (CREB).

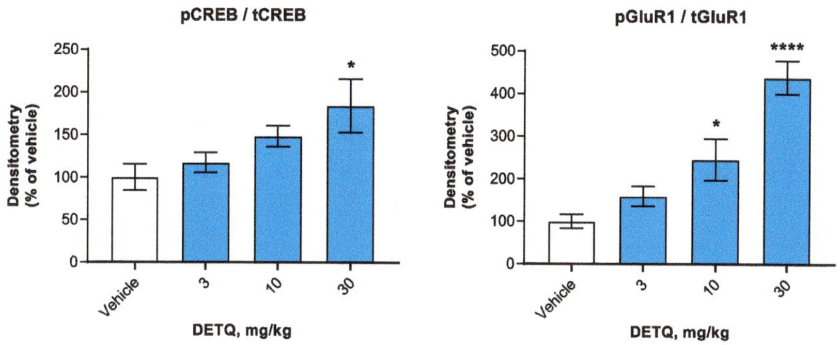

Fig. 12 Effects of DETQ (3–30 mg/kg, PO, 30 min before) on levels of pCREB and pGluR1 in the striatum of hD1 mice. Levels of pCREB and pGluR1 were measured using Western analyses, $n = 6$/group. *From Bruns, R. F., Mitchell, S. N., Wafford, K. A., Harper, A. J., Shanks, E. A., Carter, G., et al. (2018). Preclinical profile of a dopamine D1 potentiator suggests therapeutic utility in neurological and psychiatric disorders.* Neuropharmacology, *128, 351–365. https://doi.org/10.1016/j.neuropharm.2017.10.032.*

As shown in Fig. 12, DETQ produced dose related increases in phosphorylation of both CREB and GluR1 in the striatum of hD1 mice, and the effects of the highest dose were blocked by the D1 antagonist SCH39166 (Bruns et al., 2018).

The magnitude of the response for DETQ on GluR1 activation was comparable to that seen with the D1 agonist SKF82958, while the magnitude of the effect on CREB phosphorylation was lower that observed for SKF82958 (Bruns et al., 2018).

In addition to activation of the downstream marker CREB, DETQ has been shown to elevate formation of cAMP and cGMP in striatum (Bruns et al., 2018). The increased formation of cAMP and cGMP by the D1 PAM, along with activation of CREB and GluR1, both markers implicated in synaptic plasticity, provides further support for this mechanism in neurocognitive disorders.

3. Potential therapeutic applications of D1 PAMs

The importance of dopamine for a number of central functions has been known for over half a century and several CNS drugs have been shown to work through dopaminergic mechanisms. These include L-DOPA and various dopamine receptor agonists for Parkinson's disease, D2 receptor antagonists for schizophrenia, dopamine reuptake inhibitors for depression, and dopamine releasers for attention deficit hyperactivity disorder. These classes of drugs offered major therapeutic breakthroughs for debilitating disorders, in particular L-DOPA for Parkinson's disease and dopamine D2 receptor antagonists for schizophrenia, both of which were introduced in the early to mid-1960s. However, there are still areas of high unmet needs for neuropsychiatric disorders, especially with respect to the cognitive deficits that accompany many of these conditions. The strong rationale for cortical dopamine D1 receptors in higher cognitive functions has prompted interest in developing selective D1 agonists (Arnsten et al., 2017; Hall et al., 2019); however, these efforts have been hampered by a narrow therapeutic window and development of tachyphylaxis (Gulwadi et al., 2001; Vijayraghavan, Wang, Birnbaum, Williams, & Arnsten, 2007). Positive allosteric modulation of the dopamine D1 receptor represents an alternative approach that might avoid some of these disadvantages.

DETQ is the prototype of a family of D1 PAMs with pharmacology parallel to but clearly distinct from D1 agonists (Beadle et al., 2014; Svensson et al., 2017). In contrast to D1 agonists, DETQ depends on release of endogenous dopamine for its actions, since its locomotor effects are abolished by depletion of dopamine. In addition, the effects of DETQ are mediated by the D1 receptor since they were blocked by a D1 antagonist and were essentially absent in wild-type mice, in which the native D1 receptor has low affinity for DETQ (Svensson et al., 2017). A potential advantage of D1 PAMs over D1 agonists is illustrated by the observation that DETQ showed a monophasic rather than an inverted U-shaped dose response curve on locomotor activity, lacking the intense stereotyped behavior seen with high doses of D1 agonists. In addition there was no evidence of tachyphylaxis upon repeat dosing (Svensson et al., 2017). While the behavioral profile of DETQ was different from that of D1 agonists, neurochemical studies showed clear similarities that support central activation of D1 receptors. Parallels with D1 agonists included increased formation of brain cyclic nucleotides, increased release of cortical acetylcholine and histamine release, and activation of various markers of synaptic plasticity including the transcription factor CREB and the AMPA receptor GluR1 (Bruns et al., 2018).

Taken together, the pharmacological profile of D1 PAMs as exemplified by DETQ suggests potential utility in an array of therapeutic indications, as outlined below.

3.1 Schizophrenia

The introduction of atypical antipsychotics about 25 years ago offered clear improvements in therapy for patients with schizophrenia. Compared to traditional (typical) antipsychotics, newer drugs such as clozapine, risperidone, and olanzapine offered reduced extrapyramidal side effects while maintaining efficacy against positive symptoms such as hallucinations, delusions, and agitation. However, cognitive impairment, particularly attentional, working memory, and executive functional deficits, still remain an unmet medical need in these patients as these symptoms are poorly treated with the atypical antipsychotics (Désaméricq et al., 2014).

Brain imaging studies suggest elevated dopamine release in the striatum of schizophrenic patients; however, there is also evidence for a deficiency of dopamine release in the dorsolateral prefrontal cortex (Slifstein et al., 2015). This may contribute to deficits in working memory known to exist in schizophrenics (Abi-Dargham, 2003; Weinberger, 1987; Weinberger, Berman, & Illowsky, 1988), a concept that is supported by evidence in non-human primates that prefrontal D1 receptor activation is required for optimal functioning of working memory (Arnsten, 2013; Goldman-Rakic, Muly III, & Williams, 2000). Pilot studies in schizophrenics with D1 agonists like dihydrexidine (Rosell et al., 2015) or SKF38393 (Davidson et al., 1990) have been reported.

The NMDA antagonist ketamine induces psychotic-like symptoms and cognitive deficits in humans (Krystal et al., 1994) and has frequently been used in animal models. Studies with ketamine in non-human primates show working memory deficits and these can be reversed by systemic administration of D1 receptor agonists (Roberts, Seymour, Schmidt, Williams, & Castner, 2010). Also, deficits induced by chronic haloperidol treatment were reversed by the dopamine D1 agonist SKF38393 (Castner & Goldman-Rakic, 2004; Roberts et al., 2010). Interestingly, data recently disclosed at the 2019 Alzheimer's and Parkinson's Diseases Congress revealed that the D1 PAM DPTQ enhanced performance in the spatial working memory model in the rhesus monkey (Castner et al., 2019), which supports a role of D1 activation in this model. Furthermore, we recently reported that the D1 PAM DETQ reverses the deficit in novel object recognition in the hD1 mouse caused by chronic treatment with the NMDA receptor antagonist phencyclidine (Meltzer et al., 2019). This model is considered to reflect episodic and working memory performance (Ennaceur & Delacour, 1988). In contrast to what has been observed with D1 agonists in this model

(Horiguchi et al., 2013), DETQ did not produce an inverted U-shaped dose response. This is in line with our findings on exploratory locomotor activity and Y-maze spontaneous alternation (Bruns et al., 2018; Svensson et al., 2017). Besides these behavioral observations, neurochemical results support the potential efficacy of D1 PAMs for the treatment of cognitive deficits. DETQ showed dose-related neurochemical evidence of forebrain activation (Bruns et al., 2018). The increased formation of cyclic nucleotides and activation of the transcription factor CREB and the AMPA receptor, GluR1, indicate enhanced synaptic plasticity, which could drive memory function (Kandel, 2012; Sheng & Kim, 2002; Shepherd & Huganir, 2007). D1 PAMs, like D1 agonists, also increase the release of acetylcholine and histamine in cortical areas, including the prefrontal cortex and the hippocampus (see Figs. 9 and 10). Also, there is evidence to support a close interaction between histaminergic and cholinergic neurons to regulate arousal and various forms of cognition, primarily learning and memory (Blandina, Efoudebe, Cenni, Mannaioni, & Passani, 2004).

As discussed below, acetylcholinesterase inhibitors offer modest but significant efficacy in treating memory deficits in neurodegenerative disorders and histamine H3 antagonists have been considered for several neuropsychiatric disorders (Vohora & Bhowmik, 2012). The effects of D1 PAMs on the release of these neurotransmitters may contribute to potential pro-cognitive effects, primarily in neurodegenerative disorders.

It should be noted that D2 antagonists, by blocking inhibitory autoreceptors on dopaminergic terminals, increase dopamine release and hence D1 tone (Boyar & Altar, 1987). It is possible that this indirect stimulation of D1 receptor activity may contribute to the antipsychotic spectrum of D2 antagonists.

3.2 Parkinson's disease

About 60 years after the initial discovery of its anti-Parkinson effects, L-DOPA is still the primary standard of care and most effective treatment against the debilitating motor symptoms of PD. However, L-DOPA is associated with tolerance development, motor fluctuations, hypotension, development of dyskinesias, and other side effects including hallucinations, and gastro-intestinal disturbances. Based on this, there is a need for improved therapies for the motor symptoms of PD.

The D1 receptor agonist ABT-431 has been tested clinically in Parkinson's disease and showed clear evidence of efficacy on motor symptoms. A major objective of this study was to show a lower prevalence of dyskinesias relative to standard of care; this endpoint was achieved in one study but could not be repeated in a second study (Giardina & Williams, 2001). The clinical study was terminated due to this finding and other side-effects such as hypotension and nausea. DETQ was active in the PD model pioneered by Carlsson et al. (1957) using reserpine-induced dopamine depletion. Versus a low dose of reserpine, DETQ was able to restore LMA to control levels, whereas versus a higher dose of reserpine DETQ showed a marked synergy with L-DOPA (Bruns et al., 2018). These results show promise that a D1 PAM could be used as a single agent in early PD, and could be used to improve the response to L-DOPA in advanced PD. If the dyskinesias and other side-effects seen with ABT-431 are due to overstimulation of D1 receptors, it is possible that a D1 PAM may lack these liabilities.

Parkinson's disease patients also suffer from non-motor symptoms, including cognitive impairment, mood related symptoms, and excessive daytime sleepiness (Chaudhuri, Healy, & Schapira, 2006; Poewe, 2008). Cognitive impairment in Parkinson's disease and other forms of Lewy Body dementias likely involves loss of prefrontal dopamine input, which contributes to hypo-activity of cholinergic inputs from the basal forebrain (Kehagia, Barker, & Robbins, 2013; Narayanan, Rodnitzky, & Uc, 2013; Williams-Gray, Foltynie, Lewis, & Barker, 2006). The acetylcholinesterase inhibitor rivastigmine, originally approved for Alzheimer's disease, has more recently been approved for moderate to severe dementia of PD (Emre et al., 2004) but has a relatively narrow therapeutic index (Winblad et al., 2007). As noted above DETQ showed both behavioral and neurochemical evidence for potential pro-cognitive effects with significant increases in both acetylcholine and histamine release. Also, the additive or synergistic effects between DETQ and rivastigmine in the acetylcholine release (Bruns et al., 2018) or novel object recognition (Meltzer et al., 2019) assays suggests a potential as add-on therapy for patients suffering from dementia. The close structural analog of DETQ, LY3154207, is currently in phase 2 testing for Lewy Body dementias, including patients with Parkinson's disease. Finally, as discussed below, the observed effects of DETQ in the behavioral despair (forced swim) test, and sleep EEG models imply that this mechanism could benefit additional non-motor symptoms in Parkinson's disease, such as mood related symptoms and excessive daytime sleepiness.

3.3 Alzheimer's disease

Alzheimer's disease patients show a range of symptoms from mild cognitive impairment to mild to severe dementia (Campos et al., 2016). The disease usually starts with episodic memory impairment with anterograde amnesia: the ineffective consolidation or storage of new information is a clinical hallmark of the disease (Weintraub, Wicklund, & Salmon, 2012). Alzheimer's patients also show evidence of impaired prefrontal function with reduced attention, working memory, and executive function in various tests (Waltz et al., 2004). Acetylcholinesterase inhibitors have limited efficacy and are not well tolerated by some patients (Campos et al., 2016). They are typically used in mild to moderate stages of dementia, sometimes together with the NMDA antagonist memantine. Due to the limitations of current standard of care, there is an urgent need for improved therapies as the aging population grows. Most drug discovery efforts in this area are focused on disease modifying therapies including β-amyloid and tau clearing mechanisms that potentially could slow the progression of this devastating disorder. However, there is also an urgent need for improved symptomatic therapies. Based on the enhanced hippocampal acetylcholine release with DETQ (Bruns et al., 2018; Meltzer et al., 2019), it is possible that D1 PAMs could provide symptomatic treatment of memory impairment in Alzheimer's disease in addition to effects on higher cognitive functions mediated through D1 activation in the prefrontal cortex. The observed positive interaction with rivastigmine is of particular interest regarding adjunctive therapy. The role of D1 receptor activation in synaptic plasticity is also worth considering in terms of both short and long term effects on cognition. Sustained effects on spatial working memory performance after intermittent dosing with small doses of the D1 agonist ABT-431 have been reported in aged but not young rhesus monkeys (Castner & Goldman-Rakic, 2004). Many Alzheimer's patients also show non-cognitive symptoms such as apathy and daytime sleepiness that could potentially respond to a D1 PAM (as discussed below).

3.4 Major depressive disorder

Available antidepressant drugs including serotonin and serotonin/norepinephrine uptake inhibitors have limited efficacy and typically exert their effects with a delay of several weeks (Briley & Moret, 1993), suggesting that the elevation in mood occurs at the end of a prolonged, multi-step sequence of events. In contrast, dopaminergic drugs have immediate mood-elevating effects, consistent with the well-known role of dopamine in limbic reward systems. A D1 PAM could therefore have a rapid onset of efficacy in depression, and it is possible that the more direct mode of action could provide greater efficacy than current treatments. Parkinson's patients have a high incidence of depressive symptoms (Poewe, 2008), confirming the importance of dopamine in maintaining mood, and the occurrence of depression and suicidal ideation in patients treated with the D1 antagonist SCH39166 (ecopipam) (Astrup et al., 2007) indicates that the D1 receptor plays a role. Interestingly, reduced cortical D1 binding has also been reported in depressed patients (Dougherty et al., 2006).

DETQ reduced immobility in the forced-swim test, a model in which various clinically validated antidepressant interventions acting through diverse mechanisms have been shown to be active (Petit-Demouliere et al., 2005; Witkin et al., 2016). The ability of DETQ to acutely increase formation of cyclic nucleotides and induce phosphorylation of GluR1 and CREB also suggests that D1 PAMs may be useful in major depressive disorder (Svenningsson et al., 2007). In addition, many depressed patients suffer from cognitive impairment and this can contribute to poor social functioning (Rock, Roiser, Riedel, & Blackwell, 2014). A novel therapy with the potential to enhance both mood and cognitive function could be beneficial. In summary, the current results with DETQ in the forced-swim test, GluR1/CREB phosphorylation, and in various models implicated in cognition reinforce expectations from the clinical literature that amplification of the D1 signaling system may have a beneficial effect in major depressive disorder.

3.5 Other therapeutic opportunities for D1 PAMs

Dopamine-releasing agents such as amphetamines and methylphenidate are used clinically for the treatment of narcolepsy and excessive daytime sleepiness and for attention deficit disorder (Iversen & Iversen, 2007). The ability of DETQ to cause wakefulness in hD1 mice and to stimulate release of ACh and histamine suggests that D1 PAMs may be useful in these two indications. There is also reason to anticipate that D1 PAMs would have a more benign, focused profile of action compared to dopamine releasers. The latter agents release other biogenic amines such as norepinephrine and serotonin in addition to dopamine, and would also activate all five dopamine receptors. In addition, dopamine releasers do not depend on the activation of the physiological dopaminergic system. In contrast, the actions of a selective

D1 PAM would be confined to the D1 receptor and would be under the control of the normal dopaminergic pathways. Possibly relevant to the above is the observation that amphetamines and D1 agonists impair spontaneous alternation behavior with an inverted U-shaped dose response in the Y-maze (suggesting an anti-cognitive effect) whereas DETQ increases distance traveled without decreasing alternation (Anisman & Kokkinidis, 1975; Bruns et al., 2018).

4. Conclusion

There is a strong rationale implicating central dopamine D1 receptors as a target for new therapies that could address unmet medical needs in neuropsychiatric disorders. While the development of D1 agonists over the past decades has been challenging, selective D1 PAMs could offer a path forward. By amplifying the effects of endogenous dopamine, D1 PAMs offer a new, more physiological approach to D1 receptor activation. The pharmacological profile of the D1 PAM DETQ aligns closely with that of D1 agonists, but with important differences, including lack of strong stereotypy and tachyphylaxis (Svensson et al., 2017). Overall, the behavioral and neurochemical results reported for DETQ suggest efficacy of D1 PAMs in Parkinson's disease and a range of other neuropsychiatric disorders.

Acknowledgment

The work reviewed here is a compilation of many years of hard work by a number of individuals, including past and present employees of Eli Lilly and Company as well as external collaborators.

Conflicts of interest

Authors Svensson and Hao are current employees of Eli Lilly and Company and Bruns is a retired employee of Eli Lilly and Company.

References

Abekawa, T., Ohmori, T., Ito, K., & Koyama, T. (2000). D1 dopamine receptor activation reduces extracellular glutamate and GABA concentrations in the medial prefrontal cortex. *Brain Research*, *867*(1–2), 250–254.

Abi-Dargham, A. (2003). Probing cortical dopamine function in schizophrenia: What can D1 receptors tell us. *World Psychiatry*, *2*(3), 166–171.

Alvarez, E. O. (2009). The role of histamine on cognition. *Behavioural Brain Research*, *199*(2), 183–189.

Anisman, H., & Kokkinidis, L. (1975). Effects of scopolamine, d-amphetamine and other drugs affecting catecholamines on spontaneous alternation and locomotor activity in mice. *Psychopharmacologia*, *45*(1), 55–63. https://doi.org/10.1007/bf00426210.

Arnsten, A. F. T. (2013). The neurobiology of thought: The groundbreaking discoveries of Patricia Goldman-Rakic 1937–2003. *Cerebral Cortex*, *123*, 2269–2281.
Arnsten, A. F. T., Girgis, R. R., Gray, D. L., & Mailman, R. B. (2017). Novel dopamine therapeutics for cognitive deficits in schizophrenia. *Biological Psychiatry*, *81*(1), 67–77. https://doi.org/10.1016/j.biopsych.2015.12.028.
Astrup, A., Greenway, F. L., Ling, W., Pedicone, L., Lachowicz, J., Strader, C. D., et al. (2007). Randomized controlled trials of the D1/D5 antagonist ecopipam for weight loss in obese subjects. *Obesity*, *15*(7), 1717–1731.
Beadle, C. D., Coates, D. A., Hao, J., Krushinski, J. H., Jr., Reinhard, M. R., Schaus, J. M., et al. (2014). *3,4-Dihydroisoquinolin-2 (1h)-yl compounds.* Patent Number: WO2014193781 A1.
Beaulieu, J. M., & Gainetdinov, R. R. (2011). The physiology, signaling, and pharmacology of dopamine receptors. *Pharmacological Reviews*, *63*(1), 182–217. https://doi.org/10.1124/pr.110.002642.
Blandina, P., Efoudebe, M., Cenni, G., Mannaioni, P., & Passani, M. B. (2004). Acetylcholine, histamine, and cognition: Two sides of the same coin. *Learning & Memory*, *11*(1), 1–8.
Boyar, W. C., & Altar, C. A. (1987). Modulation of in vivo dopamine release by D2 but not D1 receptor agonists and antagonists. *Journal of Neurochemistry*, *48*(3), 824–831.
Briley, M., & Moret, C. (1993). Neurobiological mechanisms involved in antidepressant therapies. *Clinical Neuropharmacology*, *16*(5), 387–400.
Bruns, R. F., & Fergus, J. H. (1990). Allosteric enhancement of adenosine A1 receptor binding and function by 2-amino-3-benzoylthiophenes. *Molecular Pharmacology*, *38*, 939–949.
Bruns, R. F., Mitchell, S. N., Wafford, K. A., Harper, A. J., Shanks, E. A., Carter, G., et al. (2018). Preclinical profile of a dopamine D1 potentiator suggests therapeutic utility in neurological and psychiatric disorders. *Neuropharmacology*, *128*, 351–365. https://doi.org/10.1016/j.neuropharm.2017.10.032.
Campos, C., Rocha, N. B. F., Teles Vieira, R., Rocha, S. A., Telles-Correia, D., Paes, F., et al. (2016). Treatment of cognitive deficits in Alzheimer's disease: A psychopharmacological review. *Psychiatria Danubina*, *28*(1), 1–12.
Carlsson, A., Lindqvist, M., & Magnusson, T. (1957). 3,4-Dihydroxyphenylalanine and 5-hydroxytryptophan as reserpine antagonists. *Nature*, *180*(4596), 1200.
Carlsson, A., Lindqvist, M., Magnusson, T., & Waldeck, B. (1958). On the presence of 3-hydroxytyramine in brain. *Science*, *127*, 471.
Castner, S. A., & Goldman-Rakic, P. S. (2004). Enhancement of working memory in aged monkeys by a sensitizing regimen of dopamine D1 receptor stimulation. *The Journal of Neuroscience*, *24*(6), 1446–1450. https://doi.org/10.1523/JNEUROSCI.3987-03.2004.
Castner, S. A., Svensson, K. A., Yang, C. R., Zhang, L., Hao, J., Marston, H., et al. (2019). The dopamine D1 receptor positive allosteric modulator DPTQ enhances spontaneous eye blink rate and spatial working memory in the rhesus monkey. In *Alzheimer's and Parkinson's diseases congress, Lisbon, Portugal, March 26–31, 2019*.
Chaudhuri, K. R., Healy, D. G., & Schapira, A. H. (2006). Non-motor symptoms of Parkinson's disease: Diagnosis and management. *The Lancet. Neurology*, *5*(3), 235–245.
Christopoulos, A., & Kenakin, T. (2002). G protein-coupled receptor allosterism and complexing. *Pharmacological Reviews*, *54*(2), 323–374.
Damsma, G., Tham, C.-S., Robertson, G. S., & Fibiger, H. C. (1990). Dopamine D1 receptor stimulation increases striatal acetylcholine release in the rat. *European Journal of Pharmacology*, *186*(2), 335–338.
Davidson, M., Harvey, P. D., Bergman, R. L., Powchik, P., Kaminsky, R., Losonczy, M. F., et al. (1990). Effects of the D-1 agonist SKF-38393 combined with haloperidol in schizophrenic patients. *Archives of General Psychiatry*, *47*(2), 190–191.

Davoren, J. E., Nason, D., Coe, J., Dlugolenski, K., Helal, C., Harris, A. R., et al. (2018). Discovery and lead optimization of atropisomer D1 agonists with reduced desensitization. *Journal of Medicinal Chemistry*, *61*(24), 11384–11397.

Day, J., & Fibiger, H. (1993). Dopaminergic regulation of cortical acetylcholine release: Effects of dopamine receptor agonists. *Neuroscience*, *54*(3), 643–648.

Désaméricq, G., Schurhoff, F., Meary, A., Szöke, A., Macquin-Mavier, I., Bachoud-Lévi, A., et al. (2014). Long-term neurocognitive effects of antipsychotics in schizophrenia: A network meta-analysis. *European Journal of Clinical Pharmacology*, *70*(2), 127–134.

Deuschl, G., & Goddemeier, C. (1998). Spontaneous and reflex activity of facial muscles in dystonia, Parkinson's disease, and in normal subjects. *Journal of Neurology, Neurosurgery, and Psychiatry*, *64*(3), 320–324.

Dougherty, D. D., Bonab, A. A., Ottowitz, W. E., Livni, E., Alpert, N. M., Rauch, S. L., et al. (2006). Decreased striatal D1 binding as measured using PET and [11C]SCH 23,390 in patients with major depression with anger attacks. *Depression and Anxiety*, *23*(3), 175–177. https://doi.org/10.1002/da.20168.

Eder, D. N., Zdravkovic, M., & Wildschiødtz, G. (2003). Selective alterations of the first NREM sleep cycle in humans by a dopamine D1 receptor antagonist (NNC-687). *Journal of Psychiatric Research*, *37*(4), 305–312.

Emre, M., Aarsland, D., Albanese, A., Byrne, E. J., Deuschl, G., De Deyn, P. P., et al. (2004). Rivastigmine for dementia associated with Parkinson's disease. *The New England Journal of Medicine*, *351*(24), 2509–2518.

Ennaceur, A., & Delacour, J. (1988). A new one-trial test for neurobiological studies of memory in rats. 1: Behavioral data. *Behavioural Brain Research*, *31*(1), 47–59.

Epping-Jordan, M., Le Poul, E., & Rocher, J.-P. (2007). Allosteric modulation: A novel approach to drug discovery. *Innovations in Pharmaceutical Technology*, *24*, 22–26.

Fell, M. J., Witkin, J. M., Falcone, J. F., Katner, J. S., Perry, K. W., Hart, J., et al. (2011). N-(4-((2-(trifluoromethyl)-3-hydroxy-4-(isobutyryl)phenoxy)methyl)benzyl)-1-methyl-1H-imidazole-4-carboxamide (THIIC), a novel metabotropic glutamate 2 potentiator with potential anxiolytic/antidepressant properties: In vivo profiling suggests a link between behavioral and central nervous system neurochemical changes. *The Journal of Pharmacology and Experimental Therapeutics*, *336*(1), 165–177. https://doi.org/10.1124/jpet.110.172957.

Giardina, W. J., & Williams, M. (2001). Adrogolide HCl (ABT-431; DAS-431), a prodrug of the dopamine D1 receptor agonist, A-86929: Preclinical pharmacology and clinical data. *CNS Drug Reviews*, 7(3), 305–316.

Goldman-Rakic, P. S., Castner, S. A., Svensson, T. H., Siever, L. J., & Williams, G. V. (2004). Targeting the dopamine D1 receptor in schizophrenia: Insights for cognitive dysfunction. *Psychopharmacology*, *174*(1), 3–16. https://doi.org/10.1007/s00213-004-1793-y.

Goldman-Rakic, P. S., Muly, E. C., III, & Williams, G. V. (2000). D1 receptors in prefrontal cells and circuits. *Brain Research Reviews*, *31*(2), 295–301.

Gray, D. L., Allen, J. A., Mente, S., O'Connor, R. E., DeMarco, G. J., Efremov, I., et al. (2018). Impaired β-arrestin recruitment and reduced desensitization by non-catechol agonists of the D1 dopamine receptor. *Nature Communications*, *9*(1), 674.

Gray, D. L., Zhang, Y., Sohur, U., Feng, G., Thayer, K., & Duvvuri, S. (2018). Safety, tolerability, pharmacokinetics, and pharmacodynamics of PF-06649751, an oral dopamine D1/D5 agonist, in Parkinson's disease: A single ascending dose study. *Parkinsonism & Related Disorders*, *46*, e20.

Gulwadi, A. G., Korpinen, C. D., Mailman, R. B., Nichols, D. E., Sit, S. Y., & Taber, M. T. (2001). Dinapsoline: Characterization of a D1 dopamine receptor agonist in a rat model of Parkinson's disease. *The Journal of Pharmacology and Experimental Therapeutics*, *296*(2), 338–344.

Hall, A., Provins, L., & Valade, A. (2019). Novel strategies to activate the dopamine D1 receptor: Recent advances in orthosteric agonism and positive allosteric modulation. *Journal of Medicinal Chemistry*, *62*(1), 128–140. https://doi.org/10.1021/acs.jmedchem.8b01767.

Hembre, E. J., Beck, J. A., Bruns, R. F., Hao, J., Heinz, B. A., Krushinski, J. H., et al. (2018). The discovery of novel dopamine D1 positive allosteric modulators for the treatment of neurodegenerative disorders. In *7th RSC/SCI symposium on GPCRs in medicinal chemistry, Verona, Italy, September 10–12, 2018.*

Hersi, A. I., Kitaichi, K., Srivastava, L. K., Gaudreau, P., & Quirion, R. (2000). Dopamine D-5 receptor modulates hippocampal acetylcholine release. *Molecular Brain Research*, *76*(2), 336–340.

Horiguchi, M., Hannaway, K. E., Adelekun, A. E., Huang, M., Jayathilake, K., & Meltzer, H. Y. (2013). D1 receptor agonists reverse the subchronic phencyclidine (PCP)-induced novel object recognition (NOR) deficit in female rats. *Behavioural Brain Research*, *238*, 36–43.

Horner, W. E., Johnson, D. E., Schmidt, A. W., & Rollema, H. (2007). Methylphenidate and atomoxetine increase histamine release in rat prefrontal cortex. *European Journal of Pharmacology*, *558*(1), 96–97.

Isaac, S. O., & Berridge, C. W. (2003). Wake-promoting actions of dopamine D1 and D2 receptor stimulation. *The Journal of Pharmacology and Experimental Therapeutics*, *307*(1), 386–394.

Ishizuka, T., Sakamoto, Y., Sakurai, T., & Yamatodani, A. (2003). Modafinil increases histamine release in the anterior hypothalamus of rats. *Neuroscience Letters*, *339*(2), 143–146.

Iversen, S. D., & Iversen, L. L. (2007). Dopamine: 50 Years in perspective. *Trends in Neurosciences*, *30*(5), 188–193. https://doi.org/10.1016/j.tins.2007.03.002.

Jutkiewicz, E. M., & Bergman, J. (2004). Effects of dopamine D1 ligands on eye blinking in monkeys: Efficacy, antagonism, and D1/D2 interactions. *The Journal of Pharmacology and Experimental Therapeutics*, *311*(3), 1008–1015. https://doi.org/10.1124/jpet.104.071092.

Kandel, E. R. (2012). The molecular biology of memory: cAMP, PKA, CRE, CREB-1, CREB-2, and CPEB. *Molecular Brain*, *5*(1), 14.

Karson, C. N., Lewitt, P. A., Calne, D. B., & Wyatt, R. J. (1982). Blink rates in Parkinsonism. *Annals of Neurology*, *12*(6), 580–583.

Kehagia, A. A., Barker, R. A., & Robbins, T. W. (2013). Cognitive impairment in Parkinson's disease: The dual syndrome hypothesis. *Neurodegenerative Diseases*, *11*(2), 79–92. https://doi.org/10.1159/000341998.

Kenakin, T. P. (2012). Biased signalling and allosteric machines: New vistas and challenges for drug discovery. *British Journal of Pharmacology*, *165*(6), 1659–1669.

Krystal, J. H., Karper, L. P., Seibyl, J. P., Freeman, G. K., Delaney, R., Bremner, J. D., et al. (1994). Subanesthetic effects of the noncompetitive NMDA antagonist, ketamine, in humans: Psychotomimetic, perceptual, cognitive, and neuroendocrine responses. *Archives of general psychiatry*, *51*(3), 199–214.

Laplante, F., Sibley, D. R., & Quirion, R. (2004). Reduction in acetylcholine release in the hippocampus of dopamine D5 receptor-deficient mice. *Neuropsychopharmacology*, *29*(9), 1620–1627.

Lewis, M. A., Hunihan, L., Watson, J., Gentles, R. G., Hu, S., Huang, Y., et al. (2015). Discovery of D1 dopamine receptor positive allosteric modulators: Characterization of pharmacology and identification of residues that regulate species selectivity. *The Journal of Pharmacology and Experimental Therapeutics*, *354*(3), 340–349. https://doi.org/10.1124/jpet.115.224071.

Luderman, K. D., Conroy, J. L., Free, R. B., Southall, N., Ferrer, M., Sanchez-Soto, M., et al. (2018). Identification of positive allosteric modulators of the D1 dopamine receptor that act at diverse binding sites. *Molecular Pharmacology*, *94*(4), 1197–1209.

Meltzer, H., Rajagopal, L., Matrisciano, F., Hao, J., Svensson, K., & Huang, M. (2019). The allosteric dopamine D1 receptor potentiator, DETQ, ameliorates subchronic phencyclidine-induced object recognition memory deficits and enhances cortical acetylcholine efflux in male humanized D1 receptor knock-in mice. *Behavioural Brain Research*, *361*, 139–150. https://doi.org/10.1016/j.bbr.2018.12.006.

Munk, C., Isberg, V., Mordalski, S., Harpsøe, K., Rataj, K., Hauser, A. S., et al. (2016). GPCRdb: The G protein-coupled receptor database—An introduction. *British Journal of Pharmacology*, *173*(14), 2195–2207. https://doi.org/10.1111/bph.13509.

Narayanan, N. S., Rodnitzky, R. L., & Uc, E. Y. (2013). Prefrontal dopamine signaling and cognitive symptoms of Parkinson's disease. *Reviews in the Neurosciences*, *24*(3), 267–278. https://doi.org/10.1515/revneuro-2013-0004.

Nemeth, E. F., Steffey, M. E., Hammerland, L. G., Hung, B. C., Van Wagenen, B. C., DelMar, E. G., et al. (1998). Calcimimetics with potent and selective activity on the parathyroid calcium receptor. *Proceedings of the National Academy of Sciences of the United States of America*, *95*(7), 4040–4045.

Nikulina, E. M., Skrinskaya, J. A., & Popova, N. K. (1991). Role of genotype and dopamine receptors in behaviour of inbred mice in a forced swimming test. *Psychopharmacology*, *105*(4), 525–529.

Papapetropoulos, S., Liu, W., Duvvuri, S., Thayer, K., & Gray, D. L. (2018). Evaluation of D1/D5 partial agonist PF-06412562 in Parkinson's disease following oral administration. *Neurodegenerative Diseases*, *18*(5–6), 262–269.

Petit-Demouliere, B., Chenu, F., & Bourin, M. (2005). Forced swimming test in mice: A review of antidepressant activity. *Psychopharmacology*, *177*(3), 245–255.

Poewe, W. (2008). Non-motor symptoms in Parkinson's disease. *European Journal of Neurology*, *15*(Suppl. 1), 14–20.

Roberts, B. M., Seymour, P. A., Schmidt, C. J., Williams, G. V., & Castner, S. A. (2010). Amelioration of ketamine-induced working memory deficits by dopamine D1 receptor agonists. *Psychopharmacology*, *210*(3), 407–418.

Rock, P., Roiser, J., Riedel, W., & Blackwell, A. (2014). Cognitive impairment in depression: A systematic review and meta-analysis. *Psychological Medicine*, *44*(10), 2029–2040.

Rosell, D. R., Zaluda, L. C., McClure, M. M., Perez-Rodriguez, M. M., Strike, K. S., Barch, D. M., et al. (2015). Effects of the D1 dopamine receptor agonist dihydrexidine (DAR-0100A) on working memory in schizotypal personality disorder. *Neuropsychopharmacology*, *40*(2), 446–453. https://doi.org/10.1038/npp.2014.192.

Sheng, M., & Kim, M. J. (2002). Postsynaptic signaling and plasticity mechanisms. *Science*, *298*(5594), 776–780.

Shepherd, J. D., & Huganir, R. L. (2007). The cell biology of synaptic plasticity: AMPA receptor trafficking. *Annual Review of Cell and Developmental Biology*, *23*, 613–643.

Shiraki, R., Tobe, T., Kawakami, S., Moritomo, H., & Ohmiya, M. (2015). *Heterocyclic acetamide compound*. Patent Number: US20150045402A1.

Slifstein, M., van de Giessen, E., Van Snellenberg, J., Thompson, J. L., Narendran, R., Gil, R., et al. (2015). Deficits in prefrontal cortical and extrastriatal dopamine release in schizophrenia: A positron emission tomographic functional magnetic resonance imaging study. *JAMA Psychiatry*, *72*(4), 316–324.

Svenningsson, P., Bateup, H., Qi, H., Takamiya, K., Huganir, R. L., Spedding, M., et al. (2007). Involvement of AMPA receptor phosphorylation in antidepressant actions with special reference to tianeptine. *European Journal of Neuroscience*, *26*(12), 3509–3517.

Svensson, K. A., Heinz, B. A., Schaus, J. M., Beck, J. P., Hao, J., Krushinski, J. H., et al. (2017). An allosteric potentiator of the dopamine D1 receptor increases locomotor activity in human D1 knock-in mice without causing stereotypy or tachyphylaxis. *The Journal of Pharmacology and Experimental Therapeutics, 360*(1), 117–128. https://doi.org/10.1124/jpet.116.236372.

Valant, C., Felder, C. C., Sexton, P. M., & Christopoulos, A. (2012). Probe dependence in the allosteric modulation of a G protein-coupled receptor: Implications for detection and validation of allosteric ligand effects. *Molecular Pharmacology, 81*(1), 41–52. https://doi.org/10.1124/mol.111.074872.

Vijayraghavan, S., Wang, M., Birnbaum, S. G., Williams, G. V., & Arnsten, A. F. (2007). Inverted-U dopamine D1 receptor actions on prefrontal neurons engaged in working memory. *Nature Neuroscience, 10*(3), 376–384. https://doi.org/10.1038/nn1846.

Vohora, D., & Bhowmik, M. (2012). Histamine H3 receptor antagonists/inverse agonists on cognitive and motor processes: Relevance to Alzheimer's disease, ADHD, schizophrenia, and drug abuse. *Frontiers in Systems Neuroscience, 6*, 72.

Waltz, J. A., Knowlton, B. J., Holyoak, K. J., Boone, K. B., Back-Madruga, C., McPherson, S., et al. (2004). Relational integration and executive function in Alzheimer's disease. *Neuropsychology, 18*(2), 296.

Wang, X., Heinz, B. A., Qian, Y.-W., Carter, J. H., Gadski, R. A., Beavers, L. S., et al. (2018). Intracellular binding site for a positive allosteric modulator of the dopamine D1 receptor. *Molecular Pharmacology, 94*(4), 1232–1245. https://doi.org/10.1124/mol.118.112649.

Weinberger, D. R. (1987). Implications of normal brain development for the pathogenesis of schizophrenia. *Archives of General Psychiatry, 44*(7), 660–669.

Weinberger, D. R., Berman, K. F., & Illowsky, B. P. (1988). Physiological dysfunction of dorsolateral prefrontal cortex in schizophrenia: III. A new cohort and evidence for a monoaminergic mechanism. *Archives of General Psychiatry, 45*(7), 609–615.

Weintraub, S., Wicklund, A. H., & Salmon, D. P. (2012). The neuropsychological profile of Alzheimer disease. *Cold Spring Harbor Perspectives in Medicine, 2*(4), a006171.

Westerink, B. H., Cremers, T. I., De Vries, J. B., Liefers, H., Tran, N., & De Boer, P. (2002). Evidence for activation of histamine H3 autoreceptors during handling stress in the prefrontal cortex of the rat. *Synapse, 43*(4), 238–243.

Williams-Gray, C. H., Foltynie, T., Lewis, S. J., & Barker, R. A. (2006). Cognitive deficits and psychosis in Parkinson's disease. *CNS Drugs, 20*(6), 477–505.

Winblad, B., Cummings, J., Andreasen, N., Grossberg, G., Onofrj, M., Sadowsky, C., et al. (2007). A six-month double-blind, randomized, placebo-controlled study of a transdermal patch in Alzheimer's disease—Rivastigmine patch versus capsule. *International Journal of Geriatric Psychiatry, 22*(5), 456–467. https://doi.org/10.1002/gps.1788.

Witkin, J. M., Monn, J. A., Schoepp, D. D., Li, X., Overshiner, C., Mitchell, S. N., et al. (2016). The rapidly acting antidepressant ketamine and the mGlu2/3 receptor antagonist LY341495 rapidly engage dopaminergic mood circuits. *The Journal of Pharmacology and Experimental Therapeutics, 358*(1), 71–82. https://doi.org/10.1124/jpet.116.233627.

Zhuong, X., Belluscio, L., & Hen, R. (2000). $G_{olf\text{-}alpha}$ mediates dopamine D_1 receptor signaling. *The Journal of Neuroscience, 20*, 91–95. RC91.

FSC
www.fsc.org
MIX
Papier | Fördert gute Waldnutzung
FSC® C083411

Kolibri 360 GmbH
Ferdinand-Jühlke-Straße 7
99095 Erfurt, Deutschland
produktsicherheit@kolibri360.de